Nursing Ethics and Professional Responsibility in Advanced Practice

Pamela J. Grace, PhD, APRN
Associate Professor
Ethics and Adult Health
W. F. Connell School of Nursing
Boston College
Chestnut Hill, Massachusetts

JONES AND BARTLETT PUBLISHERS
Sudbury, Massachusetts
BOSTON   TORONTO   LONDON   SINGAPORE

World Headquarters

Jones and Bartlett Publishers	Jones and Bartlett Publishers	Jones and Bartlett Publishers
40 Tall Pine Drive	Canada	International
Sudbury, MA 01776	6339 Ormindale Way	Barb House, Barb Mews
978-443-5000	Mississauga, Ontario L5V 1J2	London W6 7PA
info@jbpub.com	Canada	United Kingdom
www.jbpub.com		

Jones and Bartlett's books and products are available through most bookstores and online booksellers. To contact Jones and Bartlett Publishers directly, call 800-832-0034, fax 978-443-8000, or visit our website www.jbpub.com.

Substantial discounts on bulk quantities of Jones and Bartlett's publications are available to corporations, professional associations, and other qualified organizations. For details and specific discount information, contact the special sales department at Jones and Bartlett via the above contact information or send an email to special-sales@jbpub.com.

The authors, editor, and publisher have made every effort to provide accurate information. However, they are not responsible for errors, omissions, or for any outcomes related to the use of the contents of this book and take no responsibility for the use of the products and procedures described. Treatments and side effects described in this book may not be applicable to all people; likewise, some people may require a dose or experience a side effect that is not described herein. Drugs and medical devices are discussed that may have limited availability controlled by the Food and Drug Administration (FDA) for use only in a research study or clinical trial. Research, clinical practice, and government regulations often change the accepted standard in this field. When consideration is being given to use of any drug in the clinical setting, the health care provider or reader is responsible for determining FDA status of the drug, reading the package insert, and reviewing prescribing information for the most up-to-date recommendations on dose, precautions, and contraindications, and determining the appropriate usage for the product. This is especially important in the case of drugs that are new or seldom used.

Production Credits
Publisher: Kevin Sullivan
Acquisitions Editor: Emily Ekle
Acquisitions Editor: Amy Sibley
Associate Editor: Patricia Donnelly
Editorial Assistant: Rachel Shuster
Production Manager: Jenny L. Corriveau
Associate Marketing Manager: Ilana Goddess
Manufacturing and Inventory Control Supervisor: Amy Bacus
Composition: diacriTech
Cover Design: Brian Moore
Printing and Binding: Malloy, Inc.
Cover Printing: Malloy, Inc.

Library of Congress Cataloging-in-Publication Data
Grace, Pamela.
  Nursing ethics and professional responsibility in advanced practice / Pamela Grace.
    p. ; cm.
  Includes bibliographical references.
  ISBN-13: 978-0-7637-5110-4 (pbk.)
  ISBN-10: 0-7637-5110-3 (pbk.)
  1. Nursing ethics. 2. Nurse practitioners. I. Title.
  [DNLM: 1. Ethics, Nursing—United States. 2. Nurses—ethics—United States. WY 85 G729n 2008]
  RT85.G73 2008
  174.2—dc22
                                    2008011086
6048

Printed in the United States of America
13 12 11 10 09   10 9 8 7 6 5 4 3 2

Contents

SECTION II: ETHICAL ISSUES COMMON ACROSS
               PRACTICE SPECIALTIES

    Gregory Sheedy

    Introduction   339
        Ethical Theory and Problem Solving   340
        Principle-Based Ethics   341
        Case-Based Ethics   341
    Do-Not-Resuscitate Orders During Surgery   342
        DNR and the Principle of Autonomy   342
        DNR and Patient Self-Determination Act   343
        DNR and Policy   344
        DNR and Required Reconsideration   345
        DNR Orders with Incompetent Patients   351
        DNR Orders in Pediatric Patients   352
    The Jehovah's Witness Patient   353
        Doctrine on Blood Transfusions   353
        Informed Consent with the Jehovah's Witness Patient   354
    Truth Telling in the Operating Room: The Obligation of Veracity 358
        Veracity in Therapeutic Relationships   359
        Veracity in Anesthesia Care   359
    Conscientious Objection in Anesthetic Practice   363
        The Conflict Between Fetal- versus Maternal-Focused
            Ethical Obligations   363
    Anesthesia and Distributive Justice   368
        The Principle of Justice   368
        Distributive Justice   369
        Distributive Justice in Anesthesia Practice   370
    Protecting Patients from Incompetent and Impaired
        Healthcare Providers   373
        Fidelity and Advocacy in Anesthesia Practice   373
        Incompetent and Impaired Healthcare Providers   375
    Summary   379
    References   379
    Suggested Reading   381

13. Nursing Ethics and Advanced Practice: Gerontology and
    End-of-Life Issues   383
    Pamela J. Grace

    Introduction   383
    Gerontological Advanced Practice   384
        Definitions and Cautions   384
        Multidisciplinary Approaches   385

Preface

There are many excellent bioethics and nursing ethics textbooks. However, none to date effectively captures the nature of many of the ethical issues that can arise in the daily work of advanced practice nurses (APNs). Although I am not sure of the reason for this relative dearth of ethics content that is salient to advanced nursing roles, my experience is that either these roles are (rightly) taken to be nursing roles, and thus a *nursing ethics* text will suffice as an appropriate resource, or the roles are more akin to medical practice (a distortion of the role), and thus a medical ethics or bioethics text is appropriate. However, advanced practice nursing roles are associated with unique problems for which both basic nursing ethics and bioethics texts may be helpful adjuncts but inadequate sole resources.

The augmented responsibilities of the APN role demand a book that is specifically dedicated to exploring the types and complexities of issues faced by this set of nurses. It has become increasingly clear to me over time, and as a result of a variety of experiences, that this book is needed. I became an APN nearly 20 years ago. Since that time, I have taught advanced practice nursing courses, gained a doctorate in philosophy with a concentration in medical ethics, and for the past 8 years taught among other courses one entitled "Ethical Issues in Advanced Practice Nursing." Over this period of time, I have continued to be somewhat frustrated by the lack of a comprehensive resource that is dedicated to exploring professional and ethical issues related to expanded nursing roles. It occurred to me that I was in as good a position as any to embark on such a project, and an opportunity arose for me to devote the time needed for its development. In the spring of 2007, I was granted a sabbatical semester by my institution, Boston College, which permitted the realization of this endeavor.

Students in the courses I teach are in a variety of specialty tracks and for the most part are concurrently immersed in advanced practice clinical practica within their specialties. Thus, they have access to issues that are prevalent in those practices and bring these issues for their classmates to explore as pertinent to the content being covered. I have drawn on these contributions in places to illustrate points. Additionally, I was able to utilize the expertise of faculty colleagues and graduates with whom I have maintained contact to corroborate that certain problems remain salient areas of difficulty for APNs. Some colleagues, former students, and current students have contributed chapters or collaborated with me on chapters.

The aim of this book, then, is to provide a consistent thread that relates advanced practice both to nursing practice and to the need for the provision of good health care. It is unique in its application to professional issues and advanced practice roles. Although this book is specifically directed to APNs, much of the content is applicable to allied healthcare professionals who practice in expanded roles. As with any textbook concerned with practice, supplementary reading materials may be needed to gain in-depth or extant knowledge of a specific problem.

The underlying assumption of this book is that the development of confidence in moral decision making is possible and that this is facilitated by practice in moral reasoning. Nurses already possess clinical knowledge and expertise, but they also need the tools to identify and articulate to others the requirements for good care in their practice settings and they need the motivation to provide good care in the face of obstacles. Facilitators of confidence in moral decision making are exposure to contemporary ethics literature, seriously listening to the views of others with whom one would normally disagree in an attempt to understand why the person thinks the way he or she does, practice in exploring difficult cases and articulating salient aspects to others, and understanding the sources of one's own biases and prejudices. Exercises for practicing these skills are offered at the end of most chapters.

The methods I use for teaching the "Ethical Issues in Advanced Practice Nursing" course are eclectic and depend to some extent on the size and makeup of the class. However, it is usually quite interactive, so I do set ground rules that have proved to be invaluable for getting input from all class members, whether this is in the large group discussion or in smaller group discussions. That these ground rules facilitate participation by even the most timid is evidenced both in class interactions and course evaluations. Ground rules for discussion are that persons should consider their points carefully, articulate them succinctly (this skill can take time to learn), be nonjudgmental in any challenge to the point of view of others, consider all sides of the issue carefully, and be willing to try and understand the other person's perspective even when disagreement exists. In the small group case, discussion members take turns leading the group and reporting the group process.

The book is divided into three sections. The first section lays a foundation for understanding what is ethical advanced practice nursing. The chapters in this section build upon one another. Chapter 1 traces the development of professional ethics back to its origins in moral philosophy, that is, in the development of theories about what it is good for human beings to be or do. Chapter 2 explores the idea that nursing ethics is both an area of study about what are good nursing actions and why and is also an appraisal of nursing actions.

The second section investigates common issues in advanced practice that occur regardless of setting or in most settings and provides resources and strategies for dealing with these. Chapter 3 explores the characteristics needed for good advanced practice, decision-making issues as these relate both to patients and advanced practice nurses, concerns about privacy and confidentiality, and the importance of truth telling. Chapter 4 explores the tensions for APNs between attending to the needs of individuals and the needs of the larger society. It discusses human rights and the idea of professional advocacy for ethical healthcare environments. Chapter 5 examines the nature of APN relationships with colleagues and allied health professionals. It is particularly concerned with the nature of collaborative relationships as a means of ensuring ethical patient care. Chapter 6 discusses advanced practice roles related to the ethical treatment of persons who are human subjects of research or who are considering whether they should enroll in a research study.

The third and final section consists of seven chapters, each of which is dedicated to a separate area of specialty practice. The chapter authors each hold advanced practice qualifications in the specialty area and/or have knowledge of the ethical issues peculiar to the content area. The specialty areas are neonatal, pediatrics, women's health, adult health, psychiatric, nurse anesthesia, gerontology, and end-of-life issues.

Acknowledgments

The idea for this book built slowly over time and for its realization depended upon the support, insights, and experiences of countless past and current patients, nurses, colleagues, students, friends, and family. I owe especial thanks and praise to guest authors, who each provided "true" accounts and illustrations of issues faced in their specialties and without whose contributions this book could not achieve its purpose. Additionally, the editorial and marketing staff at Jones and Bartlett Pulishers proved superb at keeping me on track. They quietly, diligently, and encouragingly did their work, paying attention to every detail.

From a lack of scholarly focus earlier in my early life it could not have been foreseen that I would complete any endeavor requiring concentrated effort—so that this book has reached completion is somewhat remarkable even to me. The turnaround was enabled by the incredible people whose lives have collided with mine over the years. My mother—a nursing role model for me—was the first nurse in her family. She had a quiet exterior that belied the toughness she could exert on behalf of her patients. An important influence was the late David Roberts, who urged me to do more and would be smiling now. I am grateful to both my English and West Virginia families, including the IROTI group, for their ongoing encouragement and unconditional acceptance of me as a member.

Thanks must go to current and past students—their experiences are sprinkled throughout the chapters, indeed they authored several. Of my colleagues present and past many deserve mention. Scholarly discussions, debates, and collaborations are a privilege of academic life, and in nursing help us to stay grounded in our professional purposes. Nan Gaylord and I have collaborated, published, and presented together since 1992. She is responsible for the idea of having a textbook that specifically addresses problems of advanced practice and has become a treasured friend. Additionally, I am grateful to work in an environment that supports and encourages scholarly growth. Former and present Boston College colleagues Sara Fry, Lois Haggerty, Dorothy Jones, Sr. Callista Roy,

Danny Willis, and Ellen Mahoney, along with many others, have proved an invaluable source of new insights, ideas, and critique. Their interest in nursing's responsibilities for patient and societal good is unwavering. Collaborative relationships with Martha Jurchak, Ellen Robinson, and Elizabeth Tracey, who are all nurses and clinical ethics experts, informed much of the content. Martha Jurchak thoughtfully reviewed some of the book content.

Besides nursing colleagues, my thanks go to faculty in the philosophy department at the University of Tennessee–Knoxville who helped me to develop and hone philosophical skills—although they didn't completely succeed in getting me to exchange my "nursing hat" for a philosopher's. Glenn Graber deserves a special mention for his steadfast support of my desire to apply the fruits of philosophical study to nursing problems. I have also benefited from the lasting friendships of my philosophy student cohort.

Finally, thanks to MLB Chris Hayford, without whom these last two years would have been much more arduous and less joyful.

Contributors

Jane Flanagan, PhD, APRN, BC
Assistant Professor
William F. Connell School of Nursing
Boston College
Chestnut Hill, MA

Nan Gaylord, PhD, RN, CPNP
Associate Professor
College of Nursing
University of Tennessee
Knoxville, TN

Debbie Giambanco, RNC, MSN,
    NNP, BC
Neonatal Nurse Practitioner
Children's Hospital Boston
Boston, MA

Peggy Doyle Settle, RNC, PhD(c)
Doctoral Candidate
Boston College
Chestnut Hill, MA

Gregory Sheedy, CRNA, MS
Anesthesia Associates of
    Massachusetts
Clinical Instructor
William F. Connell of Nursing
Boston College
Chestnut Hill, MA

Katharine T. Smith, RN, MS, ARNP
Women's Health Nurse Practitioner
Planned Parenthood of Western
    Washington
Seattle, WA

Pamela A. Terreri, MS, APRNBC
Clinical Assistant Professor
William F. Connell School of Nursing
Boston College
Chestnut Hill, MA

FOUNDATIONS OF ADVANCED PRACTICE NURSING ETHICS

CHAPTER 1

Philosophical Foundations of Applied and Professional Ethics

Pamela J. Grace

Believe those who are seeking the truth. Doubt those who find it.
Andre Gide, 1869–1951

INTRODUCTION

This chapter explains that the roots and strength of advanced pract
nurses' (APNs') professional responsibilities are in philosophical understa
ings about what constitutes good human action and why. From this founda
we are able to trace the development and nature of professional responsibili
the population served by the nursing profession. A clear argument is prese
about why membership in a profession that provides an important servi
individuals and society involves stronger obligations to further the human
than exists in civilian life. Finally, an exploration of the place of philoso
skills, theories, and principles in decision making about good action pro
basis for examining the complex issues encountered by APNs. This is an
tant first step for developing and enhancing APNs' confidence in their
decision-making skills.

GROUNDWORK

The Problem of Professional Responsibility

Most nurses and allied professionals understand that the p
professional healthcare practice is accompanied by both mora
accountability for professional judgments and the resulting action
many are not confident that they are adequately equipped to addre
to good practice or the complex ethical problems that can ar
care situations. Yet good patient care is reliant on all of the fo
cian characteristics: knowledgeable, skillful, and experience
about inadequacies in the caregiving environment; willingness t

3

'vidual needs of the patient in question; and motivated to resolve problems
variety of levels as necessary. These listed characteristics are important
ɔvious reasons and are discussed in more detail in Chapter 2, but less
ɪs is the idea that those in need of healthcare services are often not
ɪdgeable about what is required to meet their current or future health
ɪren't qualified to evaluate the quality of the services offered, and/or
ɪocate effectively to receive the care needed (Newton, 1988). The
of unmet or even unrecognized health needs makes people more
arily vulnerable to the ups and downs of life. The effects of unad-
ɪlth needs on human functioning and flourishing make it crucial
are professionals can be trusted to maintain their primary focus
' and societal healthcare needs even when faced with economic,
ɔr time pressures.

ice
ɪnd-
tion
ty to
ɪnted
ce to
good
phical
ɪides a
impor-
ethical

ɪtionships

s have argued that the healthcare professional–patient rela-
ɪy (Grace, 1998; Pellegrino, 2001; Spenceley, Reutter, & Allen,
That is, it is based on trust. People with healthcare needs
ɪn clinicians to understand, anticipate, and provide what
question professionals about their responsibilities, how
ɪe are, or about the basis for claiming that professionals
ɔd practice, we get varying and inconsistent answers or
ɪuestion is even being raised. Chambliss (1996), in the
ɪrses working in institutional settings, notes that when
ɪowerless to influence change in a setting where there
ɪ, they can become numbed to the ethical content
ɪ it. Others have also documented the problems for
Besides the issue of ceasing to respond to unethical
ɪ the setting or seek other types of employment
' unease also called *moral distress* (Corley, 2002;
ɔbs, 2005; Jameton, 1984; Mohr & Mahon, 1996).
believe that some nurses do not understand the
(Grace, Fry, & Schultz, 2003). Thus, recogni-
ractice responsibilities requires the nurse to
fashion in order not to become anesthetized
ɪs that at best fail to focus on optimal care
' patient. Throughout this book, reasoning
a that professional responsibility exists to
ɪ more deeply rooted systemic or societal

ɪivilege of
ɪ and legal
ɪs. However,
ss obstacles
ɪse in direct
lowing clini-
ɪ; perceptive
ɪ focus on the

Good Practice

From a philosophical stance, *good practice* is equivalent to ethical practice. *Ethical practice* is the use of disciplinary knowledge, skills, experience, and personal characteristics to conceptualize what is needed either at the level of the individual or of society. Ethical professional practice uses the goals and perspectives of the given profession to direct action. Although it is true that various healthcare professions share common goals such as promotion of health, cure of disease, and relief of suffering, they nevertheless have different practice philosophies and draw on different knowledge bases to achieve these goals.

Even when professionals understand the strength of their responsibilities, many factors can interfere with accomplishing good care. This is especially true in contemporary healthcare settings where competing interests can make it difficult to provide good patient care to individuals even when the clinician's judgment about what is needed is sound. Barriers to autonomous practice are frequently encountered and can include economic interests, institutional priorities, and provider conflicts. Some obstacles to practice are recurrent and arise out of underlying contextual or societal conditions that disadvantage groups of people and thus require a broader understanding of professional responsibility as relating to individuals, institutions, and society (Ballou, 2000; C, 2001; Spenceley et al., 2006). The broad scope of professional responsibility is discussed in more detail in Chapter 4.

As noted, this and the next three chapters are designed to provide the basis for APNs, and perhaps others in advanced practice roles, to understand the origins, scope, and limits of their responsibilities to patients and to society. They provide the APN with the knowledge, tools, and skills for ethical practice. Included in the necessary skill set is an understanding of the language of clinical ethics. This is because all nurses—but especially APNs—collaborate with others on behalf of their patients and need a common language with which to articulate their concerns about the issues they face in practice.

Philosophy, Professional Responsibility, and Nursing Ethics: What's the Connection?

Nursing ethics and *professional responsibility* are equivalent. This idea is reinforced throughout the book. However, one cannot say this is so and expect the reader to agree; the assertion has to be backed by discussion and evidence. This is one of the techniques of

mentation. As a starting place, it is important to grasp that the idea and
bility of ethical practice lie in philosophical understandings about human
and their relationship to the world in which they live.

race the development of professional responsibility from its origins in
hy, it is helpful to rely on an analogy commonly seen in primary care
that of a family tree. The tree and its branches are traced here to give
w, and then pertinent aspects are discussed in more detail. A word
The branches are made distinct for the purposes of clarity, but there
eas of overlap or shared space.

Family Tree

ne of philosophy is the starting point where all theorizing about
world and our place in it begins. There are several branches of
phy. These branches represent particular areas of philosophical
s, ethics, epistemology, logic, and metaphysics" (Flew, 1984,
in Figure 1-1. They all share some common characteristics.
oning and reasoning (the methods of philosophy) to try to
ionship of human beings to the world. However, their theme
different. For example, *aesthetics* is philosophical inquiry
thics is philosophical inquiry about the good and is also
hy (everyday definitions of *ethics* differ from this, as
istemology* is philosophical inquiry about knowledge,
ble it is.

s, our interest is in Ethics viewed as philosophical
Philosophical inquiry about what is good in human
to areas of applied ethics. *Applied ethics* are the
oretical ethics. Branches of applied ethics include
ics (what is good human action with regard to
thics (how should we treat animals and why?),
tions of biological advances and how should they
hics (what is the nature of a given profession's
ns of this for those served?).

as of overlap. For example, bioethics is inquiry
technological advances on humans and what
related to healthcare professions has to do
ed for good professional action. Because
chnology to provide good care, these areas
estion might be "How do we decide who
r people who urgently need it?" Nursing
professional responsibility toward my

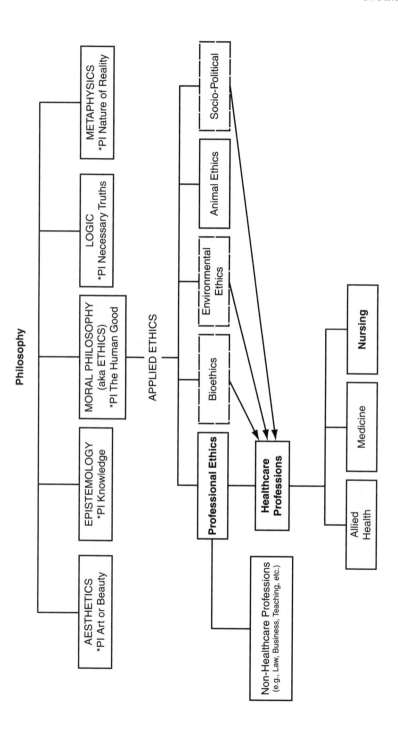

*PI = Philosophical Inquiry about
Dashed-line boxes = Areas of applied ethics impacting the healthcare professions in various ways.

Figure 1-1 The relationship of philosophy to nursing ethics

patient whether or not he receives the heart? What is needed for his good care?" When Ethics or philosophical inquiry about good action is coupled with an area of human practice of some sort, for example, health care, business, or the law, it is called applied ethics. That is, theoretical understandings about what is good and/or the methods of philosophy (analysis and reasoning) are brought to bear upon a situation to both understand it and, if necessary, resolve it.

Ethics: A Few Necessary Distinctions

For the most part, in daily life when people discuss *ethics* they mean something very different from *ethics* as we have been using the word. In common language, *ethics* can merely mean how persons act in their daily lives and whether these actions accord with community values. In professional practice, *ethics* are sets of rules or standards, developed within the profession, that guide the actions of the professionals while working in their professional capacity. The American Nurses Association (ANA) *Code of Ethics for Nurses with Interpretive Statements* (2001) is an example of this latter meaning of ethics. These senses of *ethics* might be grasped more easily if we notice that we could add a modifying term to them. So, for example, *personal* ethics is related to personal conduct, *nursing* ethics is related to the conduct of nurses as they engage in practice, *medical* ethics has to do with the conduct of physicians, *bio*ethics is concerned with the use of technological advances (and so might include a variety of health professionals, researchers, and technology professionals involved in using or propagating these).

Additionally, many people make a distinction between ethics and morals. They view *morals* as personal conduct reflecting personal values, whereas ethics is associated with critical reflection of the values we hold (Weston, 2002). In fact, the root meaning of both terms is the same: "customs, mores, . . . conventions, institutions, laws" (Bahm, 1992, p. 8). For our purposes— considerations of professional judgment and action—the terms *ethical* and *moral* are used interchangeably to mean those actions most likely to further the goals of the profession.

PHILOSOPHY

The term *philosophy* (philosophy with a lowercase *p*) can be used in a variety of ways. It can simply mean one's personal view of a particular thing, as in "what is your philosophy about always telling the truth?" "What is your philosophy on balancing leisure and work?" Philosophy can mean a group's view of the nature and purposes of its work; for example, there are a variety of philosophies of nursing practice. Philosophies of practice use the tools of philosophy to answer important questions about that practice. Florence Nightingale wrote hers as early as 1859 in *Notes on Nursing*. Her ideas were that nurses attended to the patient's environment, making it conducive to natural healing. However, here by *philosophy* I mean the overarching discipline of Philosophy under which more particular philosophies belong.

Philosophy as a discipline encompasses the centuries-old endeavors of thinkers and scholars to find answers to the questions of existence. Philosophy, in this sense, has been concerned with a "search for wisdom about the universe and its workings" as well as the place and role of humans within the universe (Grace, 2004c, p. 280). The Presocratic (meaning before the time of Socrates) Greek philosophers such as Thales, Heraclitus, and Parmenides (around the 6th century B.C.) are considered the first philosophers (Russell, 1972). It is thought that before this time period people relied on mythological explanations for the mysterious and seemingly unpredictable workings of nature. The Presocratics, however, sought explanations using reason and observation.

For our purposes, the discipline of philosophy uses reason and analysis to examine questions that are not answerable or not completely answerable by empirical science. As Nagel (1987) notes, "The main concern of philosophy is to question and understand very common ideas that all of us use every day" (p. 5) but often without giving much thought to their meanings. As an example, empirical science investigates the causes and effects of heart disease in the interests both of prevention and cures. Philosophical inquiry, however, would be concerned with questions such as "Is it possible to have a stable definition of health? Is health measurable?" If the answer to the question of "what is health?" is at all dependent on a subjective interpretation by a given individual, then it is not measurable by science.

Another way to look at this is to say philosophical inquiry highlights what cannot be true but does not necessarily give us truths. In fact, one major question of philosophy concerns "what is truth?" The main methods of philosophy are thinking and questioning. Reason is used to formulate and pose questions, seek out and examine possible answers, anticipate what objections could be made to the answers, or question whether counterexamples exist that would reveal a theory to be false. Philosophy also helps us to understand the limits of our knowledge.

The discipline of philosophy, then, can be seen to be the enterprise of inquiry itself. The major subareas of philosophical inquiry were presented earlier. The branch of philosophy most pertinent to the current discussion of healthcare professional responsibility is that of moral philosophy, also known as Ethics. From now on, when referring to that branch of philosophical inquiry about human good, I refer to it either as moral philosophy or Ethics with a capital *e* to distinguish it from the idea of ethics as rules or standards for action.

Moral Philosophy: The Study of Ethics

Ethics as a term used to describe the area of philosophical inquiry about what it means to say something is good, bad, or neutral in human activity is also often referred to as moral philosophy. As you have seen, this is a different view of ethics from that apparent in the term's use in everyday language. Philosophical inquiry is a theoretical endeavor; therefore, Ethics is also a theoretical endeavor. Ethics or moral philosophy is concerned with understanding human values. In fact, moral philosophy often leads to the development of theories of value.

Value theories, often also called *moral theories*, try to answer such questions as "what do we mean when we say something is good, bad, praiseworthy, or blameworthy? What makes something, someone, or some action good or bad? Is something good because it is in line with divinely given rules using certain people as intermediaries (for example, Moses and the 10 commandments), or because it helps humans live a satisfying life? Are qualities of goodness and badness inherent in human nature? Are there some things that are absolutely right or wrong? Or are the understandings we have about right and wrong, good and bad just conventions developed over the years to make it easier for humans to live in relative harmony with others?" Moral philosophers have different answers to these questions. The answers they give are meticulously thought through and provide important insights into the meaning and purposes of human life. It is, however, important to remember that these insights are always necessarily influenced by the lives and political times in which the philosophers engaged in their analyses. Different theories can give conflicting directions and often urge us to take different actions depending on their premises and assumptions. What follows are examples of moral theories along with a critique of their role and limits in healthcare decision making.

Applied Ethics

As noted, the term *moral philosophy* is synonymous with Ethics viewed as a theoretical endeavor. When philosophical and theoretical concepts, suppositions, and skills are applied to practices or human action, the tendency is to refer to this as applied ethics rather than applied moral philosophy, although there is no particular reason for this—it is a convention. Applied ethics takes the theoretical knowledge and assumptions gained as a result of ethical theorizing as well as the skills and tools of moral philosophy (analysis) to solve difficult problems of living. Applied ethics, as its name implies, is the application of moral philosophy to actual situations where it is important to determine good or appropriate actions and where a person or group can be held responsible for these actions. Thus, branches of applied ethics are many and varied and include such entities as ecoethics (good human actions related to the ecosystem), animal ethics, bioethics, and professional ethics.

The appropriate ethical conduct of a profession such as nursing is determined by a synthesis of philosophical inquiry about the ontology of the profession (what nursing is, why it exists, and what its goals are), what constitutes good practice for the discipline (moral philosophy), and what is the force of the responsibility of the profession both as an organized body and via its individual members to engage in actions that further its goals (applied or practice ethics). The result of this synthesis is *nursing ethics*. Nursing ethics is an applied ethics. It is the study of what constitutes good nursing practice, what obstacles to good nursing practice exist, and what the responsibilities of nurses are related to their professional conduct. Nursing ethics can be exploratory, descriptive, or normative (also called prescriptive). Chapter 2 discusses both senses of nursing ethics in more detail.

MORAL REASONING IN HEALTH CARE: TOOLS

"Ethics as a field of inquiry studies the foundation for distinguishing good from bad and right from wrong in human action" (Grace, 2004a, pp. 299–300). "The theoretical interest is concerned with knowing; the practical interest is concerned with doing" (Melden, 1967, p. 2). Thus, moral reasoning in health care uses theoretical understandings, reasoned assumptions, and proposals about what is the good for humans and applies these theoretical explanations to problematic or complex situations where it is not clear what actions should be taken. Besides the tools of philosophy, personal characteristics and abilities are needed for the application of theory to particular cases. The purpose of this section is to describe the scope and limits of various philosophical approaches in resolving ethical issues in healthcare settings. This section is designed to familiarize APNs with the language and techniques of Ethics in the interest of facilitating communication and collaboration on behalf of their patients or patient groups.

An important point that is emphasized throughout this book is that nursing goals serve as the linchpin for decision making and are related to different aspects of promoting health and human functioning as determined by the specialty practice focus. The tools of applied ethics, then, facilitate our understanding of what is required to promote professional goals. In this sense, the question of what is the good has already been answered by nursing's scholars and theorists. Unlike the larger unanswered or unanswerable philosophical question "what is the ultimate good for human beings?" the nursing profession has an answer related to its practice and existence. We have determined what the profession's good is as explored in more detail in the following chapter.

The four main types of philosophical tools that apply to morally ambiguous healthcare situations are moral theories, moral perspectives, moral principles, and analytic techniques. An extensive discussion of ethical theory and principles is not possible (or desirable) here—whole books are devoted to any one of the theories or principles and further books are dedicated to the critiques of these. However, a comprehensive summary of those aspects of previous work in moral theory that are important for our contemporary understanding of moral authority and responsibility follows. Analytic techniques are discussed in more detail in the following chapter.

Moral Theory

What is moral theory? The simple answer is that it is a systematic justified explanation of what good means in terms of how human beings *do* or *should* seek to live their lives. That is, it may be either a descriptive (*do*) or prescriptive (*should*) theory. The author of the theory has tried to formulate an answer to the unsolved question "What is the meaning of good as it relates to human lives and human living?" The theorist, using reasoning, observation, and questioning, formulates a hypothesis and systematically justifies it, all the while trying to anticipate and address possible objections that could be raised by critics of the theory or by those holding different views. Because one of the tasks of philosophy is to show what cannot logically be true (the logic branch of philosophy), every theory has many philosopher critics.

Theorizing about human lives and the nature of good has been evident since the times of the ancient Greek philosophers such as Socrates (circa 450 B.C.), Plato, and Aristotle. There has been an ongoing quest to find systematic explanations and/or unchangeable, irrefutable truths about what is valuable in human lives. One reason this has been seen as important is the human desire for stability, the need to dispel uncertainty about action, and for clarity and direction about how we should live. As stated earlier, you may also hear moral theory referred to as value theory because its subject matter has to do with what is taken to be valuable, or what should be valued. That is, if we know what it is good for humans to pursue, what sorts of lives it is good to live, and which human characteristics it is good to develop and we have sound reasons why, then we can feel that we have a relatively firm footing from which to move forward.

No theorist, however, has found a flawless answer to that question; neither have any developed theories that can completely withstand critique. Contemporarily, many thinkers argue that this quest to find the highest good for human beings, or in Latin the *summun bonum*, is misbegotten. In fact, Dewey (1980), a philosopher of the American Pragmatist School, noted the reason that philosophers have struggled so hard and long for answers is that "man who lives in a world of hazards is compelled to seek for security" (p. 3), but the nature of human life is such that it can't be found. Thus, a paradox exists.

When relatively cohesive theories have been proposed, they made sense because of the contexts and time periods in which a particular philosopher lived but may not always be relevant currently or may not be relevant in all situations. Additionally, moral theories for the most part come up with different answers to similar questions.

> The ultimate "good" for persons (or that which persons should or do strive for as an end in itself) has been conceptualized variously as happiness (Bentham, 1789/1967; Mill, 1863/1967, duty (Kant 1785/1967; Ross, 1930), the cultivation of virtue (Aristotle, trans. 1967; MacIntyre, 1984), or something else. . . . This difference is the result of fundamentally contrasting beliefs about the nature of human beings and their place and purpose in the world. (Grace, 2004a, p. 299)

Thus, it is not surprising that they will give us different answers to the hard questions of life. We will not spend a lot of time discussing the different moral theories here because we do not tend to rely on one or another of them in clinical or healthcare settings although, from my experiences in teaching ethics, it is evident that people often *want* to use a moral theory to frame a question or justify action. This desire, arguably, stems from the mistaken idea that theories such as utility or Kantian deontology are authoritative—they give us the security that Right answers and Right actions are knowable and possible. However, we can only ever be *reasonably* sure that our actions will have good consequences.

Moral theories can be useful in clarifying an issue or highlighting underlying assumptions. They may give us some structure with which to examine an issue, but we must always be clear about why we think this is a pertinent theoretical perspective to use for the task at hand. That is, we must understand the limits of the theory and what its flaws are, rather than uncritically relying on theories to answer difficult issues in health care.

More frequently, we use ideas from an assortment of moral theories to help us clarify our thinking. These ideas are referred to as *principles*. Principles that are particularly pertinent to use in health settings are discussed shortly. However, as noted earlier, the goals of decision making in advanced practice situations are usually concerned with the well-being of a patient, or patient group, directly in our sphere of practice. This is true even when we are in supervisory, collaborative, or consultative relationships with other providers—decisions being made are ultimately with the interests of the patient in mind. Finally, the tools of moral reasoning also prompt us to ask questions about underlying conditions that give rise to the problem in front of us and help us to recognize the wide scope of professional responsibilities.

Descriptive versus Normative Theories

Moral theories such as David Hume's (1777/1967) are based on observations of what people seem to believe with regard to good actions and what reasons they give for their decisions or actions. Such theories do not prescribe what people ought to do. They are observational and explanatory rather than having any moral force. They make no claims about the existence of some universal underlying purpose that human beings should strive to fulfill, but rather aim to describe human action. Lately, a number of research studies have looked at how nurses practice, what they think is good care, what characteristics are important, and/or how they address obstacles (Corley et al., 2005; Doane, Pauly, Brown, & McPherson, 2004; Hardingham, 2004; Peter, Lunardi, & Macfarland, 2004; Varcoe et al., 2004). These result in *descriptive* conceptions of ethical practice. That is, they don't say what is right or wrong but rather what people think is right and wrong and the reasons they give for their actions.

Normative theories, on the other hand, direct action. "They are either, reasoned and logically explored explanations of the moral purpose of human interactions, or they are divinely revealed truths about good action (religious ethics)" (Grace, 2005, p. 102). Essentially they argue that because this or that is the ultimate good for human beings, then we should pursue that good; we have a responsibility to do so. So, for example, whereas the ANA's *Code of Ethics for Nurses with Interpretive Statements* (2001) is not a theory as such, it is a normative document. It tells nurses how they ought to practice and what their behavior or conduct should be. It has moral force.

Normative Moral Theories: Some Examples

Two types of normative moral theory familiar to most people are (1) consequentialist, that is, good consequences are the focus of action, and (2) duty-based or deontological, where what matters more than actual consequences is that one acts according to what is one's duty. Perhaps the best-known consequentialist theories are those of the utilitarians. Jeremy Bentham (1748–1832) and John Stuart Mill (1806–1873) both were instrumental in the development of utilitarianism. Both were social reformers reacting to the injustices of the time period in which they lived. The Industrial Revolution, which started around 1760 according to Ashton (1961/1997), caused oppression of the new working classes and mass poverty—it resulted in vast inequities in wealth. A few industrialists held all the power and wealth (Engels, 1845/1987).

Bentham was heavily influenced by Hume's descriptive moral theory that proposed that most human values are socially constructed and stem both from intrinsic human characteristics such as the ability to sympathize with others and the pleasurable effects of benevolent acts as enacted, experienced, or observed (this is a greatly simplified explanation of Hume's work). Hume is credited with introducing the idea of a utility principle into the English language. It represents the idea that human responses are fortified in relation to perception of the usefulness of their actions to others and the pleasure gained from this (Hume, 1748/1963).

Bentham, a peer and friend of John Stuart Mill's father James Mill, further developed the principle of utility and presented it as one having moral force. That is, if it is true that humans desire happiness and shun pain and suffering, then that is the good toward which human beings *should* strive. Giving these ideas moral force allowed the social reformers to criticize inequities caused by the Industrial Revolution and to push for reform. Many reforms, "legal, political, social, and educational" (Flew, 1984, p. 41), did occur as a result of utilitarian ideas. As Melden (1967) notes, "Hume's principle of Utility was transformed (by Bentham) with unwavering consistency into 'the greatest happiness principle' " (p. 367).

Following Bentham, Mill (1861/1965) wrote that "pleasure and freedom from pain are the only things desirable as ends, . . . all other desirable things (which are as numerous in the utilitarian as in any other scheme [*sic*]) are desirable either for the pleasure inherent in themselves, or as a means to the promotion of pleasure and the preventions of pain" (p. 281). Pleasure is qualitative in nature for Mill, so he does distinguish between mere physical pleasures and higher level intellectual ones. Further, the goals of action are to maximize overall happiness for a society and minimize overall pain or suffering. Each person's happiness is to count the same as everyone else's; in this sense, the theory presents an impartial view. "Because of their focus on overall good, there are implications to these theories that many would find troubling" (Grace, 2004a, p. 300) and not in tune with our intuitions about good actions. For example, it would be permissible to cause harm to one innocent person if this would relieve 100 other sufferers from pain.

There are other critiques of utilitarianism, but the most salient for our purposes is that APNs are interested in the well-being of each patient, and this requires understanding who the patient is. Context and details, the *who* of our patients, are important. Utilitarian considerations might require us to ignore individual details in the obligation to provide an overall good. Nevertheless, in social policy and justice settings, the ideas behind utilitarianism are important. We do not tend to think that social arrangements need benefit only a few when the majority is living in poverty. In healthcare settings, we obviously do think that the possible consequences of our actions are crucial considerations in planning actions—however, particular consequentialist theories do not provide a stable framework for us because of their flaws.

Neither are deontologic or duty-based theories suitable as blanket frameworks for decision making in health care. Immanuel Kant's (1724–1804) moral philosophy is deontologic. It focuses on the idea that something other than consequences is the most important consideration in decision making. That something is duty. The main philosophical assumption underlying Kant's (1785/1967) theory is that human beings are rational animals. We have the ability to reason and therefore the capacity for self-governance. Indeed, "the hallmark of human beings is their innate reasoning ability" (Grace, 2004a, p. 300). Because humans have this capacity, Kant goes further to say that we have a duty to do the action that our reason tells us is the most rational. How do we do this? We ask ourselves whether in all similar circumstances we would agree that people could act in the same way that we are proposing to act and whether we would be willing to support a rule to this effect. If the answer is yes, then it is permissible for us to act in this way. If the answer no, then duty forbids us from the action. Duty forbids us because it would be irrational for us to act as we would not wish others to act. Kant calls this principle the Categorical Imperative because it is unwavering in its moral force. We must act from duty regardless of consequences. For Kant, interestingly, it is this capacity of human beings to determine right from wrong actions that makes them worthy of respect as individuals and underlies the principle of autonomy, which I discuss in more detail shortly.

Other versions of duty-based theories are derived from religious traditions. Kant's exquisitely argued and detailed theorizing was an attempt to avoid the criticisms leveled at religious theories by basing the idea of moral duties on human capacity to reason. For Kant (1785/1967), then, there are absolute rules, such as truthfulness. He wrote that deviating from the truth even when it might not be convenient for us would be irrational. It would be irrational because if we could not rely on the sincerity of others with whom we are conversing, then meaningful communication would be impossible. Interestingly, Kant did not think that women and children had the same capacity for reasoning as men.

Criticisms of duty-based theories include (1) the rules are too abstract to apply in practice, for example, how specific should we be in determining whether a situation is similar to another? What is truth telling and does it include withholding information that might be unpleasant to us and yet not necessary for us to know? (2) What if telling the truth might cause harm to another and yet reason (Categorical Imperative) tells us we should not harm another? How do we decide between equally compelling duties?

Ethical Principles

So, we have seen that although moral theories exist as attempts to describe how human beings act or propose how human beings should act and additionally provide justification for the soundness of the theory, we should not treat them as authoritative frameworks for action in healthcare settings. Nevertheless, they do provide some important insights about human values and characteristics: utilitarianism for its ability to critique social injustices and deontology for its implications that there are general rules that we could all rationally agree upon.

Our job is to determine both what are good professional actions in situations that require attention to nuance and particularities and what is needed to identify and address more entrenched problems related to inadequacies in the healthcare system. A key point is that certain principles derived from moral theories together with analytic philosophical techniques have proved helpful in healthcare settings for separating out aspects of complex situations, illuminating hidden assumptions and factors, and revealing gaps in information. Also, they are helpful in assisting clinicians as they reflect on why they feel uneasy about certain situations. It is important for collaboration and communication that the implications of certain principles are understood. Yet there is often confusion about the origins, definition, and implications of a given ethical principle. The next section explores some important principles in a little more depth. Many of the ensuing chapters discuss these principles further in the context of specialty settings and situations.

What Are Ethical Principles?

Ethical principles are rules, standards, or guidelines for action that are derived from theoretical propositions (different moral theories) about what is good for humans. Important principles emerge over time as their usefulness in imposing order on a situation, highlighting important considerations in problem solving complex issues, locating the proper object of decision making, or enhancing social harmony is realized. They reflect philosophical, cultural, religious, and societal beliefs about what is valuable. Thus, what are considered priority principles in one society may not be taken as important in another society. In Western cultures, and related to problems of healthcare delivery, several principles have retained importance over the last few decades. The most prominent examples have been explored and described in detail by Beauchamp and Childress (2001) and include autonomy, nonmaleficence, beneficence, and justice. We are charged with determining if they apply in a given situation. If they do, then the principle must be translated into appropriate prescriptions for action. By that I mean in healthcare practice professional judgment is still needed to determine whether a given principle applies and, if it does, how it will be honored. For example, most of us understand that respect for a person's autonomy is an important ethical principle, and that, all things being equal, is likely to serve the person's good. However, if the issue that the APN encounters is related to an incompetent colleague, then the pertinent principle to use as a guide is nonmaleficence (or how we prevent this patient from being harmed by our incompetent colleague).

In nursing practice, advocacy, caring, engagement with the patient, and knowing the patient within his or her context are also important principles derived from the profession's philosophies of practice, goals, and the roles of nurses. These principles are explored further in the next chapter.

Usefulness and Limits of Ethical Principles

Ethical principles are useful in helping us identify salient issues, clarify important factors, uncover hidden assumptions, and affirm appropriate actions. However, the goals of nursing drive the principles used rather than the other way around. For example, the principle of beneficence (in general) exhorts us to provide a good, but the goals of nursing describe what that good is (e.g., promotion of health or relief of suffering), and nursing knowledge, skills, and experience provide the recipe for achieving the good. Motivation provides the impetus for action.

We need to understand that principles alone cannot solve healthcare problems because two or more principles pertinent to a situation can give conflicting direction. Additionally, principles tend to be too abstract and nonspecific to be practical. For example, no one is ever completely autonomous; we are all influenced by conscious and unconsciously experienced pressures—so, what degree of autonomy is acceptable and how do we determine this? Principles are not always sensitive to context. For example, what does *autonomous choice* mean when the patient is from a culture where family, not individual, decision making is the norm? Finally, human decision making and the actions that flow from this process involve values and emotions as well as reasoning, so these are also considerations.

In the next few paragraphs, Beauchamp and Childress's (2001) four major principles are explored in more detail. I highlight both the useful and problematic aspects of using these principles in nursing practice settings. Other helpful philosophical perspectives on solving practice problems include feminist ethics approaches, caring ethics, and virtue ethics. In later chapters, these concepts are illustrated in the specialty cases and case analyses.

The Principle of Autonomy

If we randomly polled 20 people and asked them for their understanding of the term *autonomy*, we would probably get several related but different answers. It is a term that is susceptible to a variety of interpretations. The word *autonomy* comes from Greek and literally means self-rule. It was originally used to describe the nature of governance in Hellenic cities (Beauchamp & Childress, 2001) rather than to describe individual capacities or rights. Subsequent understandings of autonomy are related to persons as individuals. Among the various meanings are self-determination, independence, freedom of the will, and ability to regulate one's own conduct using reason. It has become one of the more powerful moral principles in framing Western social and political systems and underlies ideas of universal human rights.

Because all of these different if overlapping meanings exist, it is important that clinicians clarify what definition of *autonomy* they are using when engaged in collaborative discussions or when presenting the patient's point of view. Transparency is needed to avoid miscommunication. In current healthcare practice, the recognition that patients have rights to self-determine both acceptable treatment and with whom information may be shared is derived from the ethical principle of autonomy.

So, in healthcare settings, what is meant by the principle of autonomy, where does it come from, and what are the implications for clinicians? Immanuel Kant (1724–1804) is perhaps the best-known proponent of autonomy as a moral principle. He wrote that because human beings have the capacity to reason, decide, and act, they should be free from the interference of others at least as far as personal decision making is concerned. Moreover, "reason is the ruler of our will" (Kant, 1785/1967, p. 322). Our will is good in and of itself. This is evident to Kant because of "the common idea of duty and moral laws" that is evident in social life (p. 319). Kant gives the example that people know lying is wrong—they can reason this out for themselves—because lying works against social interests in being able to communicate and interact. Thus, it is self-evident for Kant that morality is an a priori condition, inherent in us. For Kant, because man has the inherent capacity for moral decision making, he should never be used as a means to an end but always respected as having dignity and being equally worthy of moral consideration as any other man. Interestingly Kant did not view women and children as having the same capacity to reason.

So, for Kant there are two aspects to autonomy. Men, at least, are (1) capable of making their own decisions using reason, and (2) have the inherent structure to permit them to act morally (create moral rules) using the Categorical Imperative described earlier. Like Kant, "John Stuart Mill also argued that human beings—women included—have the capacity and the right to make their own decisions" (Grace, 2004b, p. 33). For Mill, diversity and creativity are to be welcomed. Freedom is in the interests of society—it allows people to flourish and makes for better societies. Indeed, for Mill the only conditions under which it is permissible to interfere with the actions of persons is when their actions pose a serious threat of harm to another person, including restricting the other person's freedom. For Mill, restricting an individual's actions for that person's own good is not permissible. In healthcare settings, both theoretically and ideally, the proscription against overriding the autonomy of another does not go to this extreme. There are occasions when the ethical action is to stop a person who is at risk for serious harm from an action, at least until we can determine whether the person's act is informed, reasonable, and in line with his or her own values and preferences. Whether in actuality we always intervene when there is ambiguity about a person's decision-making capacity is a different issue and is discussed later in this book in relation to obstacles to good practice.

Contemporarily, there is agreement among moral philosophers that the reasoning process of human beings is never completely free from the influence of such things as culturally determined beliefs, emotions, lack of information, or other environmental conditions (Grace, 2004b). Autonomy is always a "more or less" condition: the more powerful and complex the influences we are subjected to, the less likely we are to be able to exercise our autonomy effectively. Decisions may seem to be autonomous when in actuality they are heavily influenced by overt or hidden influences. Therefore, in terms of Kant's ideas we do not possess the absolute freedom to exercise our reasoning divorced from emotional or other influences.

Nevertheless, we do in general accept that people know themselves better than other people do, and thus given certain conditions they have the right to exercise this freedom without interference. Indeed, this moral right has been legislated as a legal right under the Patient Self-Determination Act of 1991 (PSDA). Patients have the right to decide whether they will accept or refuse health care including treatment and interventions. The PSDA is discussed again in relation to various specialty areas later in this book.

Two questions related to professional responsibility arise here. First, and besides the possibility of overt and hidden influences on decision making, some people are not capable of autonomous decision making because they either lack the developmental or cognitive skills necessary. This lack may be temporary or permanent. What is our responsibility in such cases? The short answer is that where possible we try to discover what is known about the person and what his or her wishes would most likely be so that actions are still predicated on the individual. However, in cases where we are not able to determine what a person would have wanted, we use a *reasonable person* standard. We try to decide what a reasonable person would want under similar circumstances. This issue of proxy decision makers is discussed in later chapters and also as related to specialty practice.

The second question relates to the shifting nature of factors influencing the exercise of autonomy. This is often also referred to as *decision-making capacity*. For APNs, related questions are (1) how do we decide when and under what circumstances a person might be deemed capable of autonomous decision making? and (2) what is necessary to facilitate autonomous decision making? Criteria have been proposed that facilitate judgments about whether a person has sufficient decision-making capacity to make a decision that is likely to serve his or her interests. These criteria present their own challenges, but nevertheless they provide a framework for judging and thus for addressing impediments to decision making.

The President's Commission (1982) formulated from the pertinent literature, commission members expertise, and discussions a minimum set of capacities needed for competent decision making. These are as follows:

- Possession of a set of values and goals
- The ability to communicate and to understand information
- The ability to reason and deliberate about one's choice (President's Commission, 1982, p. 57)

This means that for a voluntary choice to be made, professionals need to evaluate the cognitive maturity and abilities of the person. They must assess what information the person needs and how best to provide this—thus, a process of informing (rather than a singular presentation of information) is often needed. An evaluation of influences that might interfere with information processing is important. Interfering influences could include any of the following: unconscious or conscious psychological pressures; physiologic factors such as hypoxia, fever, pain; contextual issues such as economics (personal and institutional), provider pressures, or wishing to please a provider. Finally, the patient should be able to describe how a given course of action is likely to map on to his or her own life trajectory.

Perhaps the most important thing to understand is that patients who obviously do not grasp the implications of proposed actions for their own goals and future life are not in a position to act autonomously. Thus, respecting autonomy in health care means something else besides letting a patient make his or her own mistakes. Finally, in respecting autonomy there is a tendency not to interfere with people's decisions if we are sure these are informed and/or if the risks are low. However, if the risks of a proposed course of action chosen by a patient are high, then we must make a more concerted effort to ensure that these are autonomous decisions. Overriding a person's autonomy is a serious business but is sometimes necessary to serve the patient's own interests. The rationale for overriding a patient's decision is that this is most likely to serve the patient's own interests and preserve autonomy (if the person dies—then no further autonomy is possible in this life anyway).

The Principle of Nonmaleficence

Of the ethical principle nonmaleficence, Beauchamp and Childress (2001) note that "in medical ethics it has been closely associated with the maxim *primum non nocere:* 'Above all [or first] do no harm' " (p. 113). Some scholars have said that nonmaleficence means do no *intentional* harm. In healthcare practice and especially in APN practice settings, nonmaleficence is a nuanced principle with several implications. Some scholars treat nonmaleficence as a subcategory of beneficence. However, exploring it separately permits conceptual clarity.

First, it is not always clear what is meant by harm. Does psychological, spiritual, or economic distress count as harm, or does only physical distress count? Beauchamp and Childress (2001) construe harm as "thwarting, defeating, or setting back some party's interests . . . (A) *harmful action* by one party may not be wrong or unjustified *on balance, although acts of harming in general are prima facie wrong*" (italics as in the original) (pp. 116–117). *Prima facie* means on first sight. So, this means that harms are generally wrong but occasionally may be justified. In civilian life, this means a robber may be harmed by incarceration, but this harm is justified. In healthcare settings, harms are not justifiable unless they set back the patient's interests temporarily to provide a longer term benefit. For example, inserting an intravenous catheter to provide fluids and antibiotics to someone in septic shock may be permissible even if the patient objects because the risks of not doing so are irreversible and we don't have time to evaluate the person's decision-making capacity.

For our purposes, it is best to think of harm as either any avoidable distress caused to the patient in the course of providing care, or avoidable distress that is observed by the professional and/or experienced by the patient and brought to the attention of the professional but which is ignored or left unaddressed. We can do harm in several ways, mostly *unintentional* but often avoidable:

- We might fail to adequately understand a patient's needs and thus not protect from preventable harms related to unmet needs.
- Our skills and competence might be inadequate to care for the needs recognized, yet we don't seek qualified assistance.

- We neglect to anticipate foreseeable harmful effects from a proposed course of action.
- We fail to intervene to protect a patient against the actions of an impaired, incompetent, or careless colleague.

In advanced practice, we can also cause harm by referring patients to inappropriate colleagues or not adequately training or supervising others who are caring for the patient under our direction. Patients can also be harmed by ongoing interventions that are not likely to achieve their desired effects (for example, chemotherapy that can only minimally prolong life but cause suffering in the process). Nonmaleficence, then, is closely aligned with ideas of accountability for one's own practice and for practice actions. Accountability means that we take responsibility for trying to anticipate foreseeable harms so that these can either be minimized or are balanced against the good that the actions are intended to achieve. The APN can inadvertently cause harm through ignorance, incompetence, or failure to understand the patient's unique needs and desires. Harm can also be caused to patients when we can't get them what we know to be optimal treatment.

The Principle of Beneficence

The principle of beneficence in many ways is a more active principle than nonmaleficence because it is the duty to provide a good or to benefit persons. In public life, the term *beneficence* "connotes acts of mercy, kindness, and charity" toward others (Beauchamp & Childress, 2001, p. 166). It concerns the duty one person has to provide benefit to another. Beneficence is unlike nonmaleficence in that it is not morally required of societal members except in special circumstances such as parents or guardians toward their wards. "Whether beneficence is viewed as a moral requirement of societal members very much depends upon (the) philosophical beliefs," culture, and values of the individual or prevalent societal values (Grace, 2004a, p. 317).

In healthcare settings, though, beneficence is viewed as the duty to maximize benefits and minimize harms to patients. The goals of healthcare professionals are beneficent—they are inherently for the patient's good, or more broadly, to further societal health. As argued earlier, healthcare professions exist because they provide a critical good for persons. Therefore, beneficence underlies all actions of the professional while engaging in role-related activities. In the next chapter, this basis for action is discussed in more detail.

Conflicts Between Beneficence and Autonomy

Sometimes ensuring beneficence seems to be in conflict with the principle of autonomy. For example, our patient with impending sepsis refuses to have a cannula inserted so that treatment with fluids and antibiotics can begin. At first sight, it seems as if there is a dilemma: honor her autonomy or override it and give the fluids because this is what will save her life. The conflict, however, may be false. If our patient does not meet all of the criteria for voluntary informed consent, then she is not capable of exercising her autonomy. She is not adequately aware of the risks and benefits of refusal. Thus, the beneficent action is to treat but to minimize the harms that may stem from overriding her decision. She may, for instance, feel disrespected or have her trust undermined. Additionally, beneficence supports the idea that as soon as the patient regains decision-making capacity, she resumes her right to make her own decisions as long as these are adequately informed and align with her own life values and goals. Beneficence does not, as some have assumed, mean that we know what is best for the patient but rather that decisions are made based on the individual patient and his or her values, beliefs, and what is known about the patient's life and preferences. So, in overriding a person's autonomy, we are still charged with formulating actions that accord with an understanding of the patient as an individual with unique characteristics.

Paternalism

Paternalism is a term that is often linked to ideas of beneficence. That is, in ethics language, paternalism is the overriding of someone's choices or preferences in that person's own interests. As Beauchamp and Childress (2001) assert, it "is the intentional overriding of one person's known preferences or actions by another person, where the person who overrides justifies the action by the goal of benefiting or avoiding harm to the person whose preferences or actions are overridden" (p. 178). Thus, the patient's own interests are the main focus of paternalistic actions. In viewing paternalism this way, we can see that knowledge of the patient in context and as an individual with a life history, beliefs, and values, where this is possible, is a crucial goal of paternalism.

Paternalism is sometimes understood differently in healthcare settings and has assumed negative connotations in many instances. People, nurses and others, have used it to label the condescending, arrogant, or even self-interested behavior of healthcare providers toward patients who they think are making bad decisions. Patients may be persuaded to accept certain treatments, important information may be withheld from them, or a competent patient may have his or her decision overridden. Understanding the real nature of paternalistic actions as both beneficent (patient's best interests) and supportive in the long run of autonomy (restoring the patient to a state where autonomy can be exercised) keeps us focused on the needs of the patients and away from the lure of expediency.

The Principle of Justice

Several different conceptions of justice exist. In Western societies, retributive justice has to do with punishment for problematic actions, restorative or compensatory justice has to do with restoring to people what they lost in being harmed by another or others, and distributive justice has to do with the distribution of benefits and burdens across a society. For healthcare and healthcare delivery purposes, distributive justice, also understood as social justice, is an important ethical principle. Social justice, then, refers to formal systems that exist to decide who gets what in terms of social goods such as education, food, shelter, and health care. Buchanan (2000) reports that social justice has been an important concept for centuries and continues to be "central to human understandings of socially significant values" (p. 155).

> There are two broad socially-oriented ideas regarding justice. One perspective views justice as being based on desert—those who are more worthy of merit or who contribute more, are viewed as deserving of better social benefits. The other perspective views justice as equalizing benefits across society regardless of merit. This latter view is "justice as fairness." (Grace, 2005, p. 120)

In the literature related to health care, the predominant accounts are of justice as fairness. However, when discussion is about the ethics of rationing scarce resources, one can often detect a justice perspective that favors merit rather than fairness or the treating of people as being equally worthy of moral concern.

John Rawls's *A Theory of Justice* (1971) is a systematic look at the sort of social structures that would need to exist for justice as fairness to prevail. Rawls takes as a starting point Kant's ideas about people as rational and able to divine which actions are morally permissible, obligatory, or forbidden. Rawls's method is a hypothetical device. That is, he wants to show what the underpinnings of a just social system would be and what just institutions would look like. Because man is his own lawmaker, as we have seen from the idea of the Categorical Imperative (the right action is the one that I could agree everyone else *should* take in similar circumstances—that is, it is ethically sound), the design of the system will be dependent on a "group of persons" in the "original position" (Rawls, 1971, p. 12) who don't know their standing in society, or what physical characteristics or material goods they would possess, nor what their "natural assets, and abilities" (p. 12) would be. The hypothesis is that such a group would come up with the rules and standards necessary for the initiation and arrangement of institutions that would ensure everybody is served fairly.

Rawls identifies two rules of justice that he believes would emerge from the group's deliberations taking place as they are behind this "veil of ignorance" about their individual states and traits (Rawls, 1971, p. 136). "First: each person is to have an equal right to the most extensive liberty compatible with a similar liberty for others. Second: social and economic inequalities are to be arranged such that they are both (a) reasonably expected to be to everyone's advantage, and (b) attached to positions and offices open to all" (Rawls, 1971, p. 60).

As might be expected, Rawls's theory is subject to a variety of criticisms, including that the nature of human beings is such that this wouldn't eliminate jockeying for power and advantage and thus upset any ethical system initiated. However, the salient aspects of the theory for our purposes are that justice in this sense means that we need to be alert to inequities and be willing to address them. Any inequities within a society's arrangements should be slanted toward benefiting the least well off. In contemporary U.S. health care, most would agree that justice as fairness might be accepted in spirit but not in reality. Nevertheless, for APNs the ideas behind justice as fairness cohere with the premises of the ANA's (2003) *Social Policy Statement* and its *Code of Ethics for Nurses with Interpretive Statements* (ANA, 2001). Therefore, it is among our professional responsibilities to promote justice in health care because without this, the most vulnerable will remain most at risk for not receiving good care. Chapter 4 presents a more in-depth discussion of this issue.

Justice is an important concept related to research, managed care, and health disparities. The important thing to keep in mind about justice as fairness is that it is an impartial look at inequities. It might be a requirement of justice as fairness that the special needs of a disadvantaged group are considered, but each member of the group is impartially and equally accorded that consideration. The nature of justice in health care, then, is that in some circumstances it might give rise to tensions for the APN. For example, a nurse's clinical judgment leads her to believe that her patient needs an expensive drug that is not on formulary, perhaps because of prior sensitivities to other drugs or because current drugs are detrimental in some other way. She feels that she must advocate for her patient to get this, and other patients might also benefit but not to the same degree. In advocating for this treatment, resources may be diverted away from others in her care.

Other Approaches

Several other helpful approaches can assist in ethical decision making. These are discussed briefly in this section. They are not theories, rather they are added dimensions that permit us to look more deeply into the underlying conditions that give rise to practice problems.

Feminist Ethics and the Ethic of Care

Over the past few decades, feminist philosophers have criticized analytic philosophical theory and its methods as these are applied in healthcare settings (Donchin & Purdy, 1999; Tong, 1997; Warren, 2001). They suggest that beside moral theory and reasoning, ethical decision making in health care requires the "unearthing of buried assumptions about the influence of power in relationships and situations" (Grace, 2004a, p. 302). Feminist ethics, then, is not a singular approach but an assortment of perspectives. "A feminist approach is defined by taking as its starting point the experience of women, by acknowledging that this experience is characterized by oppression and domination" (Peter & Liaschenko, 2003, p. 33). Feminist ethics approaches do not limit themselves only to the concerns of women but address oppression and domination wherever they occur. So, other issues of concern are "race, class, class, disability, sexual orientation, and so forth" (Peter & Liaschenko, 2003, p. 37).

This is different from the focus of many of the theories we have explored so far. The traditional moral theories tend to view persons as isolated individuals with the right to have their autonomous actions protected or to pursue happiness. Davis, Aroskar, Liaschenko, and Drought (1997) note that Gilligan's research on moral development revealed women's moral concerns to be focused more on "care and responsibility in relationships rather than on the application of abstract principles such as respect for individual autonomy and justice" (p. 58). This is an important insight for nurses because their work is most frequently with individuals and the goals of the profession include caring for the individual as a unique being in all of his or her complexity. Chapter 2 explores the ethic of care in more detail as it applies to nursing practice. Good nursing care involves engagement with the patient and a willingness to focus on the whole person in context. This means that nurses understand the place and importance of significant others in the patient's life.

Feminist perspectives are also helpful in looking at the contexts within which nurses work. Feminist ethics supports the idea that "moral decision-making must include an investigation of both hidden and overt power relationships implicit in ethical problems" (Grace, 2005, p. 105). Questions to pose from a feminist perspective, when involved in ethically challenging situations include: What are the power structures—social, institutional, or interpersonal? Is there an imbalance? Who has an interest in keeping a power imbalance? How is this affecting the patient or the decision making? How can we change the focus of power or empower the person who is the primary focus of the issue?

Narrative Ethics

Narrative ethics represents another contemporary approach to addressing ethical issues. Narratives are stories of people's lives or situations told with rich detail and often from different perspectives. They are most frequently used either in a teaching/learning environment or as an after-the-fact exploration of a difficult case. In narrative ethics, stories are used to explore hidden facets of morally worrisome cases. They may portray the experiences of different persons involved in the story, giving fuller dimensions than usually available in a clinical case presentation. Narrative explorations permit the fleshing out of nuances in a given situation as well as stimulating further questions to be asked. Stories also permit people to vicariously engage in the experience of another although from their own subjective stance. This can enhance empathy and compassion, which in turn facilitates understanding of how the person or situation got to a certain point in time. Stories are attentive to context and evolve over the time period of the narrative rather than being a static time slice. Narrative ethics is also a way of learning from situations that have already occurred. Criticisms of narrative ethics include the problem that it is difficult to apply ethical norms or determine what the good action would be.

SUMMARY

This chapter systematically introduces the idea that professional nursing practice is intimately related to philosophy, moral philosophy, and applied ethics. Theories and principles of Ethics were introduced. These will be put into context and become more familiar as they are used to explore or analyze cases in the latter part of this text. The following discussion questions are designed to help you understand your own professional values in preparation for the next chapter. There are no right or wrong answers, only thoughtful and interesting ones.

DISCUSSION QUESTIONS

1. Preventive ethics is the anticipation of potential problems, followed by actions taken to stop their further development. So, for example, a patient diagnosed with a terminal condition is not aware of end-of-life options. In what ways do the methods and content discussed in this chapter permit early identification and thus facilitate addressing potential problems?

2. Virtue ethics is another approach that was not discussed in this chapter but that is addressed in Chapter 3. In virtue ethics, the idea is that a person can cultivate a good character. The argument is that "a person of good character will engage in good actions." So, the actions of a good nurse would necessarily be good.

Do you think a good character can be cultivated?
Does the ANA code of ethics support this idea?
Would a good nurse necessarily be a good person?
What characteristics would a good nurse possess?
Present counter examples (examples that would point to flaws in the theory) and discuss these with your peers.

3. How has this chapter changed what you understand ethics to be?
4. Knowledge of theories and principles is necessary for dialogue and collaboration with other professionals in the interests of good care for the patient. Do you agree or not? Defend your answer.

REFERENCES

American Nurses Association. (2001). *Code of ethics for nurses with interpretive statements.* Washington, DC: Author.

American Nurses Association. (2003). *Social policy statement.* Washington, DC: Author.

Aristotle. (1967). The Nichomachean Ethics, Books I, II, III (chapters 1–5), VI & X. In A. I. Melden (Ed.), W. D. Ross (Trans.), *Ethical theories: A book of readings* (2nd ed., pp. 88–142). Englewood Cliffs, NJ: Prentice Hall. (Date of original work uncertain.)

Ashton, T. S. (1997). *The Industrial Revolution, 1760–1830.* New York: Oxford University Press. (Original work published in 1961.)

Bahm, A. J. (1992). *Why be moral?* (2nd ed.). Albuquerque, NM: World Books.

Ballou, K. A. (2000). A historical-philosophical analysis of the professional nurse obligation to participate in sociopolitical activities. *Policy, Politics, & Nursing Practice, 1*(3), 172–184.

Beauchamp, T. L., & Childress, J. F. (2001). *Principles of biomedical ethics* (5th ed.). New York: Oxford University Press.

Bentham, J. (1967). An introduction to the principles of morals and legislation. In A. I. Melden (Ed.), *Ethical theories: A book of readings* (pp. 367–390). Englewood Cliffs, NJ: Prentice Hall. (Original work published in 1789.)

Buchanan, D. R. (2000). *An ethic for health promotion.* New York: Oxford University Press.

Chambliss, D. F. (1996). *Beyond caring: Hospitals, nurses, and the social organization of ethics.* Chicago: University of Chicago Press.

Corley, M. C. (2002). Nurses' moral distress: A proposed theory and research agenda. *Nursing Ethics, 9*(6), 636–650.

Corley, M. C., Minick, P., Elswick, R. K., & Jacobs, M. (2005). Nurse moral distress and ethical work environment. *Nursing Ethics, 12*(4), 381–390.

Davis, A. J., Aroskar, M. A., Liaschenko, J., & Drought, T. S. (1997). *Ethical dilemmas and nursing practice* (4th ed.). Upper Saddle River, NJ: Appleton & Lange.

Dewey, J. (1980). *The quest for certainty: A study of the relation of action knowledge and action.* New York: Perigree Books. (Original work published in 1929.)

Doane, G., Pauly, B., Brown, H., & McPherson, G. (2004). Exploring the heart of ethical nursing practice: Implications for ethics education. *Nursing Ethics, 11*(3), 240–253.

Donchin, A., & Purdy, L. (Eds.). (1999). *Embodying bioethics: Recent feminist advances.* Lanham, MD: Roman & Littlefield.

Engels, F. (1987). *The condition of the working class in England.* (Edited with an introduction by V. Kiernan). Middlesex, UK: Penguin Books. (Original work published in Germany in 1845.)

Flew, A. (1984). *A dictionary of philosophy* (Rev. 2nd ed.). New York: St. Martin's Press.

Gide, A. (1959). *So be it; or, The chips are down (Ainsi soit-il; ou, Les jeux sont faits).* New York: Knopf.

Grace, P. J. (1998). *A philosophical analysis of the concept 'advocacy': Implications for professional–patient relationships.* Unpublished Dissertation. University of Tennessee Knoxville. Available at http://proquest.umi.com. Publication number.AAT9923287, Proquest Document ID No. 734421751.

Grace, P. J. (2001). Professional advocacy: Widening the scope of accountability. *Nursing Philosophy, 2*(2), 151–162.

Grace, P. J. (2004a). Ethics in the clinical encounter. In S. K. Chase (Ed.), *Clinical judgment and communication in nurse practitioner practice* (pp. 295–332). Philadelphia: F. A. Davis.

Grace, P. J. (2004b). Patient safety and the limits of confidentiality. *American Journal of Nursing, 104*(11), 33, 35–37.

Grace, P. J. (2004c). Philosophical considerations in nurse practitioner practice. In S. K. Chase (Ed.), *Clinical judgment and communication in nurse practitioner practice* (pp. 279–294). Philadelphia: F. A. Davis.

Grace, P. J. (2005). Ethical issues relevant to health promotion. In C. Edelman & C. L. Mandle (Eds.), *Health promotion throughout the lifespan* (6th ed., chap. 5, pp. 100–125). St. Louis, MO: Elsevier/Mosby.

Grace, P. J., Fry, S. T., & Schultz, G. (2003). Ethics and human rights issues experienced by psychiatric-mental health and substance abuse registered nurses. *Journal of the American Psychiatric Nurses Association, 9*(1), 17–23.

Hardingham, L. (2004). Integrity and moral residue: Nurses as participants in a moral community. *Nursing Philosophy, 5,* 127–134.

Hume, D. (1963). *An enquiry concerning human understanding and other essays.* New York: Washington Square Press. (Original work published in 1748 by A. Millar, London.)

Hume, D. (1967). An enquiry concerning the principles of morals. In A. I. Melden (Ed.), *Ethical theories: A book of readings* (pp. 273–316). Englewood Cliffs, NJ: Prentice Hall. (Original work published in 1777.)

Jameton, A. (1984). *Nursing practice: The ethical issues.* Upper Saddle River, NJ: Prentice Hall.

Kant, I. (1967). Foundations of the metaphysics of morals. In A. I. Melden (Ed.), *Ethical theories: A book of readings* (pp. 317–366). Englewood Cliffs, NJ: Prentice Hall. (Original work published in 1785.)

MacIntyre, A. C. (1984). *After virtue: A study in moral theory* (2nd ed.). Notre Dame, IN: University of Notre Dame Press.

Melden, A. I. (1967). On the nature and problems of ethics. In A. I. Melden (Ed.), *Ethical theories: A book of readings* (pp. 1–19). Englewood Cliffs, NJ: Prentice Hall.

Mill, J. S. (1965). *Mill's ethical writings.* (Edited with an introduction by J. B. Schneewind). New York: Macmillan. (Original work published in 1861.)

Mill, J. S. (1967). Utilitarianism. In A. I. Melden (Ed.), *Ethical theories: A book of readings* (pp. 391–434). Englewood Cliffs, NJ: Prentice Hall. (Original work published in 1863.)

Mohr, W. K., & Mahon, M. M. (1996). Dirty hands: The underside of marketplace health care. *Advances in Nursing Science, 119*(1), 28–37.

Nagel, T. (1987). *What does it all mean?* New York: Oxford University Press.

Newton, L. H. (1988). Lawgiving for professional life: Reflections on the place of the professional code. In A. Flores (Ed.), *Professional ideals* (pp. 47–56). Belmont, CA: Wadsworth.

Nightingale, F. (1859). *Notes on nursing: What it is and what it is not.* London, England: Harrison. (Reprint Philadelphia: Lippincott)

Pellegrino, E. D. (2001). Trust and distrust in professional ethics. In W. Teays & L. Purdy (Eds.), *Bioethics, justice, and health care* (pp. 24–30). Belmont, CA: Wadsworth. (Reprinted from *Ethics, trust, and the professions: Philosophical and cultural aspects*, by E. D. Pellegrino, R. M. Veatch, & J. P. Langan, Eds., 1991, Washington, DC: Georgetown University Press.)

Peter, E., & Liaschenko, J. (2003). Feminist ethics. In V. Tschudin (Ed.), *Approaches to ethics: Nursing beyond boundaries* (pp. 33–44). New York: Butterworth-Heinemann.

Peter, E., Lunardi, V. L., & Macfarland, A. (2004). Nursing resistance as ethical action: Literature review. *Journal of Advanced Nursing, 46*(4), 403–413.

President's Commission for the Study of Ethical Problems in Medicine and Biomedical and Behavioral Research. (1982). *Making health care decisions.* Washington, DC: U.S. Government Printing Office. 33. PB83236703.

Rawls, J. (1971). *A theory of justice.* Cambridge, MA: Harvard University Press.

Ross, D. (1930). *The right and the good.* Oxford, England: Oxford University Press.

Russell, B. (1972). *A history of Western philosophy.* New York: Simon & Schuster.

Spenceley, S. M., Reutter, L., & Allen, M. N. (2006). The road less traveled: Advocacy at the policy level. *Policy, Politics, and Nursing Practice, 7*(3), 180–194.

Tong, R. (1997). *Feminist approaches to bioethics: Theoretical reflections and practical applications.* Boulder, CO: Westview Press.

Varcoe, C., Doane, G., Pauly, B., Rodney, P., Storch, J. L., Mahoney, K., et al. (2004). Ethical practice in nursing: Working the in-betweens. *Nursing Philosophy, 45*(3), 316–325.

Warren, V. L. (2001). From autonomy to empowerment: Health care ethics from a feminist perspective. In W. Teays & L. Purdy (Eds.), *Bioethics, justice, and health care* (pp. 49–53). Belmont, CA: Wadsworth.

Weston, A. (2002). *A practical companion to ethics* (2nd ed.). New York: Oxford University Press.

Zaner, R. M. (1991). The phenomenon of trust and the physician–patient relationship. In E. D. Pellegrino, R. M. Veatch, & J. P. Langan (Eds.), *Ethics, trust and the professions: Philosophical and cultural aspects* (pp. 45–67). Washington, DC: Georgetown University Press.

CHAPTER 2

Nursing Ethics

Pamela J. Grace

The professional must respond . . . if practices in his field are inadequate at any stage of the rendering of the service: if the client the ultimate consumer is unhappy; if he is happy, but unknowing, badly served by shabby products or service; or if he is happy and well served by the best available product but the state of the art is not adequate to his real needs.

—L. H. Newton, "Lawgiving for Professional Life:
Reflections on the Place of the Professional Code"

Let whoever is in charge keep this simple question in her head not, how can I always do this right thing myself, but how can I provide for this right thing to be always done?
—Florence Nightingale, Notes on Nursing: What It Is and What It Is Not

INTRODUCTION

The purposes of this chapter are several. The primary intent is to reinforce both advanced practice nurses' (APNs') understanding of the different senses of nursing ethics, its conceptual origins, relationship to practice, and the importance of this understanding for good patient care. It locates the foundation of APN responsibilities securely within the goals of the profession. To accomplish this it is necessary to trace the historical development of nursing into a contemporary profession with expanding professional roles that reflect knowledge development within the discipline. Some characteristics and concepts that have gained importance in professional nursing and in nursing ethics are discussed. Finally, a decision-making heuristic (helpful device) is applied to a deceptively simple case to demonstrate how all of the following are essential elements in meeting nursing goals of good patient care. The essential elements include (but perhaps aren't limited to) nursing knowledge, a basic understanding of the language of ethics, certain personal characteristics discussed later, personal and professional experiences, and the philosophical tools of exploration, analysis, and clarification.

Table 2-1 describes some habits that are vital for critical appraisals both of practice situations and reading material. Many of you will have already acquired such habits as a result of your life and practice experiences; if so, these tips will

33

Table 2-1　Habits of Critique

Questioning Authority	**Assumptions:** Authorities are human beings. Authoritative texts are the interpretations of human beings. The orders of superiors, managers, and leaders can be mistaken or misinformed. Important details of the situation may have been missed, time may be an issue, or conflicts of interest may be misplacing goals.
	Case: The chief nursing officer (CNO) is under pressure to cut costs and urges her clinical nurse specialists (CNSs) to limit the time spent mentoring new staff in favor of completing more administrative work. The CNSs understand that in the long run spending the time to mentor staff will result in better patient outcomes and be more likely to meet professional goals.
	Actions: CNSs should ask themselves what assumptions the CNO is making in proposing the plan and whether these are supportable given available data, not supportable for other reasons, or require more data. CNSs must gather needed data and present to the CNO. They should consider eliciting peer support weighing risks and benefits of this.
Self-reflection	It follows from the above that the APN's authority and expertise are also subject to critique. So, a second important (and sometimes painful) habit is that of genuine self-reflection. By *genuine* I mean the willingness to recognize and admit that we may not have things quite right and that others may have equally valid positions even though they radically differ from ours.
	Many people believe themselves to be self-reflective although actually they are more interested in molding the facts and details to fit their original belief (rationalization).
	Self-reflection allows one to both assume that biases and prejudices exist and try to discover what these might be related to a particular situation in the interests of controlling for them. More on this topic in Chapter 3.

| **Logical Critique** | This book uses reasoned argument to support positions taken. A reasoned argument is not a dispute; it is the presentation of concept, or an assertion that results from a chain of reasoning about a specific entity. It entails questioning underlying assumptions, discarding irrelevant information, and ensuring that the tentative conclusion can be supported by facts, logical reasoning, and/or sound assumptions. Sound assumptions are those that have stood up to critique and for which no counterexample can be given. There is an area of philosophy that actually studies the logic of arguments. A logically sound argument is one whereby if the premises are true, a conclusion derived from the premises will be true. A simple example of a sound argument is this:

Premise: Human beings need nutrition for survival.

Premise: Mr. Jones is unable to eat and refuses to take in nutrition by any other route. (Assuming this is true . . .)

Conclusion: Mr. Jones will not survive.

For example, sometimes in the course of presenting an argument, one discovers that an important aspect has been overlooked or that an assertion is made that is not true of all situations. So if some persons were known to have survived without nutrition we could not conclude that Mr. Jones will not survive. |
| **Reading Critically** | As you read, ask yourself, "Does this ring true?" If it does not, then try to isolate what is troubling you. Are there counterexamples that would disprove the statement being made? Is the author missing some important facts? Discuss your thoughts with your peers. Refuse to take anything at face value. There are no moral experts in health care. No group of professionals has the superior ethics knowledge; someone might have superior technical or content knowledge, but this is no preparation for ethical reasoning. |

continues

Table 2-1 Habits of Critique (*continued*)

Living with Nuance	There will always be some uncertainty in ethical decision making because of the complex nature of human beings. Absolute security in having the right answer is not possible. Dewey's (1929/1980) insight is, "The distinctive characteristic of practical activity, one which is so inherent that it cannot be eliminated, is the uncertainty which attends it" (p. 6).
Keeping Professional Goals in Mind	However, nursing ethics assumes that the application of nursing judgment and action can positively influence patient well-being and reduce the likelihood of harm. A basic foundation for ethical professional action is the knowledge developed by the practitioner's discipline and/or knowledge from other sources that is then filtered through the discipline's lens and modified to meet the discipline's goals. Additionally, the possession or development of certain characteristics is important to good practice, as discussed later. In nursing, these include the willingness to be self-reflective, reflect on practice, and engage with the patient as an individual whose needs differ in important ways from those of others. The process of furthering nursing's goals often also requires willingness to tackle difficult systemic problems arising from unjust societal healthcare arrangement. Thus, the political skills of negotiation and collaboration are also crucial to hone.

serve as a refresher and hopefully a reinforcer. Our first task, though, is to be clear about what is meant by the term *nursing ethics*. This is necessary because, although the term is used widely in the nursing literature, it is not always clear from the topic or content discussed exactly what is meant.

Two Senses of Nursing Ethics

For many people working within health care, the term *Ethics* has come to be associated with bioethical dilemmas or with other extremely difficult situations. A dilemma is a special sort of problem in which a choice must be made among two or more equally undesirable options. The origin of the term is in the Greek *di*, meaning two, and *lemma*, meaning premises or assumptions (Brown, 1993). One reason for this association is that the sorts of problems typically brought to public attention are those raised by technological or biological innovations. Nurses may well be involved in decision-making situations involving dilemmas; however, these situations are far from the most common issues that nurses face in daily practice.

In Chapter 1, I said that professional responsibility and nursing ethics may be understood as equivalent concepts. But some further explanation is necessary. The term *nursing ethics*, like the term *ethics* (as described in Chapter 1) can represent *either* a field of inquiry about nursing's responsibilities *or* nurses' actual practice-related actions (that is, those actions nurses undertake in the role of nurse and the extent to which these both flow from nursing knowledge and are anchored in nursing goals). *Nursing ethics* as a field of inquiry and *nursing ethics* viewed as professionally responsible actions are, of course, closely related and inform each other. To give a common example from my experience, if an intensive care nurse is being asked to provide care for three critically ill patients during the same shift, each of whom realistically requires the attention of one nurse, she cannot fulfill nursing goals for all or, probably, for any of the patients. No matter how experienced a nurse, the situation is impossible.

Nursing ethics as a field of inquiry is concerned, for example, with exploring the following: an individual nurse's responsibility in such situations, the persistence of such problems and the conditions that give rise to them, the profession's collective responsibility to address underlying or accompanying environmental concerns, and so on. Fry (2002) has succinctly summarized the main concerns of nursing ethics as being about "describing the characteristics of the 'good' nurse, and identifying nurses' ethical practices" (p. 1). Implicit in this definition is the further political task of critiquing environments of practice and describing the necessary educational strategies to prepare ethical nurses. However, for the nurse involved in the situation given previously, *nursing ethics* is her professional responsibility to recognize the ethical nature of the problem while trying to minimize possible harms and maximize patient good using available resources and within the limits of the immediate situation. It may also mean working after the fact (probably in concert with others—see Chapter 4 for further discussion) to address the conditions that led to this patient care problem.

So, *nursing ethics* as a field of inquiry explores why the nurse is being asked to do the impossible, what this means to the nurse, what this means to individual patients and society, and what the legitimate avenues of response are. These are questions for nursing's philosophers, scholars, and other interested parties to address (with input from practice). Whereas *nursing ethics*, viewed as professional responsibility to further nursing's goals of practice in individual situations, pertains to the nurse being and acting within the context of actual practice or perhaps in the interests of actual practice (for example, political action to change inadequate practice settings as discussed in Chapter 4). Elsewhere I have termed this *professional advocacy* (Grace, 1998, 2001). Professional advocacy is the nurse's responsibility both to address immediate situations of inadequate practice and to be active in addressing the environmental condition that gave rise to the practice problem. Professional advocacy is addressed in more detail later in this chapter as well as in other chapters.

From now on, and where it is not obvious to which I am referring, I will use the convention of capitalizing the term *Nursing Ethics* when I am referring to the field of inquiry and will leave in lowercase the term *nursing ethics* when I am talking about the ethical conduct of nurses. Nursing Ethics, then, is a field of study involved in theorizing about, or researching, what nursing practice is, what good it provides, and how nurses should or do act. It has exploratory, descriptive, and prescriptive interests. The exploratory task of Nursing Ethics includes philosophical and theoretical investigations about professional goals and ways to further these. The descriptive task involves the use of research or observation to understand how nurses act in practice, what nurses think are good ways of acting, and how they recognize and address problems. Finally, the prescriptive or normative aspect provides guidelines for nurses about what actions are expected of the nurse. For example, the American Nurses Association (ANA) (2001) *Code of Ethics for Nurses with Interpretive Statements* (Table 2-2) or the International Council of Nurses (ICN) (2006) *Code of Ethics for Nurses* both provide guidelines for ethical conduct that are derived from disciplinary goals. The development of a code of ethics is one of the hallmarks of a contemporary service profession and is an especially important characteristic of what are often called crucial professions (Windt, 1989), or those that address an important societal need such as health care. The ANA code of ethics and its implications for advanced practice are discussed again later and referred to throughout the book.

Table 2-2   American Nurses Association *Code of Ethics for Nurses*

1. The nurse, in all professional relationships, practices with compassion and respect for the inherent dignity, worth and uniqueness of every individual, unrestricted by considerations of social or economic status, personal attributes, or the nature of health problems.
2. The nurse's primary commitment is to the patient, whether an individual, family, group, or community.
3. The nurse promotes, advocates for, and strives to protect the health, safety, and rights of the patient.
4. The nurse is responsible and accountable for individual nursing practice and determines the appropriate delegation of tasks consistent with the nurse's obligation to provide optimum patient care.
5. The nurse owes the same duties to self as to others, including the responsibility to preserve integrity and safety, to maintain competence, and to continue personal and professional growth.
6. The nurse participates in establishing, maintaining, and improving healthcare environments and conditions of employment conducive to the provision of quality health care and consistent with the values of the profession through individual and collective action.
7. The nurse participates in the advancement of the profession through contributions to practice, education, administration, and knowledge development.
8. The nurse collaborates with other health professionals and the public in promotion of community, national, and international efforts to meet health needs.
9. The profession of nursing, as represented by associations and their members, is responsible for articulating nursing values, for maintaining the integrity of the profession and its practice, and for shaping social policy.

Source: Reprinted with permission from American Nurses Association, *Code of Ethics for Nurses with Interpretive Statements*, © 2001 Nursesbooks.org, Silver Spring, MD.

NURSING AS A PROFESSION

Characteristics of Professions

Before embarking on the discussion of nursing viewed as a profession, it might be helpful to review briefly what professions are and what purposes they are supposed to serve. It is commonplace to describe almost any vocational group as a profession. For example, dry cleaning businesses advertise themselves to be professional. In the business section of any phone book one can find many instances of plumbers, carpenters, and others all advertising their professional status. However, historically *profession* meant something very particular. The earliest organized occupational groups were the craftsmen's guilds. They are noted to have formed in medieval times and perhaps earlier (Carr-Saunders & Wilson, 1933). They consisted of groups of technically accomplished artisans who banded together to hone and protect their skills and knowledge in order to make a living. Out of these beginnings some groups began to affiliate themselves with the Church, which besides engaging in ministerial duties often also had educational and intellectual aims. Much of university education in medieval times and later was ecclesiastical in origin.

The original professions were ministry, medicine, and the law. These three disciplines often required members to take a vow to be accountable for actions, to profess their sincerity, abilities, and/or motivations. These Church-affiliated groups supposedly had altruistic motivations behind their educational endeavors and a service focus. They were less inclined toward substantial monetary awards and more inclined toward developing virtues than many other occupational groups (Carr-Saunders & Wilson, 1933). Thus, a distinction evolved that separated the artisan or tradesman from the professional. Gradually professions such as medicine and law withdrew from their theological origins while maintaining their service goals and mission.

Contemporary professions emerged from this background. Perhaps the most well-known attempt to describe the essential characteristics and purposes of professions emerged from Flexner's (1915) extensive study of medical education in the United States and Germany, which resulted in major reforms in medical education in the United States and elsewhere. Flexner, an educator, proposed that professions have an extensive and specialized knowledge base, take responsibility for developing and using their knowledge, have a practice or action orientation that is used for the good of the population served, and autonomously set standards for and monitor the actions of their members.

Following Flexner, further attempts have been made to identify essential characteristics of professions. Kepler (1981) notes that "professions are organized . . . (and) a high level of education is necessary to provide knowledge not readily available or capable of being understood by all. Professions normally interact with clients for whom they provide services rather than goods" (pp. 17–18). The profession is also self-reflective so that it can adapt to changing needs. It is, however, the possession of not readily available knowledge that persuades societies to grant a certain level of prestige and autonomy to professions (Grace, 1998). Perhaps the aspect of contemporary professions that is both the most important to those served and to the membership has been the explicit formulation of codes of conduct or ethics.

In reviewing historical accounts of the traditional professions, ministry, law, medicine, and later the professoriate, less noble accounts of their purposes emerge. Some have argued that professions are self-serving and deliberately protective of their knowledge in order to benefit their memberships. My doctoral dissertation (Grace, 1998) investigates such claims in more detail than there is room for here. However, a synthesis of the literature reveals that, though historically some disciplines were protective of their power and prestige, modern helping professions do not see their goals as being primarily self-serving. Nor do they view themselves as engaged in promoting the interests of their membership. Rather we can see from their published codes of ethics that they view themselves as existing for the primary purpose of serving the public good via their areas of knowledge, skills, and expertise.

Codes of Ethics

The codes of ethics of contemporary healthcare professions in essence represent the discipline's promises to society (Grace, 2004b). These codes are developed over time and are periodically revised by the profession's leadership, with membership input, in response to how well they continue to address professional goals and the evolution of societal needs. Although they tend to be abstract rather than specific (the exception to this is lawyers' codes of professional conduct, which are more specific and directive), they provide general direction and guidance to their membership related to professional conduct and the scope of practice. Some, such as the ANA *Code of Ethics for Nurses with Interpretive Statements*, are accompanied by interpretive statements that provide more detailed explanations of each provision or tenet.

Importantly, professions and their members can be held accountable by the public through such agencies as professional licensure boards for the promises (Grace, 2004b, p. 284) made. Curtin (2001) notes that historically "codes of ethics came into being—as did almost all early laws—to protect the vulnerable from the powerful; the unwary from the unscrupulous" (p. 1). However, the public is typically not cognizant of the existence, never mind the content, of professional codes of ethics. Nevertheless, were these to be broadly publicized, they could serve as a potent tool for political action. This idea is discussed later.

Helping Professions and the Public Good

Codes of ethics, formulated as they are from within the profession, also serve as the profession's check on what it expects of its members related to the primary foci of actions. For example, the Preamble to the American Medical Association's *Principles of Medical Ethics* (2001) asserts that "a physician must recognize responsibility to patients first and foremost, as well as to society." The ANA (2001) and ICN (2006) codes of ethics for nurses likewise assert that nurses' primary interest is the service of individual and societal well-being. The National Association of Social Workers (1999) in its preamble promises, "A historic and defining feature of social work is the profession's focus on individual well-being in a social context and the well-being of society."

In an earlier work, I noted that "the philosophical roots of the helping professions are imbedded in the idea that humans are not solely self-interested individuals but also have the capacity for altruism" (Grace, 2004b, p. 283). Altruism is the ability to understand that others have aims, projects, and life ambitions just as we do and to feel sympathy for someone who is suffering as a result of being unable to fulfill his or her own needs. We understand that others sometimes require assistance in achieving their aims and are willing to assist even if we won't necessarily gain direct or primary benefit (Nagel, 1970). That is, the philosophical aims of the helping professions are directed not primarily at furthering the needs of the professional to make a living (as they might be in retail or business settings) but toward the well-being of the individuals served. This is one meaning of altruism. It has been extensively documented as well as supported in the research literature that what draws many people to a profession such as nursing is the desire to contribute to the well-being of others.

Societal Importance of Professions

As has already been pointed out, nursing, medicine, and other professions such as law and education provide services that are crucial in some way to the functioning of individuals and the societies in which they live. So, if we look at the relationship of what Windt (1989) terms a crucial profession to the population served, it might shed some light on the persistent importance to society of having professions, given the existence of ongoing debates about what exactly these are and what groups qualify for the designation.

The explanation for the importance of professions hinges on the idea of human vulnerability. Crucial professions serve a specific human need that left unserved would make people as Sellman (2005) terms it "more-than-ordinarily vulnerable" to the environment in which they live. Moreover, this vulnerability is widespread. Lack of education (teaching profession) disadvantages people in all sorts of ways. An inability to hold people accountable for infringing on the property or other rights of people (law) would cause security and safety problems for civilians, and everyone is susceptible to ill health or less than optimal functioning. Healthcare professions, such as nursing and medicine, supply services that promote human functioning and flourishing albeit they have different perspectives on this.

Society should be able to trust professions to provide the service that they profess to be capable of delivering (see the discussion in Chapter 1 related to trust and fiduciary relationships). The existence and privileges of certain professions are sanctioned by society in exchange for their specialized services.

> In return for these services, society awards professions and professionals a certain standing. It places a high value on the information and skills that professionals contribute . . . and supports the education of professionals (often) by subsidizing their training costs. They are trusted to provide what they promise in exchange for financial or other types of compensation. In return, professionals are held to standards of practice that support the betterment of society as a whole. (Grace, 2004b, p. 284)

Some philosophers, sociologists, and political commentators have worried about the dangers to society should crucial professions lose their professional status. This phenomenon has been termed *deprofessionalization* (Bruhn, 2001; Dougherty, 1990; Sullivan, 1999). In deprofessionalization, the professions lose the ability and right to control their own practice—two of the most *essential* aspects of professions. These are essential aspects, for many reasons but most especially that professionals understand what is needed to meet individual and societal goals. Professional goals are focused on a good that is not *primarily* economic or business oriented, and the results of inadequate services are generally more immediately perceived and more concerning to the professional than to others with commercial rather than service interests.

The advent of managed care in the United States, as well as cost-containment initiatives in other countries that have a variety of healthcare financing arrangements, lead many to worry that those not directly involved in the care of the patient and who may have a different agenda than good patient care are actually determining what interventions are permissible (Bruhn, 2001; Dougherty, 1992; Mechanic, 1998). To make this point a little clearer, for a person such as a professional to be held accountable for his or her clinical judgments and the actions that follow from them, there must be a choice of action. If someone else is dictating what will or can be done, and what cannot, then there is no such thing as responsibility for action. There is no choice to be made.

In philosophical circles this is termed the problem of "ought implies can," meaning that, if we say someone *ought* to provide the appropriate care for a patient, then the care needed must be available. We cannot hold someone responsible for carrying out an impossible task. We might be warranted, however, in holding responsible that professional who does not attempt to locate and remedy the source of a problem after the fact. What I am saying here is that although sometimes we do not have a choice of action in a problematic situation, we must still try to work with others after the fact to ensure better options are available in the future. For example, in the case of the critical care nurse who is asked to care for three patients, she must do what she can until reinforcements arrive; however, she also has a responsibility to try to change the underlying conditions that led to this current situation. The idea is that professionals, perhaps especially healthcare professionals, understand the end results and implications of poor care for their population perhaps better than any other group. Chapter 4 explores in more detail the relationship between human rights and healthcare professional responsibility for influencing healthcare policy.

The Status of Nursing as a Profession

Concerns

Why should nurses be concerned with the quality and intent of *all* clinical judgments and the actions that follow from them? Aren't some actions purely routine? Why should everything about nursing practice be subject to ethical appraisal (nursing ethics)? The answer lies partly in the idea that nursing is one of those professions that caters to the sorts of human needs that left unmet make subjects more than ordinarily vulnerable to their environments and partly in the idea that all actions are in some way directed toward the care of a human individual with unique needs. Thus, even tasks that on first face seem simple, such as giving an intravenous (IV) medicine or taking a blood pressure, will have a different meaning for that patient than for any other. We are responsible for responding to patients as unique individuals with unique needs. And when circumstances don't allow for this, for whatever reason, we are responsible for recognizing the ethical nature of the obstruction to what we know to be good care. Also problems that have often been assumed as out of the purview of nurses, such as institutional obstructions to patient care, inadequate staffing, poor inter- and/or intradisciplinary communication about a patient, all have ethical aspects for the same reason: they obstruct efforts to provide good care.

Therefore, we can assert now that besides responsibilities related to direct care there is logical support for the idea that nurses have broader societal responsibilities as outlined in the ICN (2006) and ANA (2001) codes of ethics and in the ANA (2003) *Social Policy Statement*. In addition, individuals on entering a profession and achieving professional status are implicitly promising to fulfill the goals of the profession. The profession's code of ethics applies to the practice of each professional. It is considered to supersede all other institutional policies and cannot be negated by other professions, by administrators, or by the demands of the workplace (ANA, 1994). In advanced practice settings, where APNs so often find themselves working side by side and on a par with colleagues from other disciplines, they may find it hard to resist the "pull" of the other profession's particular aims, or of economic interests, and lose sight of the importance to individual and societal health of prioritizing *nursing* goals (Bryant-Lukosius, DiCensio, Browne, & Pinelli, 2004; Hagedorn & Quinn, 2004).

Therefore, it is critically important that APNs understand that advanced practice, although it may bring with it augmented responsibilities, is nevertheless advanced *nursing* practice and be able to articulate what this means. One way to think about this is that further education enables nurses to meet professional goals of good patient care more comprehensively because they are then able to provide for a wider array of patient needs. This lessens the fragmentation that can occur with multiple providers attending to different problems or systems and makes it easier to elicit the real needs of patients both for care and information.

Changes in Contemporary Healthcare Settings

Changes in contemporary healthcare settings both in the United States and elsewhere, resulting from a shift of emphasis to the economic bottom line and expediency and away from the patient and/or societal good, lend urgency to the need for all professional nurses to understand that the basis for their work is firmly attached to the goals of their profession. Unless this is taken seriously, the goals of other professions or institutions will dominate nursing work at all levels—this is a problem for the reasons given in more detail shortly but mostly because nursing serves a distinct purpose and has a distinct perspective that is crucial to the well-being of individuals and for societal health. Should nursing merge with another healthcare profession or its goals become subsumed under the goals of the other profession, the gains that have been made over the last century in professional autonomy, and thus the ability to directly influence nursing care, will be lost.

Not only do contemporary healthcare delivery systems both in the United States and elsewhere present a danger that nursing will lose its hard-won autonomy, but the autonomy of other professions is also at risk. So, it is more vital than ever that the healthcare professions in general, including nursing, retain their societal status as professions—they are, arguably, the last line of defense against the business interests of contemporary health care (Bruhn, 2001; Dougherty, 1992; Mechanic, 1998).

Interdisciplinary work and action are becoming more common because collaboration is often needed to address or research complex health issues. The danger is that a blurring of professional boundaries will occur. Nursing is perhaps more vulnerable to this than other professions are, yet nursing's perspective is important because of its unique emphasis on the person as contextual and continuously evolving.

Ambiguity About Nursing as a Profession

The question of whether nursing is a fully fledged or mature profession is still somewhat open for debate. One reason for this is that a settled definition of the concept profession does not exist. A second reason is that other more established professions have ignored or are unaware of nursing's particular knowledge about, and contributions to, the health of persons and the larger society. The troubled history of nursing as a female profession, the progress of which "has echoed the status of women in society" (Grace, 2004b, p. 285) as an oppressed group, is well documented (Andrist, Nicholas, & Wolf, 2006; Group & Roberts, 2001). Nursing as a predominantly female discipline has been subject to "gender discrimination" (Andrist et al., 2006, p. 1), lessening its ability either to see its political potential or be taken seriously by others as a political force. Wuest (2006) highlights the paradox that a key factor of professions historically is that they excluded women. When women did enter professions such as nursing, their motivations did not tend to include the acquisition of power. This has led to relatively easy domination by other groups working within the same environments, such as physicians and administrators. I do not mean by this to denigrate the significant contributions of some eminent members of the profession who managed Herculean tasks of nursing and healthcare reform.

Multiple Entry Levels

A further problem for the development of the nursing profession is lack of internal cohesiveness caused in part by its multiple levels of entry. A registered nurse in the United States may have completed a 2-year associate degree program, a 3-year diploma program, a baccalaureate degree, or have entered nursing as a second-career nurse with degrees in another field. This lack of a unified entry level is suspected to have contributed to the delayed progress of nursing as a power for change in health care. Nursing's scholars and leaders continue their struggle for disciplinary unification. By using insights from nursing's history, the feminist movement, sources of nursing knowledge development, and a changing professional body with its increasingly more highly educated membership, it is hoped nursing will be more equipped to meet its goals related to the health of individuals and society.

Nursing Possesses the Essential Characteristics of a Profession

So, although no agreement has been reached about the precise nature of professions, nevertheless, there is general consensus that professions serve an important purpose in democratic societies, and they have certain characteristics in common. The discipline of nursing possesses these characteristics and thus answers the description of a profession. Professions have responsibilities to society that cannot be circumvented by economic or business interests. Professions direct and monitor their own activities independent of those who might wish to subvert professional goals. The loss of professional status would not bode well for the population nursing serves for reasons highlighted later. And yet there is great concern among nursing scholars that nursing, instead of realizing its potential for societal good, is in danger of becoming weakened by lack of attention to, or concern for, the philosophical and theoretical work that draws upon and contributes to nursing practice (Fawcett, Newman, & McAllister, 2004).

The Relationship of Nursing's Goals and Nursing Ethics

In the preceding discussion, I do not make much of a distinction between medicine and nursing in regard to goals because the point I make is about the importance of certain professions to individuals and society. This section concentrates more on laying out the distinct nature of nursing goals and nursing perspectives as they have developed over the last century or so.

There is an inevitable relationship between nursing's goals and nursing ethics that has not always been as well recognized as it is currently. Nursing's philosophers and scholars over the past 150 years or so have been diligently involved in trying to determine and describe what the purpose of nursing is, who is served, what knowledge is needed for addressing these goals, and the responsibilities of nursing's membership in keeping these goals as the focus of their endeavors. This quest to define nursing and its unifying purpose is well documented in nursing literature (Donaldson & Crowley, 1978; Milton, 2005; Newman, Sime, & Corcoran-Perry, 1991; Packard & Polifroni, 1992) and represents the self-reflective nature of the discipline. Interestingly, medicine as a discipline has not been so self-reflective—much of what has been written about the nature and goals of medicine has come from philosophers and historians who for the most part are not physicians.

Fowler (1997) draws attention to the fact that ethics has "been at the foundation of nursing practice since the inception of modern nursing in the United States in the late 1870s" (p. 17). Fry (1995) has documented the development of nursing ethics. She describes its evolution as "paralleling the development of nursing as a profession" in that early nursing ethics resembled rules of etiquette and duties that included such things as "neatness, punctuality, courtesy, and quiet attendance to the physician" (p. 1822).

So, we can see that nursing ethics in the early days was less about nurses' autonomous actions than it was about good personal conduct in carrying out physician orders. Part of the reason for this was that a hierarchy existed. Nurse educators in the United States and elsewhere were drawn from an elite group of privileged women from the higher classes. They were influenced by Florence Nightingale's ideas about nursing as a virtuous activity. Coburn (1987) notes that it was difficult to attract the numbers of refined women to institutional nursing that were needed. Working-class women were attracted because they had limited work options. Thus, nurse educators attempted to instill in the women from the lower classes the characteristics thought necessary for the care of the sick.

On a personal note and in support of the historical account, my own mother, who was from a working-class family in Manchester, England, told her family that she wanted to become a nurse. She was 18 years old at the time. Her parents refused to sanction this because of the long working hours (72 hours per week) and the arduous nature of the work. So, for 4 years she worked as a secretary in a factory, at which point she applied for nurse training, was accepted in 1942, and graduated in 1945. Later she became a midwife (perhaps the earliest version of advanced practice nursing). Anecdotal accounts of her training period echoed historical accounts.

The reason that ladylike characteristics were promoted, nevertheless, was directly related to the interests of the patient. It was thought that quiet diligence and competence in the tasks of caregiving would provide the most beneficial environment for a patient's recovery. This view of nursing conduct was heavily influenced by Nightingale's (1859/1946) theory of good nursing. As evidenced in her writings, she believed that the right environment was crucial to the healing process and nursing's job was to manage the environment to facilitate healing.

Since Nightingale's era the nature and substance of nursing ethics literature has, not surprisingly, closely followed developments in the profession and in nursing education. As nursing has evolved and become increasingly differentiated from medicine in terms both of goals and of practice autonomy, the subject matter of Nursing Ethics has evolved and nurses' understanding about what constitutes good practice actions (nursing ethics) has developed.

Evolution of Nursing and Consolidation of Nursing Goals

Important Questions

What is nursing's particular knowledge base and how does this differ from that of other professions? The question of whether nursing has a unique knowledge base continues to be argued in contemporary nursing literature. Many scholars believe the question has been answered; however, many more practicing nurses remain unsure of the theoretical bases for their practice. This is a problem at all levels of nursing but most especially at the level of advanced practice. Cody (2006) notes,

> The practice of nursing at an advanced level requires a deep understanding of theory and the ability to apply theory effectively in providing healthcare services to people. Indeed, if such understanding and ability is not found within a given nurse, in any specialty whatsoever, his or her practice *cannot* be considered to be advanced at all. (p. ix)

The acceptance and proliferation of advanced nursing roles makes an understanding of the particular and unique nature of nursing concerns ever more critical if individual and societal needs for holistic nursing care are to be met. The latest move for acceptance of a Doctor of Nursing Practice (DNP) as *the* advanced practice qualification has exacerbated concerns that the importance of understanding nursing's unique nature may become diluted or lost (Dracup, Cronenwett, Meleis, & Benner, 2005; Silva & Ludwick, 2006). Concerns exist about the possibility that instead of advanced *nursing* practice, DNPs will be used to make up for shortages of physicians in both specialist and generalist medical settings. There are concerns that the control of these clinicians will fall under the department of medicine rather than belong to nursing's services. The worry is that if DNPs are accepted at all by the healthcare delivery system, they will be co-opted to a medical model of practice.

A further anxiety is that a proliferation of DNP programs will lead to a reduction in the number of PhD-educated scholars involved in research that expands and supports nursing's knowledge base. Additionally, there are fears that there will be a reduction in numbers of APNs because of the extra credit hours that will be required. These and other concerns are at the root of the current and potentially divisive crisis in nursing and nursing education, which cannot be investigated in detail here but which will require ongoing attention to facilitate ethical *nursing* practice.

> Contemporary developments in nursing and the movement of nursing toward professional maturity have occurred partly because nursing's scholars, theorists, and even researchers have been willing to ask the hard questions about nursing. They have been willing to ask, "What is it we are doing when we are doing nursing? How is what we do different than what other professionals do? What is our unique purpose?" (Grace, 2004b, p. 288)

Present-day APNs will have an important role in keeping and promulgating a nursing perspective. Most readers engaged in higher nursing education are exposed to nursing's conceptual bases for practice and will have had courses or modules that trace and critique the theoretical works of nursing's scholars. This chapter does not explore these works in detail for that reason. However, a brief overview will help those who have not yet been exposed, or it can serve as a refresher for those who have, and will allow an understanding of the inevitable link between theory development and the evolution of nursing ethics.

Nursing Theory and Disciplinary Knowledge Development

Florence Nightingale is generally considered the first person to have asked and answered the question "What is nursing?" In her *Notes on Nursing: What It Is and What It Is Not* (1859/1946), she clearly articulates her philosophy of nursing. Her philosophy has to do with the idea that nurses, in appropriately manipulating the patient's environment, "put the patient in the best condition for nature to act upon him" (p. 75). She uses previous knowledge, research, and current conditions to conceptualize what good nursing actions are. Thus, her particular focus proves very different from those followed by the medical and surgical establishments of the era. The foci of the medical professions actually did very little to change conditions in spite of gains in empirical knowledge about disease and illness that were available. Nightingale's influence both on public health and on the education of nurses was significant and led to the development of schools of nursing in Europe and eventually the United States.

Nursing for several decades after Nightingale, as noted earlier, was vocational rather than professional. Cody (2006) writes that it was not until Hildegarde Peplau published *Interpersonal Relations in Nursing* as a theory of nursing in 1952 that a shift in the development of nursing into a more professional endeavor commenced in earnest. This development coincided with the post–World II implementation of tax-supported college education for veterans funded by the G.I. Bill of Rights of 1944. More opportunities arose for nurses to receive baccalaureate-level or higher nursing education.

In the 1950s and 1960s, "additions to the literature on philosophy and theory in nursing began to appear" (Cody, 2006, p. 2). The important idea that nursing was concerned with "the *whole person* and *health in all its dimensions*" (Cody, 2006, p. 2) emerged. In 1961, Virginia Henderson's definition of nursing was published by the ICN. She notes that the definition represents the crystallization of her ideas about nursing over a period of time.

> The unique function of the nurse is to assist the individual sick or well, in the performance of those activities contributing to health or its recovery (or to peaceful death) that he would perform unaided if he had the necessary strength, will or knowledge. And to do this in such a way as to help him gain independence as quickly as possible. (Henderson, 1991, p. 21)

In 1970, Rogers's account of human beings as consisting of more than the sum of their parts and inseparable from their environments was published. She termed this view of persons *Unitary Man*. Cody (2006) points out that over the next 20 years or so "at least 20 significant frameworks intended to guide practice were published" (p. 3). Thus, he asserts, "The distinctiveness of nursing's disciplinary knowledge base is a reality that cannot be ignored" (p. 3). Nursing's knowledge base constitutes a science in this sense—that is, it is a developed body of knowledge about a phenomenon. The development of nursing's knowledge base has been directly informed by practice. Nursing's scholars and philosophers, almost all of whom have at some point been immersed in practice, have in turn used the questions and problems of practice to theorize about what it is that nurses do and how they might do it to meet professional goals more effectively.

"The (foundational) goal of the nursing profession is generally agreed to be that of promoting a 'good' which is health. Health may be variously defined depending on philosophical and theoretical perspectives guiding practice" (Grace, 2001, p. 155) and on the particular contexts of practice. Nevertheless, nursing has espoused a perspective of human beings that grounds the discipline's activity in the assumption that human beings are contextual beings whose needs cannot be conceptualized in isolation from the larger contexts of their lives, histories, relationships, projects, and values. Additionally, many of nursing's philosophers have noted the importance of the nurse–patient relationship and engagement with patients to facilitate meaning-making in difficult and fluid circumstances. The relationship and engagement are important even in cases of those who have profound cognitive challenges that prevent the individual's direct input.

Some have criticized nursing's perspective, noting that certain allied professions could also lay claim to this perspective. Indeed, in the past 20 years or so, some physicians have moved to adopt what they call the "new medicine" or an "integrative medicine" approach to patient care (Blumer & Meyer, 2006). This is good for patients. Even so, the new medicine fails to draw on the copious previous work done in nursing, and "new medicine" practitioners cannot necessarily be found in all the disparate settings where nurses practice in advanced roles, and neither do they stand in the same relationships to patients. Additionally, it is doubtful that many physicians see integrative medicine as a realistic approach, given the limits of current healthcare environments and their emphasis on cure along with a narrow view of what constitutes a good outcome. Nevertheless, it is an encouraging movement and one where nurses are well equipped to provide leadership.

Revisiting Nursing Ethics as Professional Responsibility

In light of the preceding discussion, we can now claim that an examination of nursing ethics is appropriately addressed "via the explications of nursing's theorists and scholars" (Grace, 2006, p. 68). In turn, nursing's theorists and scholars can realistically be called nursing philosophers because their theories or thoughts emerge from their philosophical attempts (informed by practice experiences) to find reasonable answers to the following questions: What is nursing? Why is nursing necessary? How can it best be done? What is needed to do it (including knowledge, characteristics, and skills required of practitioners as well as the environments in which it can be done)? From this, we can see that the two main goals of theorizing in nursing are "(1) To describe and explain (all levels of) nursing" (Grace, 2006, p. 68), and (2) to provide a structure or framework that facilitates practice, guides research endeavors aimed at expanding nursing's knowledge base, and underpins practitioner development and education.

The use of philosophies, models, and theories as guides for nursing practice and the reverse influence of practice experiences on theory development are factors critical to the development of nursing's knowledge base and thus to the maturation and evolution of the discipline. However, it is the discipline's explicit aim of contributing both to the health of individuals and the overall health of society that makes nursing itself a moral endeavor. Flaming (2004) has argued that because theories of nursing say what nursing is (ontology), they can be said to represent ethical imperatives. Take, for example, the goal of nursing to promote an individual's health. Because nursing views of health all include the understanding that human beings are complex entities, inseparable from the environment in which they live, and connected to countless important others in their lives, then promoting health means taking into account the person-in-context. Failure to do this represents a failure of nursing ethics or, alternatively stated, a failure of professional responsibility.

Critical Questions

At this point, the diligent reader might well raise the question, given that there are quite a few nursing philosophers and theorists and as many philosophical, conceptual, or theoretical approaches to nursing knowledge development in the interests of nursing care, how does the APN know which perspective to follow to ensure professionally responsible care? The answer is that the perspective and knowledge brought to bear on a practice issue will to a certain extent depend upon the nature of the problem, the patient or group involved, the nature of the practice setting, and the personal and professional characteristics and experiences of the clinician. The point is not so much that following a particular theory or perspective will result in ethical action, although having a structure to one's practice definitely helps with consistency of data gathering and approach to care and so forth, but rather that much work has been accomplished in identifying nursing's goals, and that there is agreement among nursing scholars on certain key points.

There is implicit or explicit agreement that nursing's metaparadigm concepts, or the overarching concepts of the discipline, include person, environment, health, and nursing (Fawcett & Malinski, 1999). What this means, roughly, is that there is unity about the fact that "nursing has to do with assisting humans, who are viewed as complex individuals who interact with their environment and have health needs that nursing can address" (Grace, 2004b, p. 288).

The Goals of Nursing

The authors of the current ANA *Code of Ethics for Nurses with Interpretive Statements* (2001) synthesized historical and contemporary literature and present, in the Preface, the goals of nursing as follows: "The prevention of illness, the alleviation of suffering, and the protection, promotion, and restoration of health." Similarly, the ICN affirms the goals of nursing in terms of the responsibilities of nurses and nursing "to promote health, to prevent illness, to restore health and to alleviate suffering" (ICN, 2006). Given agreement on the goals of nursing, we can keep these in mind as we examine skills and characteristics needed to practice ethically.

However, there are other factors important to ethical practice that apply regardless of what philosophical or theoretical approach to care is used. These factors include understanding the role of bias in data gathering or relationships, the boundaries of knowledge and skills possessed, moral development and motivation to engage with patients and to act (see also Table 2-1).

Nursing Ethics: State of the Science

Three Phases

To recap, the status of Nursing Ethics as a field of inquiry can be categorized into three phases as described by Sara Fry (2002). The first phase covers the early days of nursing's formal development via training or apprenticeships and in line with Florence Nightingale's vision. Fry (2002) notes that "during the early days of the 20th century, nursing ethics was understood as the articulation of the customs, habits and moral rules that nurses follow in the care of the sick" (p. 1). The transition to the second phase began after World War II, as described earlier. During this time, more nurses were able to gain access to university education, started to become more independent (from physicians) in their practice, and thus assumed more accountability for actions that resulted from their clinical judgments. "This new expectation of accountability created changes in how nurses' ethical duties and behaviours were understood" (Fry, 2002, p. 1). Much earlier, nursing leaders had begun to recognize the need for a formalized code of ethics (that would serve as a unifying guide for action.) However, it took 53 years between recognition that a code was needed and the actual adoption of the 1950 *Code for Nurses* (Fowler, 1997). Following the ANA, in 1953 the ICN, a federation of nursing groups from several countries (now more than 128), also developed and published a document entitled *The Code for Nurses* that reflected the "shared values of nurses" across borders (Curtin, 2001).

Finally, the current or third Nursing Ethics phase is concerned with exploration and analyzing contemporary nursing practice for its ability to meet nursing goals. The concerns of contemporary Nursing Ethics reflect the maturing of the discipline. Nursing Ethics explores the meaning of being a good nurse and good nursing practice in increasingly complex settings. This contemporary phase has seen an increase in research activities. See Table 2-3 for a synopsis of nursing ethics research phases.

Table 2-3   Phases of Nursing Ethics Empirical Research

Earliest Nursing Ethics Research	1935 Rose Vaughan studied the diaries of student and graduate nurses related to ethical problems encountered for her dissertation (Fry & Grace, 2007)
1980s Ethics Research Expands	Content related to nurses' ethical reasoning, judgments, and behaviors
1990s Nursing Ethics Research Focus	As above plus concepts such as advocacy, participation in end-of-life decision making, patient values, influence of education on moral reasoning, nurses' experiences of ethical issues
1994 Inception of the *International Journal of Nursing Ethics* (Tschudin, 2006)	Early issues featured research on advocacy, quality care, nurses' decision making, and ethical issues experienced by nurses. There was an increase in qualitative studies: reflective practice, experiences of moral unease and moral distress
Contemporary Nursing Ethics Research	Qualitative and Quantitative studies: Obstacles to care, the meaning of experiences, nurse–patient relationships, characteristics of good nurses, patient decision making, collaboration. Some studies on advanced practice: conflicts of interest, collaboration, specialty practice

Important Concepts

Fry (2002) identifies four concepts that are important to contemporary practice and that apply also to advanced practice. These concepts are "cooperation, accountability, caring, and advocacy" (p. 2). These four related concepts are discussed in more detail in the following chapters. They are especially important in advanced practice because of the expanded nature of such practice and the leadership roles assumed by APNs. Briefly, cooperation and collaboration are responsibilities to work with others within and outside the profession to get what is needed for patient care on the individual as well as the societal levels. The problem for APNs in collaborative relationships is how to maintain their disciplinary perspective while taking into account other perspectives. That is, how do nurses ensure that the collaboration is egalitarian in view of nursing's history of subservience? *Accountability* has already been discussed in detail in the body of this chapter related to autonomy of practice and accompanying responsibilities. I use a modified conception of advocacy I term *professional advocacy* (Grace, 2001) to denote actions required to ensure good care at the level of the individual and at increasingly broader levels as necessary to demolish obstacles to good practice. This is a panoramic conception of advocacy that goes beyond mere protection of human rights. Many argue that the political activities required by conceiving the scope of professional responsibilities this way are not possible for most nurses who do not possess the knowledge, skills, energy, or necessary supports. Chapter 4 presents rationale to counter this argument.

Finally, *caring* requires a little more discussion here because contemporarily it has received a lot of attention both within and outside the discipline. Indeed, nursing has been heavily criticized by feminists and other ethicists for using caring as an ideal of practice. Defining what is meant by caring provides an important grounding for the ensuing section.

Care and Nursing Practice: Ethical Implications

Care is a concept that highlights the relational aspects of human interactions. As an ethic of nursing practice, it has its origins in insights from feminist ethics and related research (Gilligan, 1982). These insights expose the idea that women take contexts and relationships to be important in reasoning about ethically difficult situations. They do not rely purely on principle-based reasoning.

For example, a nursing home patient, Mr. Jones, wants to be allowed to walk to the bathroom unattended even though he is unsteady on his feet and has been evaluated as a falls risk. The gerontologic nurse practitioner (GNP) reasoning about his autonomy and how best to facilitate this request would do a risk–benefit assessment and make a decision that balances protecting Mr. Jones's autonomy against the likelihood of a fall—this is the same assessment that would be made of any other patient whose autonomy was threatened. However, from a care perspective, the GNP is interested in knowing about Mr. Jones within this particular context, what it means to him to walk unaided, and how his wishes could be accommodated in a way that makes sense to him. The GNP would engage with Mr. Jones in the decision-making process. "The ethic of care means a responsibility to attend to the individual as individual in all of his or her complexities" (Grace, 2005, p. 105). Indeed the goals of nursing practice require that the clinician has, or cultivates, a predisposition to engage with the patient to understand that person's particular needs. Benner, Tanner, and Chesla (1996) note that care facilitates "the alleviation of vulnerability;

the promotion of growth and health; the facilitation of comfort, dignity or a good and peaceful death" (p. 233).

Care as a facet of nursing requires engagement on the part of the nurse with the patient in a relationship that permits the meaning and context of the person's need to be exposed. This is not a purely emotional sense of care; it is not, for example, the same meaning as "I care about my friend." Rather, knowledge, skills, and motivation are all needed for an engaged knowing of the person. In their research, Benner and colleagues (1996) note that it appears as "the dominant ethic found in (nurses') stories of everyday practice" (p. 233).

Of course, there are criticisms of the ethic of care. Nelson (1992), a bioethicist, notes the problem of moral predictability. That is, she wonders how one could determine right actions from within the nurse–patient care relationship. Another criticism is that a care ethic does not permit a critique of morally suspect environments. Further, feminists have cautioned that adoption of an ethic of care as *the* nursing ethic could further jeopardize nursing's power to effect change on behalf of patient care and even that nurses could be manipulated by powerful patients. One other important criticism has to do with the fact that nurses have responsibility for more than one patient, so excessive care for one might disadvantage another.

These are all valid criticisms and worrisome if the ethic of care is taken to be the only important consideration in clinical decision making. However, an ethic of care is an important concept where knowledge of the patient as individual is needed for the goals of the profession to be furthered. Ethical decision making, like sound clinical judgment, requires nurses to take into account both the larger context and the context of the individual. It includes determining which tools are appropriate to employ in identifying the ethical content of everyday practice.

ETHICAL DECISION MAKING AND ACTION FOR GOOD CARE

Clinical and Moral Reasoning

So far, we have traced the development of nursing into a profession and made the argument that membership in the profession leads to responsibility and accountability for practice actions and that all practice actions are subject to critique related to how well they are likely or able to fulfill the profession's goals as these have been developed over time. At this point, then, it is appropriate to gain clarity about practical applications. As articulated so far, the argument can be made that in many ways clinical and moral (ethical) reasoning are inseparable concepts. "Good or 'ethical' nursing practice results from the use of theoretical, conceptual, and practical knowledge in formulating clinical judgments, and evaluating ensuing actions for their ability to meet patient needs" (Grace, 2004a, p. 296). The "conceptual or theoretical knowledge may be derived from other disciplines as well as nursing" (Grace, 2004a, p. 296); however, this knowledge should still be filtered through a nursing lens (perhaps by asking "How will this facilitate the patient's good in the context of nursing practice?" or "How should I work to influence needed practice or societal changes?").

So, I make the case for viewing *clinically good* actions as synonymous with *ethically good* actions. However, we can go one step further and say that when clinically good actions (those most likely to further the patient's good) are obstructed in some way, good clinical judgment would conceptualize what nonclinical actions are needed to circumvent or tear down the obstruction—these actions highlight what professional responsibility requires of us. Strategies for addressing obstacles are suggested and proposed throughout the following chapters. As synthesized from extant nursing, philosophical, and research literature, good or ethical practice requires all of the following:

- An ongoing focus on the goals of the discipline and the ethical nature of these goals
- Disciplinary knowledge and skills related to the practice setting and role assumed
- Adherence to the scope and limits of nursing or nursing specialty practice as well as one's own knowledge and experience (entails knowing your own limits and being willing to seek assistance from knowledgeable or skilled others)
- Ability to communicate a nursing perspective using the language of ethics to convey a patient's or group's needs
- Understanding of personal and professional values (self-reflection and reflection on practice)
- Willingness and capacity to engage with patients (there may be some patients with whom one cannot engage related to prior personal life experiences; in this case, good practice would permit turning care of the person over to another)
- Motivation to act
- Ethical action

The next section explores in more detail the cognitive and affective processes that underlie ethically appropriate actions. By *ethically appropriate* I mean those actions that are required by nursing's goals and the role responsibilities of nurses.

Processes of Moral Action

James Rest gleaned his views on the cognitive and affective processes that must underlie moral behavior from the contemporary theory and literature of disparate disciplines. His insights cohere, for the most part, with the list of attributes given earlier as synthesized from nursing and allied literature. Rest (1982, 1983), an educational psychologist, notes that research or inquiry about cognitive and affective processes underlying moral action is in its infancy. Approaches tend to be scattered or fragmented, often focused on only one of the following: moral thought, moral emotion, or moral behavior, but not the interfaces among these. Additionally, the different disciplines tend to be concerned only with their perspective, causing further fragmentation. Yet we need a coherent understanding of the processes of moral behavior to know what can and cannot be fostered and what strategies are most likely to work. To be clear Rest's quest was *not* about discovering absolute or universal truths; it was about the psychology of human action, that is, about what cognitive and affective factors are in play when a person acts morally, given some predetermined moral goal of action.

The assumption of all professional education is that it is, for the most part, possible to foster the sorts of characteristics needed for moral practice and moral decision making. Therefore, future studies should look at how these processes are integrated or integral to each other for us to know more about *how* to foster moral behavior. Rest's assumption, derived from a thorough review of work done so far in a variety of sciences and disciplines, is that the processes are interrelated with each other, and all are necessary for a moral action or moral behavior to result. A failure in just one area or one process may result in a failure to behave morally. Many disciplines have undertaken ongoing research related to moral behavior, including nursing (see Table 2-3 for examples of contemporary nursing ethics research). Although integrative approaches that look at the relationships of all processes are included, the state of the science remains immature.

Nevertheless, Rest's tentative framework is also helpful to us in artificially delineating important aspects of moral action while understanding the necessary interdependence of them. Appreciating that there are limits and hindrances to moral decision making and moral action permits us to remain alert to those factors that can interfere with our decision making and to guard against these. Rest suggests four questions that have been partly addressed by contemporary philosophical and empirical research and that correspond to the probable internal processes behind moral decision making and action: "(1) How does the person interpret the situation and how does he or she view any possible action as affecting people's welfare? (2) How does the person figure out what the morally ideal course of action would be? (3) How does he or she decide what to do? and (4) Does the person implement what he or she intends to do?" (Rest, 1982, p. 28).

There are both affective (emotion) and cognitive (thought) components to these processes that may not be separable for the purposes of studying how people actually act. An implication is that good action results from all of these processes working together and that emotion and reason are both crucial elements. This is helpful for us in defining the characteristics of good clinicians. I have taken Rest's explanations of the nature of each process or aspect and modified these by applying them to direct patient care situations so that you can perhaps get a clearer idea of what is meant, as shown in Table 2-4. This illustrates how a nursing ethics course or book, together with group reflections on practice, might facilitate the development of or highlight already possessed attributes that are supportive of an APN's confidence in moral decision making and action. I have also synthesized the research and theoretical literature to present some factors that have been discovered to obstruct each process. The list of obstructing factors is not meant to be exhaustive.

Table 2-4 Four Aspects of Moral Action and Interfering Factors

Rest's Processes (1982)	Practical Implications	Interfering Factors
1. Interpretation of the situation	APN's understanding of the inherently ethical nature of any practice situation Assessment of this particular situation and what is needed	Personal troubles Energy level Time available Knowledge level No understanding of the inherently moral nature of practice Lack of connection with the patient/inability to engage Perception/sensitivity affected by age and life experiences Lack of self-reflection

Rest's Processes (1982)	Practical Implications	Interfering Factors
2. **Discerning the morally ideal action. What** *ought* **to be done**	Using appropriate tools, methods, and resources for decision making Identifying the beneficiary, the goal, appropriate actions	Level of moral development Level of independence Level and types of education Personal values conflict with patient/significant other/other professionals' values Lack of reflection on practice
3. **Deciding what to do**	Deciding among competing courses of action What *ought* to be done may not always be possible or consensus not reachable	Situational ambiguity Theoretical ambiguity Uncertainty about outcome Lack of institutional or peer support
4. **Implementation and perseverance**	Envisioning the steps and anticipating problems Addressing and overcoming problems and barriers Taking sociopolitical actions to get what is needed Keeping sight of the goal Reminding others of the goal	Too many obstacles Fear of personal consequences, peer/colleague disapproval Fatigue Frustration Lack of resources and supports

Self-Reflection, Values Clarification, and Reflection on Practice

Gaining confidence in one's moral decision making is admittedly a slow process. Nursing research studies and scholarly literature reveal that many nurses at all levels of practice remain unsure of the validity or importance of their point of view in ethically difficult situations (Ceci, 2004; Dodd, Jansson, Brown-Saltzman, & Wunch, 2004; Duffy & Currier, 1999; Hardingham, 2004; Kelly, 1998; Varcoe et al., 2004; Whitney et al., 2006). I believe one reason for this is the idea that ethics belongs in the realm of the obscure or difficult. There is the belief that ethics in healthcare settings is about difficult dilemmas that require esoteric knowledge brought to bear by high-minded individuals. What I realized as a result of my studies in philosophy and medical ethics is that most ethical issues arise in daily healthcare practice and are the result of lack of focus on either the goals or the recipient of care. Thus, nurses as the clinicians who tend to spend the most time with patients are often the ones who have the most comprehensive version of the patient's story. Moreover, nurses probably have the best opportunity to defuse situations that have the potential to develop into crises, in some cases simply by gathering important parties together to talk about goals in view of patient desires and preferences. APNs can serve as important resources both within institutional settings and in primary care settings.

CASE STUDY: MS. KNIGHT

Although this chapter clearly states that all practice actions, from the simple to the complex, are subject to ethical appraisal, that is, they can be judged good or bad according to whether they are focused on furthering nursing's goals, I use a slightly more complex case to demonstrate how one approaches moral decision making using the tools and skills described throughout the chapter as well as in the accompanying tables. Table 2-5 lists some key factors in any healthcare decision-making process. This table is used to guide decision making in later chapters also. However, there are many different frameworks available in the literature, and you may well find one of these is more in concert with your style of analysis. The important thing to remember is that we can probably never get enough information to be confident that our decisions are flawless, but we can gain reasonable clarity on most situations by asking the questions posed in Table 2-5.

Table 2-5   Ethical Decision Making in Difficult Situations: Important Considerations

In the course of *daily practice*, what is needed for ethical action is the thoughtful exercise of knowledge, experience, and skill together with a constant focus on the good of the patient or group in need of services and an understanding of one's own biases.

In more *complex* situations, where what is good is not so clearly seen, a more in-depth analysis may be needed. This is not necessarily a linear process nor will all of the following considerations always be pertinent. There are other decision-making models available, but all have similar considerations.

Steps	Questions
Identify the major problem(s)—relate these to professional goals.	• What are the facts: clinical, social, environmental? • What implicit assumptions are being made? • What ethical principles or perspectives are pertinent? Examples: autonomous decision making is in question, conflict of values among providers and patient/significant others, economic versus patient good. • Are there power imbalances? What are these? Who has an interest in maintaining them?
Identify information gaps.	• Do you need more information? • From whom or where might you get this information?
Determine who is involved.	• Who is the main focus? Is there more than one important party? Who has (or thinks they have) an interest in the outcome (relatives, staff, other)? Who will be affected by the outcome?
Decide what the prevalent values are. Determine if an interpreter is necessary (for cultural or language issues). Who would be the most appropriate interpreter (knowledgeable and neutral)?	• Values held by patient, staff, institution • Are there value conflicts? Interpersonal, interprofessional, personal versus professional, patient versus professional. • Are there cultural perspectives? Who can help with these?
Identify possible courses of action and probable consequences.	• Which course of action is likely to be the most beneficial and the least harmful to those involved, including you? • Can safeguards be put in place in case of unforeseen consequences?

continues

Table 2-5   Ethical Decision Making in Difficult Situations: Important Considerations (*continued*)

Steps	Questions
Implement the selected course of action. Conduct an ongoing evaluation.	• Does the actual outcome correlate with the anticipated outcome? What was unexpected? Was this foreseeable given more data? • Do similar problems keep reoccurring? If so, why (requires a look at underlying environmental or societal issues perhaps)? Does this point to the need for policy changes or development at the site, institution, or societal level? What further actions might be needed? • Are there continuing staff provider education needs related to the issue?
Engage in self-reflection, reflection on practice (individually, in an interdisciplinary group debriefing session, or in a specialty group forum).	• Could you have done things differently? What would you have liked to understand better? • Would a consultation with colleagues or an ethics resource person have altered your conception of the issue or the course of action taken? • What valuable insights did you gain that should be shared with others and may be applicable to the approach used for future problems?

Ms. Knight

Ms. Jean Knight is an 80-year-old patient 5 years post successful treatment for breast cancer. Her cancer has returned, and she now has bone and liver metastases. She was admitted 2 days ago from a local nursing home, to Clarion, a medical floor, for pain management and pneumonia. She is being treated with IV antibiotics and fentanyl patches for her pain. She occasionally experiences breakthrough pain for which she is prescribed oral hydromorphone. Her IV site has become obstructed and she is refusing to have a new IV inserted.

Gina Jenks is Ms. Knight's primary nurse. She has been working as a staff nurse for only 8 months and sometimes is not very confident in her skills. However, this is her second day with Ms. Knight, and she thought that she had developed a good rapport with her patient. She tries to reason with Ms. Knight about the importance of receiving the IV antibiotics, but Ms. Knight remains firm that she will not have the IV inserted.

Ms. Sandy Norton is the clinical nurse specialist (CNS) for this busy unit. Recently, Sandy Norton has been trying to encourage some of the newer nurses like Gina to take a more active role in presenting their patient's point of view to physicians, allied providers, and family members as needed. Gina seeks Sandy out to ask her advice. She tells her that Ms. Knight's exact words were, "I don't want any more medicines and I don't want any more fluids. I am ready to die. Just let me die, won't you?" Gina appears shaken.

Discussion

The decision-making considerations from Table 2-5 are italicized in the following discussion because, as with explorations of many difficult issues, they do not proceed in a linear fashion, but considerations or questions suggest themselves as the story unfolds. Not all considerations are pertinent in all cases; however, a cursory review of them permits relative confidence that no important aspect of analysis overlooked.

The main problem seems relatively straightforward: Ms. Knight is refusing care that her providers deem to be in her best interests. Providing IV antibiotics is the standard treatment for her immediate medical problem of pneumonia and can also be used to give pain medicines if needed. The *underlying assumptions* being made are that (1) Ms. Knight will physically benefit from the IV antibiotics (beneficence), (2) without the antibiotics she will worsen and die (nonmaleficence), and (3) death is a bad outcome for Ms. Knight.

Although premise 1 is true, premises 2 and 3 are more questionable. Premise 2 depends on there being no alternative treatments for the pneumonia, and premise 3 requires more information about *Ms. Knight, her preferences, and values*. Additionally, Ms. Knight wants her autonomy respected. She appears to understand that she might die and, if her understanding is adequately informed as discussed in Chapter 1, she has both the moral and the legal right to decide for herself what treatments she will or will not accept.

However, our responsibilities do not end even if a determination of decision-making capacity is made. *Professional goals* require that we find out more about how the patient feels and what alternatives are available that might be acceptable to her, thus not abandoning her to her autonomy. We are not told whether there are any overt *power imbalances*; however, implicit in most provider–patient relationships is an imbalance related to knowledge. The fact is that the provider serves as a gatekeeper for further care and interventions, and sometimes to setting. Power influences are likely present in the case of Ms. Knight, who is dependent upon the nurses and institution to meet all of her other daily living needs. She has no relatives in the local area, and she has lost touch with many of her friends since entering the nursing home 2 years prior because of mild mobility issues. This power differential does need to be taken into consideration in our communication with her. We must keep in mind that she might be susceptible to caregivers' influence if she thinks they will neglect her other needs, the most salient of which may be pain control.

Sandy (CNS) talks to *Gina (novice nurse)* about her feelings in the situation because Gina is visibly shaken by the event. Sandy's responsibilities as a CNS include staff support and education, both of which ultimately affect patient care. Gina says she is worried that Ms. Knight will deteriorate just when the nurses feel she is doing better. She hopes that there is something more that can be done—she doesn't want to "have to watch her die needlessly." Gina and Sandy must try to ascertain what Ms. Knight's understanding of the situation is, that is, what information gaps exist and how these could be filled in.

Gina and Sandy are charged with discovering whether Ms. Knight does actually have decision-making capacity. If decision-making capacity is impaired, then her ability to understand the implications of the choices she makes will be limited. Autonomous action depends on her ability to take in information, digest it, and convey that what she understands and wishes is in line with her previous life choices and desires for the future. Sandy decides that the best way to proceed is to role model for Gina how such an assessment can be made, acknowledging the need for discussion later. First, she talks to Gina about her feelings, reassuring her they are normal, that she knows more than she thinks she does, and that increased experience in handling such situations will help her develop confidence in decision making.

Before approaching Ms. Knight, Sandy emphasizes the importance of first making sure that there are no obvious physiologic or psychological impediments to information processing. Gina reports that although Ms. Knight did have some confusion the previous day when her oxygen saturation levels were borderline and her temperature was 101.4° F, today she has been lucid and oriented. Additionally, her pain is being well controlled with the fentanyl patch with only one additional dose of hydromorphone needed during the night. However, she did tell Gina that the management of her nursing home had changed and the residents were not getting the same quality of attention as they were previously. This made her very unhappy and she was worried about the quality of her care on her return. Sandy asked Gina to consider how this information might be relevant to the current situation and something to investigate further.

Sandy and Gina approach Ms. Knight and find her crying. Sandy says, "Ms. Knight, Gina tells me that you don't want to have your IV reinserted. I am so sorry that you are experiencing these problems. I am here to help figure out what can be done to ensure that you are comfortable and your needs are taken care of. Tell me more about what you are thinking."

Ms. Knight accurately recounts what went on and in response to further questions admits that she does not *necessarily want to die but is not happy with her life lately*, is afraid that if she goes back to the nursing home she will not get her pain needs met, and thinks that if this is the way it has to be then she is prepared to die. She turns to Gina and says, "I am sorry I yelled—you have been so good to me—you didn't deserve it, but I am at the end of my rope. I really do not want any more IVs sticks—they always have trouble with my IVs."

Sandy talks to Ms. Knight about some of the *alternatives* both to having the IV reinserted and to ongoing care in the nursing home. She also asks about her mood, suspecting that she may be depressed. They discuss the possibility of oral antibiotics and the need for Ms. Knight to drink plenty of fluids. Sandy also talks about other options that can be explored such as having hospice or palliative care services visit her at her nursing home. They can provide staff education related to pain management as well as extra patient care services. She suggests having a social worker come and talk to Ms. Knight so that arrangements can be made in advance of her discharge.

During the conversation, Ms. Knight stops crying and is agreeable both to the idea of oral antibiotics and a visit from the social worker. She admits to feeling "down what with the cancer coming back and everything, but isn't that to be expected?" Gina says, "Ms. Knight, I remember you talking to me about the pastor from your church and how she had visited you in the nursing home and been very helpful. Would you like me to contact her and ask her to visit?" Ms. Knight says, "That is a great idea. I had forgotten about Ellen—I would like that."

Back in Sandy's office, Sandy and Gina revisit the interaction. Sandy reassures Gina that her actions were appropriate, and that it was important that she recognized the limits of her experience and knowledge and sought appropriate advice, but that it was also apparent that she had her own resources to draw on—she indeed knew Ms. Knight better than anyone else. In Sandy's experience, events could have gone very differently if, for example, there had been an urgent need to restart the IV (for example, a dehydration issue) before anyone had talked to Ms. Knight about her preferences for care and interventions in the event of an emergency. Because the situation was not an emergency, Ms. Knight's wishes could be accessed and conveyed to the physician. Gina said she would be comfortable phoning Ms. Knight's attending physician and explaining the situation, what had been discussed, and what Ms. Knight wanted. However, she thought that it would be helpful for the floor nurses to have a meeting to discuss the situation. Additionally, in her college classes they had discussed the problems of advance directives and how to talk to patients about their preferences should an emergency arise and thought this would be good time to reinforce the importance of these.

SUMMARY

This chapter explores the status of nursing as a profession with its accompanying responsibilities. The relationship of clinical and moral reasoning was highlighted and supported. Finally, the exercise of clinical and moral decision making in advanced practice was exemplified by a case study and case analysis. An important facet of moral decision making in difficult situations is processing the event after the fact. This is a time when reflection and self-reflection can be crucial to the development of confidence in decision making and when the insights of others can broaden one's perspectives. Yet, perhaps understandably, this is often the most neglected part of ethical practice. Time constraints, fiscal constraints, and the relative isolation of many advanced practice settings all conspire against collegial meetings of these kinds. Important tips for the conduct of such meetings include neutral settings, confidentiality, and sensitivity to the feelings of those presenting so that they aren't made to feel "that they did it wrong." Rather, the emphasis should be on the idea that such sessions help further professional goals by facilitation of new tools, strategies, and approaches.

DISCUSSION QUESTIONS

1. Think of a simple case in which you were involved but which left you troubled. Explore this with colleagues using Table 2-5 or another decision-making heuristic (helpful framework). What new insights do you have? Would you have done things differently in light of what you learned in this chapter?
2. Preventive ethics is the process of anticipating and addressing potential problems before they arise. Many of the issues in health care that progress to the dilemma stage (choice between two or more equally bad alternatives) started off as minor communication problems. Think of one or more occasions from your practice when recognizing or addressing something early on would have defused an incipient difficult situation. For example, in my past experience in the case of a patient critically ill with toxic shock syndrome, I believe that early honest conversations with her family would have prevented the loss of trust with its subsequent suspicion and anger.

REFERENCES

American Medical Association. (2001). *Principles of medical ethics.* Retrieved May 28, 2007, from http://www.ama-assn.org/ama/pub/category/2512.html.

American Nurses Association. (1994). *Ethics and human rights position statements: the nonnegotiable nature of the ANA Code for Nurses with interpretive statements.* Washington, DC: Author. Retrieved June 8, 2007, from http://www.nursingworld.org/readroom/position/ethics/etcode.htm.

American Nurses Association. (2001). *Code of ethics for nurses with interpretive statements.* Washington, DC: Author.

American Nurses Association. (2003). *Social policy statement.* Washington, DC: Author.

Andrist, L. C., Nicholas, P. K., & Wolf, K. A. (2006). *A history of nursing ideas.* Sudbury, MA: Jones and Bartlett.

Benner, P., Tanner, C. A., & Chesla, C. A. (1996). *Expertise in nursing practice: Caring, clinical judgment and ethics.* New York: Springer.

Blumer, R. H., & Meyer, M. (2006). *The new medicine.* Ashland, OH: Atlas Books.

Brown, L. (1993). *The new shorter Oxford English Dictionary.* New York: Oxford Clarendon Press.

Bruhn, J. G. (2001). Being good and doing good: The culture of professionalism in the health professions. *Health Care Manager, 19*(4), 47–58.

Bryant-Lukosius, D., DiCensio, A., Browne, G., & Pinelli, J. (2004). Advanced practice nursing roles: Development, implementation and evaluation. *Nursing and Healthcare Management and Policy, 48*(5), 519–529.

Carr-Saunders, A. M., & Wilson, P. A. (1933). *The professions.* Oxford, England: Clarendon.

Ceci, C. (2004). Nursing, knowledge and power: A case analysis. *Social Science and Medicine, 59,* 1879–1889.

Coburn, J. (1987). "I See and Am Silent." A Short History of Nursing in Ontario, 1850–1930. In David Coburn, Carl D'Arcy, George Torrance, & Peter New (Eds.), *Health and Canadian society* (2nd ed.). Markham, Ontario: Fitzhenry and Whiteside.

Cody, W. K. (2006). *Philosophical and theoretical perspectives for advanced practice nursing.* (4th ed.). Sudbury, MA: Jones and Bartlett.

Curtin, L. (2001). Guest editorial: The ICN Code of Ethics for Nurses: Shared values in a troubled world. *ICN International Nursing Review, 48*(1), 1–2.

Dewey, J. (1980). *The quest for certainty: A study of the relation of action knowledge and action.* New York: Perigree Books. (Original work published in 1929.)

Dodd, S. J., Jansson, B. S., Brown-Saltzman, M. S., & Wunch, K. (2004). Expanding nurses' participation in ethics: An empirical examination of ethical activism and ethical assertiveness. *Nursing Ethics, 11*(1), 15–27.

Donaldson, S. K., & Crowley, D. M. (1978). The discipline of nursing. *Nursing Outlook, 26*(2), 113–120.

Dougherty, C. J. (1990). The costs of commercial medicine. *Theoretical Medicine, 11,* 275–286.

Dougherty, C. J. (1992). The excesses of individualism. For meaningful healthcare reform, the United States needs a renewed sense of community. *Health Progress Journal, 73*(1), 22–28.

Dracup, K., Cronenwett, L., Meleis, A. I., & Benner, P. E. (2005). Reflections on the doctorate of nursing practice. *Nursing Outlook, 53,* 177–182.

Duffy, M. E. , & Currier, S. (1999). *Ethics and human rights in nursing practice: A survey of New England nurses. Unpublished report of the survey.* Principal investigators: Sara Fry, Henry Luce Professor of Nursing Ethics, Boston College, Chestnut Hill; & Joan Riley, Director, Department of Nursing Emmanuel College, Boston, MA.

Fawcett, J., & Malinski, V. M. (1999). On the requirements for a metaparadigm: An invitation to dialogue. In J. W. Kenney (Ed.), *Philosophical and theoretical perspectives for advanced nursing practice* (2nd ed., pp. 111–116). Sudbury, MA: Jones and Bartlett.

Fawcett, J., Newman, D. M. L., & McAllister, M. (2004). Advanced practice nursing and conceptual models of nursing. *Nursing Science Quarterly, 17*(2), 135–138.

Flaming, D. (2004). Nursing theories as nursing ontologies. *Nursing Philosophy, 5*(3), 224–229.

Flexner, A. (1915). Is social work a profession? *Proceedings of the National Conference of Charities and Correction,* 581, 584–588, 590. Retrieved May 26, 2007 from http://darkwing.uoregon.edu/~adoption/archive/FlexnerISWAP.htm.

Fowler, M. (1997). Nursing's ethics. In A. J. Davis, M. A. Aroskar, J. Liaschenko, & T. S. Drought (Eds.), *Ethical dilemmas and nursing practice* (4th ed.). Stamford, CT: Appleton & Lange.

Fry, S. T. (1995). Nursing ethics. In W. T. Reich (Ed.), *Encyclopedia of bioethics* (Rev. ed., Vol. 2, pp. 1822–1827). New York: Simon & Schuster Macmillan.

Fry, S. T. (2002). Guest editorial: Defining nurses' ethical practices in the 21st century. *ICN International Nursing Review, 49,* 1–3.

Fry, S. T., & Grace, P. J. (2007). Ethical dimensions of nursing and health care. In J. L. Creasia & B. Parker (Eds.), *Conceptual foundations: The bridge to professional practice* (4th ed.). Philadelphia, PA: Mosby, Elsevier.

Gilligan, C. (1982). *In a different voice: Psychological theory and women's development.* Cambridge, MA: Harvard University Press.

Grace, P. J. (1998). *A philosophical analysis of the concept "advocacy": Implications for professional-patient relationships.* Unpublished doctoral dissertation, University of Tennessee Knoxville. Available at http://proquest.umi.com, Publication Number AAT9923287, Proquest Document ID No. 734421751.

Grace, P. J. (2001). Professional advocacy: Widening the scope of accountability. *Nursing Philosophy, 2*(2), 151–162.

Grace, P. J. (2004a). Ethics in the clinical encounter. In S. K. Chase (Ed.), *Clinical judgment and communication in nurse practitioner practice* (pp. 295–332). Philadelphia: F. A. Davis.

Grace, P. J. (2004b). Philosophical considerations in nurse practitioner practice. In S. K. Chase (Ed.), *Clinical judgment and communication in nurse practitioner practice* (pp. 279–294). Philadelphia: F. A. Davis.

Grace, P. J. (2005). Ethical issues relevant to health promotion. In C. Edelman & C. L. Mandle (Eds.), *Health promotion throughout the lifespan* (6th ed., chap. 5, pp. 100–125). St. Louis, MO: Elsevier/Mosby.

Grace, P. J. (2006). Philosophies, models, and theories: Moral obligations. In M. R. Alligood & A. Marriner-Tomey (Eds.), *Nursing theory: Utilization and application* (3rd ed., chap. 4, pp. 67–85). St. Louis, MO: Elsevier/Mosby.

Group, T. M., & Roberts, J. I. (2001). *Nursing, physician control and the medical monopoly.* Bloomington, IN: Indiana University Press.

Hagedorn, S., & Quinn, A. A. (2004). Theory-based nurse practitioner practice: Caring in action. *Topics in Advanced Practice Nursing, 4*(4).

Hardingham, L. (2004). Integrity and moral residue: Nurses as participants in a moral community. *Nursing Philosophy, 5,* 127–134.

Henderson, V. A. (1991). *The nature of nursing.* New York: National League for Nursing.

International Council of Nurses. (2006). *Code of ethics for nurses.* Geneva, Switzerland: Author. Retrieved May 28, 2007 from http://www.icn.ch/icncode.pdf.

Kelly, B. (1998). Preserving moral integrity: A follow-up study with new graduate nurses. *Journal of Advanced Nursing, 25*(8), 1134–1145.

Kepler, M. O. (1981). *Medical stewardship: Fulfilling the Hippocratic legacy.* Westport, CT: Greenwood Press.

Mechanic, D. (1998). The functions and limitations of trust in the provision of medical care. *Journal of Health Politics, Policy and Law, 23,* 661–686.

Milton, C. (2005). Scholarship in nursing: Ethics of a practice doctorate. *Nursing Science Quarterly, 18*(2), 113–116.

Nagel, T. (1970). *The possibility of altruism.* Oxford, England: Clarendon.

National Association of Social Workers. (1999). *Code of ethics.* Retrieved May 28, 2007 from http://www.socialworkers.org/pubs/code/code.asp.

Nelson, H. L. (1992). Against caring. *Journal of Clinical Ethics, 3,* 8–15.

Newman, M. A., Sime, A. M., & Corcoran-Perry, S. A. (1991). The focus of the discipline of nursing. *Advances in Nursing Science, 14*(1), 1–6.

Newton, L. H. (1988). Lawgiving for professional life: Reflections on the place of the professional code. In A. Flores (Ed.), *Professional ideals* (pp. 47–56). Belmont, CA: Wadsworth.

Nightingale, F. (1946). *Notes on nursing: What it is and what it is not.* Philadelphia: Lippincott. (Original work published in 1859.)

Packard, S. A., & Polifroni, E. C. (1992). The nature of scientific truth. *Nursing Science Quarterly, 5*(4), 158–163.

Rest, J. (1983). The major components of morality. In P. Mussen (Ed.), *Manual of child psychology* (Vol. Cognitive Development). New York: John Wiley and Sons.

Rest, J. R. (1982). A psychologist looks at the teaching of ethics. *Hastings Center Report, 12*(1), 29–36.

Rogers, M. E. (1970). *An introduction to the theoretical basis of nursing.* Philadelphia: F. A. Davis.

Sellman, D. (2005). Towards an understanding of nursing as a response to vulnerability. *Nursing Philosophy, 6*(1), 2–10.

Silva, M. C., & Ludwick, R. (2006). Is the Doctor of Nursing Practice ethical? *Online Journal of Issues in Nursing,* March 20. Retrieved June 5, 2007 from http://www.nursingworld.org/ojin/ethicol/ethics_17.htm.

Sullivan, W. M. (1999). What is left of professionalism after managed care? *Hastings Center Report, 29*(2), 7–13.

Tschudin, V. (2006). How nursing ethics as a subject changes: An analysis of the first 11 years of publication of the *Journal of Nursing Ethics. Nursing Ethics, 13*(1), 66–82.

Varcoe, C., Doane, G., Pauly, B., Rodney, P., Storch, J. L., Mahoney, K., et al. (2004). Ethical practice in nursing: Working the in-betweens. *Nursing Philosophy, 45*(3), 316–325.

Whitney, S. N., Ethier, A. M., Fruge, E., Berg, S., McCullough, L. B., & Hockenbury, M. (2006). Decision making in pediatric oncology: Who should take the lead? The decisional priority in pediatric oncology model. *Journal of Clinical Oncology, 24*(1), 160–165.

Windt, P. Y. (1989). Introductory essay. In P. Y. Windt, P. C. Appleby, M. P. Battin, L. P. Francis, & B. M. Landesman (Eds.), *Ethical issues in the professions* (pp. 1–24). Englewood Cliffs, NJ: Prentice Hall.

Wuest, J. (2006). Professionalism and the evolution of nursing as a discipline: A feminist perspective. In W. K. Cody (Ed.), *Philosophical and theoretical perspectives for advanced nursing practice* (4th ed., pp. 85–98). Sudbury, MA: Jones and Bartlett.

ETHICAL ISSUES COMMON ACROSS PRACTICE SPECIALTIES

CHAPTER 3

Advanced Practice Nursing: General Ethical Concerns

Pamela J. Grace

Our privileges can be no greater than our obligations. The protection of our rights can endure no longer than the performance of our responsibilities.
—*John F. Kennedy, "The Educated Citizen," Vanderbilt University 90th Convocation Address, May 18, 1963*

INTRODUCTION

In the first two chapters of this book, I laid the groundwork for advanced practice nurses (APNs) to understand the basis of their ethical responsibilities in the professional nursing role. Hanson and Hamric (2003) have synthesized a definition of advanced practice nursing from several important resource documents and their own experiences of the development of advanced practice: "Advanced nursing practice is the application of an expanded range of practical, theoretical, and research-based therapeutics to phenomena experienced by patients within a specialized clinical area of the larger discipline of nursing" (p. 205).

Accordingly, this chapter distinguishes the APN role from other nursing roles only by the breadth and depth of responsibility to patients implied by the term *advanced practice*. This means, for example, that APNs often oversee the patient's total care in a given practice setting (primary care, anesthesia, midwifery, gerontology), and in alternate settings they also have expanded responsibilities. For this reason, it can be asserted that "they have greater moral responsibilities than nurses who share (patient) oversight with other health-care professionals" (Grace, 2004b, pp. 321–322). Effective exploration of ethical issues faced in advanced practice, then, should reflect the implications of these broad role obligations. That is, although the ethical substance of situations may not differ from that faced by nurses in nonexpanded roles, advanced practice nursing ethics accounts for the more extensive duties incurred in these roles.

The following inquiry focuses on a variety of ethical problems and concerns that are common across many advanced practice settings. Such concerns are also discussed in general nursing ethics textbooks and will not be unfamiliar to the seasoned clinician. However, the implications of these issues are discussed specifically in terms of the APN's augmented responsibilities. Illustrative examples used are drawn from a variety of advanced practice sources and from my experiences. A more focused application of particular ethical issues may be found in the later specialty chapters. Because it is not feasible to cover all issues that an APN is likely to encounter, it is suggested that any troubling issues that the student or graduated APN faces that are not directly addressed in this book be brought up for in-class exploration with faculty and peers or explored with colleagues using the insights and strategies provided here or in other resources.

An appropriate start to the next section is a comprehensive discussion of the demands of the nurse–patient relationship. Characteristics discovered to be essential for consistently good patient care and decision making are explored with suggestions for the development of these. These qualities are sometimes called virtues and include the use of both intellect (thinking) and affect (emotions and motivation) in decision making and ensuing action. Examples of important qualities include empathy, veracity, transparency of purpose, cultural sensitivity, and motivation to act. A further important issue for all clinical and research settings is that of adequately informing patients about their options for care, treatments, and procedures. Thus, the parameters and demands of informed consent are explicated with the exception of informed consent in human subjects' protection, which is discussed in detail in Chapter 6. Problems associated with the adequacy of informed consent to care and therapeutics include the issue of patients who lack decision-making capacity for a variety of reasons, persons who are difficult to engage with, and people who are making decisions that seem to be at odds with their own values. A further topic investigated is that of privacy and confidentiality related to patients' health information. In this highly technological age, it is becoming increasingly difficult to adequately protect patient information from entities that do not necessarily have patient good in mind when seeking it. The protection of information is multifaceted. One important aspect is transparency. The person at risk should be told for what purposes the data are required and to what uses they will be put. This is in addition to being careful about who can have access to personal data.

Additionally, APNs often have concerns about how to maintain their personal integrity. Sometimes this is related to patient or peer requests to engage in something that is at odds with a nurse's values, or it may be related to conflicts within the healthcare system such as managed care or institutional pressures to limit care. Some of the sources of these concerns along with strategies to address them are presented. Finally, because some practice problems end up as complex and extremely difficult to sort out, the issue of preventive ethics is woven throughout this section. Many so-called dilemmas actually could have been prevented or diffused by good communication or an early understanding of the likelihood that unaddressed problems might cause critical difficulties for the patient in question and/or significant others.

VIRTUE ETHICS: THE CHARACTERISTICS OF GOOD APNs

At the end of Chapter 1, I raised some questions to engage the reader in thinking about which characteristics are important for good nursing care. Many people are attracted to the nursing profession because they see it as a practice that contributes to individual as well as the greater societal good. This is true not just at the undergraduate level but also for those who choose nursing as a second career and take an accelerated route to advanced nursing practice. Thus, the personal values of nurses are often congruent with the values of the nursing profession—for example, nascent nurses are drawn to the idea of contributing to the well-being of others. The desire to contribute to the welfare of others is often considered a virtue (as opposed to the desire to hurt someone, which would be considered a vice). As Feldman (1978) writes, in acknowledging that something is good, we are noting its qualities "relative to some class of comparison . . . some feature of that thing in virtue of which (we) hold it to be good. This feature is its virtue, or good-making characteristic" (p. 234). This section explores the issue of virtue ethics as it relates to good APNs, where *good* is taken to be synonymous with ethical. Virtue ethics in healthcare practice is essentially the idea that a person can cultivate certain characteristics (virtues) that will predispose him or her to good actions related to the profession's predetermined goals.

Contemporary proponents of virtue ethics almost all trace their influences back to Aristotle, although ideas about virtue can also be discovered in ancient texts on Eastern philosophy. Aristotle's idea is that a good or virtuous person is someone who possesses practical wisdom or prudence. The Greek term for this is *phronesis*. Practical wisdom permits a man (in ancient times women were considered subordinate to men) both to understand what is a good way to live and that living a good life necessarily means developing mutually beneficial relationships with others. To act well a man must learn to habitually moderate emotional impulses by using reasoning. This is what is required to achieve the desired purpose of living a good life. Eventually, a person will habituate himself to always engaging in good action—he will become a good or virtuous person. The desirable or virtuous purpose of all human beings, according to Aristotle, is to live in accordance with their human nature. The essential characteristic of human nature—that which distinguishes human nature from the nature of all other beings—is rationality. The ability of human beings to use logical reasoning gives human beings purpose, and that purpose is the pursuit of a satisfying life. The Greek term for this is *eudaimonia*, often also referred to as happiness, although it loses something in the translation and does not mean happiness in any superficial sense of the term (Hutchinson, 1995).

Practical reason acts as a constraint on emotional and instinctual drives that can result in harmful actions on the one hand, and on the other hand in a lack of needed action or inadequate action. Reason mediates a balance between extremes of action. So, for example, for Aristotle, courage is a virtue. Unrestrained courage can cause unnecessarily risky behavior, which is therefore irrational. Alternatively, timidity in the face of doing something important is problematic and also requires reason to moderate action. Practicing the development of virtue eventually leads to the formation of a virtuous character. Additionally, a satisfying life is necessarily lived within society and in relationships with others and facilitates harmony in these relationships. It is noteworthy that for Aristotle being virtuous is primarily aimed at supporting one's own interests but a harmonious society is needed for one's life to be satisfying. Thus, the actions of a virtuous man have the serendipitous result of contributing to the good of others.

So, you may well ask, "What is the pertinence of this explanation of virtue to the current project of understanding what characteristics are necessary for good practice?" The answer is that contemporary, moral philosophers such as Elizabeth Anscombe (1958/1981), Bernard Williams (1985), and Alasdair MacIntyre (2007) have been interested in resurrecting the idea of virtue as a way to understand people's relationships to each other and to inform provider–patient relationships. This move represents, in part at least, a way around the problem that deontological and consequentialist ethical theories don't account for: the contextual and relationship-dependent nature of human life (see Chapter 1) in situations where moral decision making is needed. Neither do these theories always capture contingencies of healthcare providers' multifaceted and relationally oriented roles.

MacIntyre's work, although not resulting in a theory that can be applied directly to action, does provide some unifying ideas about the virtues (Sellman, 2000, p. 27). The constituents of virtue, or those characteristics that make a virtuous person virtuous in MacIntyre's view, are context dependent. Thus, virtues may be "seen as supporting and maintaining particular ends" (Sellman, 2000, p. 27). Because virtues are seen as those characteristics necessary to support a particular end, goal, or practice, some common objections to the idea that a virtue ethic is helpful in healthcare practice are overcome (Armstrong, 2006; Begley, 2005; Sellman, 2000). Criticisms of virtue ethics include the observation that what is virtuous in one situation or in a given culture may not be considered virtuous in another. Therefore, there is no stable footing for the idea of a virtuous person and neither is there a list of virtues a person must possess to be virtuous.

An additional and potentially serious criticism is that there is no external criterion for judging whether the actions of a virtuous person are actually good. There is no gold standard for good actions. Additionally, the actions of someone who is thought to be virtuous will not necessarily always be good; that is, they may not meet a predetermined goal. Many factors can interfere with a good person's ability to do good actions, as listed in Table 3-1.

Table 3-1 Factors That Interfere with Ethical Nursing Action

Agent Related	Level of moral development
	Capacity to recognize ethical content. Chambliss (1996, chap. 1) discusses the phenomenon "routinization of disaster."
	Openness to reflection
	Personal or emotional issues
	Energy levels
	Creativity
	Locus of control (powerfulness/powerlessness)
	Unable to connect with patient
	Fear of disapproval (peer or other)
	Disapproval of patient's choice
	Time of day—complexity of preceding workload or decisions
	Level of knowledge related to the issue
Environmental	Pressures from peers—supervisors
	Competing demands (peers/patients/relatives/ institution)
	Social sanction
	Economic and institutional conditions
	Time or resource constraints
	Conflicts of interest
	Job insecurity

However, if we view the virtues pertaining to a particular professional practice and necessary for meeting the goals of that practice, then we can evaluate a given action based on how well it addresses those goals. Because nursing is a practice profession with relatively well articulated goals, we can agree that persons who possess certain characteristics are more likely that those who do not to routinely engage in good practice. A further consequence is that, as a profession, we need to continue to investigate what the characteristics of a good nurse are to nurture these traits in the education and mentoring of nurses.

Virtues of Nursing

Nursing practice and the fulfillment of nursing goals, then, can be understood to require the development of certain facilitative characteristics. Indeed by exploring what is needed to provide good nursing care to patients—as outlined in the literature and in our codes of ethics—we can relatively quickly compose a list of virtues that it would be good for nurses to cultivate. Additionally, nursing curricula would nurture these characteristics (Haggerty & Grace, in press). Begley (2005) has composed such a list. Included in her list are compassion, integrity, honesty, patience, tolerance, courage, imagination, perception, perseverance, self-reflection, and many more. The possession and exercise of any virtue within a nursing care setting will also rely on other interrelated virtues, the clinician's knowledge, and skills pertinent to the practice domain. Compassion for a cancer patient's suffering, for instance, without knowledge of how to mitigate it and/or the motivation to alleviate it is an empty virtue. However, theoretical knowledge of pain management without experience in patient assessment, planning, delivery, and evaluation or without understanding the meaning that suffering holds for the patient is also problematic.

For APNs, who are often required to supervise, mentor, or collaborate with others, virtues such as leadership, cooperation, and discernment of the different needs of those with whom they interact will be important to cultivate. The next section uses the idea that certain virtues are needed for interacting with patients who are faced with making decisions about their care. Patients give their consent to care either implicitly, verbally, or in written form depending on the invasiveness or risk of the proposed action. APNs are in the privileged position of assisting with, or empowering the patient to make, healthcare decisions that by their nature have some sort of effect on that patient's life. With this privilege comes added responsibility.

INFORMED CONSENT

The principle of autonomy, as discussed in Chapter 1, underlies the idea of informed consent. A brief recap might be helpful. In Chapter 1, it was noted that because human beings have the capacity to reason, decide, and act and because they might be presumed to know better than anyone else what their interests are, all things being equal, they have the right to make decisions concerning their health care. They should (barring any incapacitating factors) be free from the interference of others at least as far as personal decision making is concerned. This translates into the right of patients to accept or refuse healthcare treatments, regardless of risk, given the possession of decision-making capacity and an adequate understanding of the risks of refusal and the potential benefits of treatment. This right was legislated under the Patient Self-Determination Act (PSDA) ratified in 1991 (as part of the Omnibus Budget Reconciliation Act, 1990), which is discussed in more detail shortly.

Types of Consent

People give three types of consent in permitting healthcare professionals to evaluate and act on their health needs. The first is implicit consent, the second is verbal consent, the third is written consent. When a patient is unable to consent, as discussed later, then an informed proxy makes a decision on the patient's behalf and with the patient's best interest (where this is knowable) in mind. Informed consent, then, is *the process of interaction between a healthcare provider and person in which necessary information is exchanged and an appropriate level of understanding is gained to enable that person to make a decision about acceptable care, treatment, interventions, or courses of action in light of his or her preexisting values, beliefs, and lifestyle.*

Implicit Consent

In presenting to a healthcare delivery setting in search of assistance for health needs, a person is implicitly assenting, at minimum, to be evaluated for those needs. If the setting is an inpatient or institutional setting such as a hospital, the person might sign a form giving consent for certain routine evaluations. However, this form is general and does not detail all aspects of the evaluation, which may include tests and manual assessments such as a physical examination. Moreover, usually admitting personnel who have no medical or nursing knowledge are charged with obtaining signatures. So, implicit consent is not usually very informed, and patients may well not understand what rights they have.

In primary care sites, those who present for care do not necessarily understand the customary routines of the practice site—neither are they required to accept them, although frequently both ancillary staff and clinic nurses do not act as if they understand this. For these reasons, we need to be ready to ascertain what the patient has understood, and what it would be helpful for him or her to know. If a patient objects to some aspects of routine care, we are responsible for discovering what underlies the objection, how important it is for us to gather the data in question, and whether acceptable alternatives may be offered. For example, a faculty colleague who is also a women's health nurse practitioner (NP) reported that she was doing a breast exam on a patient as part of the patient's yearly checkup. She asked the woman if she did monthly breast exams on herself. The woman replied, "No, I don't like to touch my breasts, and for that matter I don't like anyone else to touch them either—not even my husband." At that point, my colleague realized both that she had not asked permission and had not sought to understand what, if any, meaning this particular act of assessment held for the woman. She apologized and the patient said she understood that it was part of the exam and had to be done. But my colleague wished she had thought to ask permission. She felt that this may have allowed the patient to discuss the issue with her, but now the opportunity had passed. Touching someone without that person's permission is also a legal consideration and may subject one to charges of battery.

The preceding scenario, which happened early in my colleague's professional life, made her more sensitive to the idea that patients might have good reasons for refusing even routine care and that they have a right to refuse it. However, we also have a responsibility to ensure that our patients understand the implications of refusing evaluations, tests, or treatments and try to lessen any risks from this refusal by reformulating an acceptable plan of care. To illustrate this point I give an example from my practice experience. A slightly overweight woman in her early twenties came to my primary care setting for treatment of a sore throat. It was her first visit. The office assistant, a nurse's aide, told her she had to be weighed as part of the "new patient" routine. The young woman refused. The aide tried to persuade her but to no avail.

I heard arguing in the hall, went to investigate, and saw a very upset young woman. I brought her right away into an empty room, acknowledged how upset she was, and asked her what happened. She said, "I really hate being weighed—I don't see why it is necessary—they used to do that at the other clinic." I explained that measuring a person's weight is in many cases a very useful assessment and had become a routine, but I realized from her reaction that we might need to rethink this policy. In the course of our interaction, and because she could see that I took her concern seriously, she confided that she used to be weighed weekly by her mother when she was a teenager and was physically punished for gaining weight. This opened an opportunity to help her further, and she eventually got counseling for unresolved issues with her mother.

After this, we changed our office policy and educated the medical assistants and aides about patient rights to accept or refuse some of the routines that were not important for the given patient's care. If the routine was important, for example, weighing a patient with chronic heart failure, then rationale should be given. Alternatives, such as weighing self and reporting significant changes, can be negotiated. Also, there are, of course, some cases when weighing a patient becomes crucial. For example, some drug dosages are calculated based on weight.

Verbal Consent

Although for many patients a host of routines covered by implicit consent cause neither distress nor affect their care in any perceptible way, in the cases described earlier informed consent to care was important both for the patients' immediate well-being and for determining whether follow-up care would be necessary or desired. Gaining informed verbal consent permitted the nurse to understand what else might be required to provide good care. Sound clinical judgment (see Chapter 4, Table 4-1) facilitates identification of the patient's particular needs, which in both cases proved to be more extensive than immediately understood. Obtaining verbal consent to care—including evaluation, tests, therapeutics, and decisions about the best ways of managing chronic conditions—is really synonymous with good APN practice in direct patient care and is dependent upon establishing a nurse–patient relationship that is concerned with understanding the patient's vulnerability and needs and to address these.

Written Consent

The third type of informed consent is a written consent. Written consent "is intended to protect patients from . . . ethical or legal breaches and make formal their right to all relevant information, tailored specially to them" (Grace & McLaughlin, 2005, p. 79). Experienced nurses practicing in institutional settings are mostly familiar with the term *informed consent* as it relates to invasive medical procedures and perhaps to patients who are participating in research studies (see Chapter 6 for information on informed consent to participate in research studies). In their definition of the term, Beauchamp and Childress (2001) acknowledge that "informed consent occurs if and only if a person or subject, with substantial understanding and in the absence of substantial control by others, intentionally authorizes a professional to do something" (p. 78). Although Beauchamp and Childress are explicitly discussing the necessary criteria for written and verbal informed consent rather than implicit consent, these criteria are also relevant for implicit consent.

In the case of proposed invasive procedures or surgery, the person responsible for carrying out or supervising the intervention is the one responsible for obtaining written consent. This is usually a physician, although increasingly it may be an APN. APNs who are qualified to carry out procedures or perform anesthesia are responsible for obtaining written consent. Staff nurses have responsibilities for ensuring that their patients are in a position to adequately understand what they are agreeing to. This has implications for the clinical nurse specialist (CNS) who serves as a floor resource, mentor, and educator and who sets the tone for the staff nurses on his or her unit.

Informed Consent: Ethical Problems

Informed consent, however, is a complex and tricky concept. For each person, the information needed for the person's consent to be *substantially informed* is different. For procedures or interventions that involve more than minimal risk (risk that we encounter in daily life), informing the patient should be viewed as a process because, for the most part, those faced with invasive procedures are already upset and anxious. Information processing under conditions of anxiety and stress is difficult, and studies have shown that patients do not retain information well under such conditions (Broadstock & Mitchie, 2000; Charles, Gafni, & Whelan, 1999; Kegley, 2002; Gafni & Whelan, 1999). The informing process involves understanding certain things about the patient. We need to understand the patient's beliefs, values, and goals; the patient's ability to process information; and psychological, physiological, or environmental factors that might interfere with or facilitate processing of information.

Kegley (2002) notes the "subjective substantial disclosure rule" (p. 461) is a standard that is starting to be used to understand what information is needed related to genetic testing and other complex decision-making scenarios. It "requires a substantial degree of knowledge about the patient, her context, and what is important to her" (p. 461). This represents a change from previous tests used in law to evaluate the adequacy of information given to a patient. The standards used in the legal system as a measure of adequacy either compared the knowledge possessed by the person in question against that of a knowledgeable group of physicians or against conceptions of what a reasonable person should know. Neither took into account the particular needs of a patient within the context of his or her life.

Patient-related psychological factors that can interfere with information processing are such things as denial of physical diagnosis, loss of hope, unreasonable expectations of the intervention, a desire to please the provider or significant others, lack of energy to think through possible options and how they relate to goals, and cognitive problems. Physical factors include pain, sedation, fever, and poor cerebral perfusion, among others. Provider-related problems include inadequate knowledge about the procedure and its potential side effects (for example, a lack of understanding of the full range of implications related to genetic testing—discussed later in the chapter); an inability to connect with a particular person, which can interfere with the project of tailoring information to that person's specific needs and abilities; lack of understanding of the origins or meaning of any cultural factors; lack of knowledge about existing options or objections to providing the full range of options (for example, provider beliefs about the moral status of emergency contraception); self-knowledge related to prejudice or bias. Additionally, certain situations are fraught with communication difficulties. Examples of such situations include language barriers, hearing impairments, and patients who are perceived as "difficult."

Many related issues are discussed in detail in the later specialty practice chapters. Here, three important complicating factors related to appropriately informing patients are explored: the provider's appeal to conscience in not providing patients with the full range of options legally available, cultural considerations in informing patients, and the issue of difficult patients. Early identification of potential communication problems and attempts to anticipate and address these problems have been termed *preventive ethics*, as noted earlier in the book. One important professional-related problem is that of withholding information or not offering the available range of options for a patient's situation because it is against the provider's conscience. The next section addresses this issue.

Conscience and Personal Integrity

The issue of healthcare professionals' refusal to provide patients with certain information and/or services has recently received publicity in the popular press. Consequently, the ethical implications of refusing to disclose legally available options or to offer a full range of services have elicited renewed scrutiny on the part of moral philosophers, ethicists, and scholars in the various healthcare professions. Appeals to conscientious refusal to provide certain options are usually based on one of the following arguments: (1) although legally available, the healthcare provider finds the option morally objectionable based on religious grounds or on the basis of other personal beliefs; (2) the provider believes certain options to be congruent with his or her beliefs, and others are not, and there is no obligation to reveal this bias to the patient; or (3) the provider believes some available options are inferior or have too many side effects, and thus the provider is saving the patient from confusion.

As an example of argument 1, Jacobson (2005) highlights the case of Andrea Nead, RN, who did not want to "administer emergency contraception" (p. 27) as part of her role responsibilities. She claimed the reason she did not get a position she sought in a university health clinic was related to her religious beliefs. Other examples (arguments 2 and 3) from advanced practice settings include the colleague who referred patients in need of mental health services only to a Christian mental health facility, and another colleague who neglected to offer a variety of therapeutic options available for labor pains by encouraging patients to "have an epidural—it is a woman's best friend." In palliative care settings, refusal to provide adequate pain relief may result from providers' beliefs that they may be contributing to a person's death.

The preservation of personal integrity is very important. It enables us to provide for a patient's good, sometimes against sturdy barriers. Integrity means maintaining a sense of self as a whole. It is tied into ideas of personal identity (Benjamin, 1990). Loss of a sense of self and personal integrity has been associated with the experience of moral uncertainty and moral distress as discussed in Chapter 1, especially when a nurse is unable to ensure that a patient receives the care that clinical judgment reveals is needed. These experiences can lessen an APN's confidence and resolve related to decision making. Provision 5 of the American Nurses Association (ANA) (2001) *Code of Ethics for Nurses with Interpretive Statements* upholds nurses' needs to care for the self, asserting, "The nurse owes the same duties to self as to others, including the responsibility to preserve integrity and safety, to maintain competence, and to continue personal and professional growth." Additionally, many state laws (in 45 states) have conscience clauses that allow providers to refuse treatment or recuse themselves from participating in care based on philosophical or religious objection.

Charo (2005) notes that conscience clauses in state law result from "the abortion wars" in the United States (p. 2471). That is, conscience clauses are "laws that balance a physician's conscientious objection to perform an abortion with the profession's obligation to afford all patients non-discriminatory access to services" (Charo, 2005, p. 2471). These laws are often broad enough to protect other professionals from the legal consequences of conscientious objection to certain procedures or treatments.

However, as we might imagine, legal protection is not a good reason to impose one's beliefs and values upon another. In fact, refusing to provide care because of personal beliefs requires that the nurse carefully consider the situation and understand the implications of this refusal. This is especially important when one is in a strong position relative to the person who is seeking legally available information or treatment. Our ethical responsibilities for good care may often include following the considered wishes of patients for something with which we don't agree or for which we wouldn't wish. However, it is important to keep in mind that the healthcare decision is not based on our preferences but ideally on the lifestyle, culture, beliefs, and values of the person that it will most affect. Thus, we must understand whether we have the facts straight, to what extent we are likely to be affected by going against our conscience, and how enduring the insult to our sense of identity is likely to be.

The question is, "How do we preserve integrity while fulfilling our professional duties related to informed consent?" First, it is crucial to remember the almost inevitable inequality of any provider–patient relationship. Patients are vulnerable to their lack of knowledge, skills, resources, or capacities in regard to meeting their health needs. They present to a provider trusting that their concerns will be taken seriously, the healthcare provider will be honest and transparent, and the healthcare provider will not either deliberately or unthinkingly hide available options or potential resources. In a sense, healthcare providers can be said to "hold the keys" to a wide variety of not easily available knowledge and have the necessary skills of interpretation for making distinctions clear. Such privileges should not be abused. The ANA (2006) position statement *Risk and Responsibility in Providing Nursing Care* provides important guidance. "The nurse who decides not to take part on the grounds of conscientious objection must communicate this decision in appropriate ways. Whenever possible, such refusal should be made known in advance and in time for alternate arrangements to be made for patient care." This position statement includes criteria for determining what level of personal risk is acceptable and what further responsibilities fall to the nurse involved.

Several integrity-preserving options are open to APNs in difficult situations. First, self-reflection should reveal the source and strength of the objection and whether the APN has a thorough grasp of the state of the science involved. For example, many objections to emergency contraception are based on inaccurate information related to how it works. The APN's objection may stand even after a provider has completed his or her research about the facts involved; nevertheless, fact gathering is a professional responsibility.

Second, the APN should answer the following question: "If I needed information about a healthcare issue with which I was unfamiliar, what would I want from the specialist? How would I feel if I discovered the provider had selectively withheld options or information from me?" If the APN on answering these questions nevertheless remains strongly opposed to participation in a legally available procedure or to providing certain types of information, the reason for not discussing options or not providing the requested care must be communicated to the patient. The patient should be enlightened about the fact that resources are available and/or referred to another provider who is willing to discuss the range of options or undertake the procedure (see Chapter 5 related to referral issues). APNs should be transparent about the fact that there are other options but that the APN's own beliefs do not permit him or her to discuss them.

Further, if the APN personally does not object to providing certain types of information or interventions but is restrained by the institution or practice (perhaps by working in a setting that is managed by a religiously based organization) from discussion of options or undertaking the procedure, this should be acknowledged and appropriate resources provided.

Culturally Based Communication Issues

Other issues that serve as obstacles to obtaining substantially informed consent are related to culture differences and lack of fluency in the patient's language or the patient's lack of fluency in the language of the context. Although in Western cultures the idea of autonomy is valued, in many other cultures decision-making responsibility belongs to the head of the household or is a family affair. Trying to understand the beliefs and values of someone from another culture can be a perplexing and frustrating task. It can be difficult to separate issues of coercion and undue influence from the cultural norm. Additionally, the cultural norm in some cultures can be oppressive for one group such as women or, less usually, may be age-related.

What are our responsibilities in such circumstances? There are no ready answers to such questions. It is an obligation of practice to learn more about a culture, if members of that culture are seen frequently in one's practice environment. In some cultures where there is evidence to show that certain practices are harmful, for example, female circumcision, one can join with concerned others to understand more about the practice, the underlying assumptions of the practice, and what others have done to either change the practice or provide appropriate care for the subjects of the practice. Most important, maintaining a nonjudgmental but interested affect is probably the most helpful both in ascertaining a person's needs and providing assistance.

For language difficulties, certain considerations are important. Does one have a good interpreter? Are there ways to validate understanding and ensure that the interpreter has translated the intent of your evaluation or information sharing? The following are some helpful hints synthesized from a variety of sources including my own professional experiences.

In line with viewing informed consent as a process, time and patience are needed. More than one appointment or session may be required. It is helpful to speak in short units and have all parties take turns speaking—you, the interpreter, and the patient. Ask for back-interpretations from the interpreter to ensure patient understanding and permit patient questioning/clarification.

Look at the patient while you are speaking and be aware of the patient's body language and appearances of confusion or discomfort. Validate with the patient if your perception is accurate and respond accordingly. Speak directly to the patient as in, "This will mean that you . . ." Be aware that the interpreter will interpret everything, so be careful not to say to the interpreter something that you do not want interpreted. Supplement explanations with visual materials when possible. Your practice may want to invest in video presentations in the patient's language as an adjunct, but this does not substitute for a fuller process of information gathering and giving. Try to keep your focus on meeting the patient's needs and not on any inconvenience or discomfort that you feel.

It is best not to use family members for interpretation service, especially not children. It can be a temptation to rely on a person's children because they may be more fluent in English (or the language of the provider) than their elders are, but interpreting is a heavy responsibility to place on them and inappropriately shifts family roles. A case study outlined in the Hastings Center Report (2004) describes the case of a 15-year-old daughter of a Chinese male immigrant. Her father was admitted with a cardiac problem. Circumstances were such that a Cantonese translator could not be found easily. The physician wonders if she should allow the daughter to translate for her father, among other things, the seriousness of his condition. I have included this sketch at the end of the chapter and pose questions for discussion.

Difficult Patients

We have all encountered patients that we perceive as difficult in some way. Wolf and Robinson-Smith (2007) define difficult patients "as those whom nurses perceive consume greater periods of time than their condition suggests; they impede the work of the nursing staff with demands, complaints, and lack of co-operation" (p. 74). Patients may seem or be difficult for a variety of reasons. We may experience a dislike for them for unknown reasons. Perhaps they remind us of someone of our acquaintance with whom we argue, or they question our knowledge or expertise. Perhaps they are violent, abusive, or argumentative. They may be difficult because of the complexity of their issues or the perceived hopelessness of their situation. Additionally, certain patients may be stigmatized by their lifestyle, obesity, or disease (see later chapters).

Whatever, the reason, we are still responsible for trying to meet their needs. Wolf and Robinson-Smith's (2007) study investigates strategies that are used by CNSs in "difficult clinician–patient situations" (p. 74). Two frequently used strategies were demonstrating "respect for the patient" and "focusing on the issue at hand" (pp. 79–80). This includes avoiding labeling the patient and CNSs setting an example to others. Both of these strategies avoid bias and are aimed at trying to understand who the patient is and what underlies the patient's actions and affect in order to meet the patient's needs. In addition to the preceding problems related to assessing the patient's particular needs, there may also be subtle influences on the provider to emphasize some aspects of information over others, as discussed next.

Other Influences on the Informing Process

Ensuring that patients' decision making is adequately informed for their needs also requires us to reflect on which other factors may be subtly influential such that we may not readily recognize them. The ethos of the practice environment, economic or time constraints, the influence of drug company practices, and pressures from colleagues all have the potential to cause a subtle skewing of the information we give to patients.

We know from studies, for example, that drug companies have been quite successful in influencing prescribing practices (Angell, 2004; Kassirer, 2005; Steinman, Harper, Chren, Landefeld, & Bero, 2007). An example from my experience is that of the drug company representative who provides dinner for the local APN association. He brings his samples to the office and urges us to try them with patients (Kassirer, 2005). Several studies have confirmed the suspicion that drug company gifts influence prescribing patterns (Coyle, 2002; Steinman et al., 2007; Wazana, 2000). Kassirer's book urges physicians to divorce themselves altogether from accepting drug company gifts. NP prescribing practices are perhaps not as amenable to study as physicians' are but probably would mirror those of physicians. Provider conflicts of interest are discussed near the end of this chapter.

As discussed earlier, ensuring that our patients are well informed is a difficult task not to be taken for granted. Ongoing self-reflection and reflection on our practice are crucial. Understanding the important elements of the process as well as likely problem areas necessitates vigilance. However, the other side of the problem has to do with the obstacles that exist for patients in apprehending and processing the information they need for decision making. The next section explores a concern related to informed consent, that of determining decision-making capacity. APNs in different roles and across specialties may be faced with the responsibility of determining whether a patient is reasonably capable of making an informed decision.

DECISION-MAKING CAPACITY

How do we know when a patient is not able to make an informed decision? In some cases, the answer to the question can be relatively easy. It is obvious, for example, that a comatose patient, a neonate, or a patient with an advanced dementing illness cannot process information or communicate his or her wishes directly to the provider. For such patients, an alternate decision maker is necessary. This person acts as a proxy either to convey what the person's wishes would probably have been, given knowledge of the person's beliefs, values, and life goals, or to ensure the patient's probable best interests where no knowledge is possible (neonates) or available. The issue of decision-making capacity is especially pervasive in mental health settings and is addressed in more detail in Chapter 11, "Nursing Ethics and Advanced Practice: Psychiatric and Mental Health Issues."

In other cases, determinations of decision-making capacity may be more difficult. Buchanan and Brock (1989) note that decision making in healthcare settings is almost always for the purposes of accomplishing a task and occurs along a continuum. The issue of decision-making capacity was studied in-depth by the President's Commission for the Study of Ethical Problems in Medicine and Biomedical and Behavioral Research assembled by President Carter in 1978. The formation of this commission was a response to the increasing complexity of problems caused by biological and technological advances. Examples of such problems include how and when can we determine death when we can indefinitely prolong life artificially? What is the range of possible effects caused by the application of genetic innovations in health care? What can we do about health disparities? And, important for our purposes, how do we ensure that patients are capable of making their own medical decisions and are not subject to undue interference by interested others who may or may not hold a person's best interests as primary? The commission's report (President's Commission for the Study of Ethical Behavior in Medicine and Biomedical and Behavioral Research, 1982) concludes that minimal capacities for decision making are "1. Possession of a set of values and goals, 2. the ability to communicate and to understand information, and 3. the ability to reason and deliberate about one's choices" (p. 57).

These criteria are made more stringent when the risks of choosing are high and the patient seems to be making a choice that is not in concert with his or her own values and goals. Beauchamp and Childress (2001) note that in cases where the risk of action or inaction are relatively high (the possibility of serious harm exists), it is also important to assess for the voluntariness of the decision. That is, we should evaluate whether some internal or external influence is pressuring the person to make a particular decision (see the section titled "Informed Consent: Ethical Problems" earlier in this chapter). The following case is provided as an example of considerations related to decision-making capacity.

Case Example

Jenny is a 33-year-old woman brought into the emergency room from a homeless shelter by shelter staff. She is evaluated by Pauline Hill, an emergency department NP, who, after evaluating Jenny, determines that Jenny's provisional diagnosis is pneumonia accompanied by dehydration. Jenny is also confused and keeps saying, "How did I get here?" The shelter staff person tells Pauline that Jenny had just completed detoxification for alcohol and unspecified drug abuse 2 weeks ago, was staying sober, and had just gotten a job. Currently, she is febrile with a temperature of 103.5° F and RR 36. Pauline determines that intravenous fluids and antibiotics are necessary because Jenny is in danger of sepsis. Jenny refuses treatment because she says, "I am trying to stay clean. I want to get my kids back." Pauline talks to Jenny about her worries, tells her of the proposed plan, and reassures her that she is not receiving anything that will set her rehabilitation back. At first Jenny seems to understand and acquiesces, but when it is time to insert the cannula, Jenny starts crying and yelling, "No, I don't want it! I can't have it!" When questioned further, it becomes obvious that Jenny has not retained the information that Pauline discussed with her, nor does she see the connection between treatment and achieving her goals. Pauline realizes that Jenny is not capable of making this decision because she keeps misunderstanding what is proposed.

There is a lot more that could be said about this case, including responsibilities to try to improve Jenny's ability to process information (oxygen, or a respiratory treatment) or to consider alternative courses of action that might achieve their purpose of resolving Jenny's immediate physical needs without further distressing her. However, the purpose of Jenny's case is to illustrate a problem with decision-making capacity for the task at hand. The risks of not treating are high and do not serve Jenny's goals of becoming physically capable of having her children returned to her and being able to care for them. Therefore, we do need to treat the pneumonia and dehydration because not to do so could result in Jenny's harm, perhaps even her death. So, the point is that, paradoxically, in treating her against her will, which could be seen as not honoring her autonomy, we are actually facilitating autonomous future decision making. One cannot exercise one's autonomy when one is not alive to do so.

Proxy Decision Making

Proxy decision making is the act of deciding what healthcare actions are permissible for someone who temporarily or permanently has lost decision-making capacity, never had decision-making capacity (profound cognitive deficits), or is not yet considered to have sufficient maturity to make healthcare decisions (children). When children are involved, the proxy decision maker is usually a parent or guardian who makes decisions on the child's behalf. However, if developmentally appropriate, children may assent or dissent to a course of treatment. However, a child's dissent may be overruled by a parent or guardian when the risk of not treating is high. The involvement of children in decision making is discussed more extensively in Chapter 6, "Research Ethics: Advanced Practice Roles and Responsibilities," and Chapter 8, "Nursing Ethics and Advanced Practice: Children and Adolescents."

There are three types of surrogate decision making. In the United States, what is accepted as legal differs from state to state. This necessitates that APNs familiarize themselves with the laws of the state in which they practice. (See Table 3-2.) Specific decision-making challenges are discussed in later chapters on mental health, adult health, nurse anesthesia, and gerontology. This section outlines some general issues associated with APNs' role in assisting their patients to be prepared for a variety of possibilities related to decision making.

Proxy decision making in health care may be needed for everyday healthcare decisions, for decisions related to an acute illness, and for end-of-life (EOL) issues. Although many APNs do not work in a hospital setting, understanding a little about the PSDA (OBRA, 1990) as it applies to institutions and what it was meant to achieve is helpful for the purpose of attending to the holistic needs of patients.

In the event that decision-making capacity is lost, it generally is better for patients to have considered in advance what sort of care they would like and who might best serve as a good proxy decision maker on their behalf. Although such decisions may well be made when patients are already critically ill, this is not optimal (Hiltunen, Medich, Chase, Peterson, & Forrow, 1999; Marshall, 1995; Wolf et al., 2001). Time, a low-pressure environment, and the assistance of a trusted health provider are probably the best conditions under which to process information. Thus, good APN practice means taking the opportunity to raise questions and provide necessary information related to the idea of proxy decision making if a patient appears receptive. From my experiences in both critical care and primary care settings and from the research cited, it is very difficult to discuss such issues when a person is gravely ill, already receiving highly technical care, and in a noisy and hectic environment.

Table 3-2   Proxy Decision Making

Type	Explanation

A. Autonomy based—Person's previously expressed wishes	• *Written*
	Living will, advance directives
	• *Substituted judgment*:
	  1. Durable power of attorney for health care (person appointed to provide information about a patient's previous wishes expressed while having decision-making capacity)
	  2. Informal (family member, friend, significant other)

B. Best interests	• Surrogate determines the "highest net benefit among available options" (Beauchamp & Childress, 2001, p. 192). This is a quality-of-life (QOL) evaluation—it may or may not be based on a person's previously expressed desires. Previous values, beliefs, and wishes are considered to the extent that they give information about what would constitute QOL for the person. • This may permit overriding a durable power of attorney's decision that does not seem to further patient best interests and when there are no written instructions (from the incapacitated patient) to support the proposed course of action.

C. Reasonable person	• A standard used when neither A nor B is applicable. It asks, "What would a reasonable person want?" The typical patient was never competent (e.g., baby or cognitively impaired) and/or previous wishes cannot be determined. For example:
	  1. Some permanently unconscious patients who might be said to have no interests and who cannot be "benefited" or "burdened."
	  2. Incapacitated, dying patients left on life support to preserve organs for transplantation (Medical College of Georgia, 2000).

Source: Reproduced from P. J. Grace (2004), Ethics in the clinical encounter. In S. K. Chase (Ed.), *Clinical judgment and communication in nurse practitioner practice* (pp. 295–332). Philadelphia: F. A. Davis.

Additionally, discussion about advance directives (AD) need not be limited to the older population. McAliley and colleagues (2000) studied adolescent attitudes toward living wills, or as they are alternatively known, ADs. Of the 107 participants in the study, the majority felt that it was "somewhat important" or "very important" for someone of their age to have a living will (p. 471). The advent of ADs or living wills is relatively new. According to Clarke (1998), the term *living will* was invented in 1967 by Louis Klutner "in a law journal proposal" (p. 92).

Patient Self-Determination Act

The PSDA (OBRA, 1990) was conceptualized as a result of several landmark right-to-die cases. It relies on state laws related to EOL care and "was designed to encourage communication about end-of-life issues" (Grace, 2004b, p. 310). It requires institutions that receive Medicare and Medicaid funds to inform patients in writing of their rights to accept or refuse care. It was meant to increase healthcare provider knowledge and thus affect current EOL problems arising in tertiary care institutions.

The PSDA has not been as effective as hoped, and there are many documented reasons for this. First, a large study to understand prognoses and preferences for outcomes and risks of treatment conducted over several years and initially involving observation but later adding interventions aimed at improving the communication of patients wishes failed to show that patients' preferences were respected. Marshall (1995) and others have argued that this is because institutional hierarchies and power structures had not significantly changed as a result of the PSDA.

Others have noted a variety of concerns about ADs that might make some people reluctant to draft one and some healthcare providers reluctant to comply with them. The concerns include the idea that people don't like to imagine themselves experiencing serious illness or death. Accurately predicting what might be needed out of a wide array of possibilities is difficult. Patients are afraid they might change their minds but not in time to change their AD, or that not accepting certain interventions might lead to their abandonment by caregivers (Teno, Gruneir, Schwartz, Nanda, & Wetle, 2007; Wolf et al., 2001). Additionally, there are cultural and minority fears about the untrustworthiness of predominantly white middle-class healthcare professionals (Baker, 2002).

Despite concerns about ADs, many professionals and ethicists who are involved in EOL care think that with time and custom more people will become involved in the process of advanced planning for the event of lost decision making. The most effective plan is probably a two-part initiative: the appointment of a trustworthy representative who may or may not be a relative, and written instructions to assist the proxy. Understanding both the benefits and criticisms of formal ADs allows the APN to assist patients in thinking about their specific advanced planning wishes. In advanced practice, nurses are key to interpreting a variety of EOL scenarios in terms that are tailored to a particular patient's needs and level of understanding.

VERACITY AND TRANSPARENCY

Veracity is an ethical principle underlying the idea of trust and fiduciary relationships. "Veracity or truthfulness in giving patients information about their health-care needs facilitates autonomous choice and enhances patient decision making" (Grace, 2004b, p. 315). However, veracity is a more difficult concept to apply than it appears on the surface. It is fair to say that in ordinary life rarely are we completely truthful with friends, family, and strangers. We hold information back either because we feel it could come back to haunt us or because to be completely truthful may well hurt the other person. Yet "truthfulness has long been regarded as fundamental to the existence of trust" (Fry & Grace, 2007, p. 287), and as noted earlier trust is fundamental in the nurse–patient relationship. Patients are vulnerable to their healthcare needs and must rely on us to help them meet these. If we are not able to gain a certain level of trust with patients, then our data-gathering activities are likely to be frustrated. This in turn lessens the likelihood that we will be able to give holistic care, which in turn means that nursing goals are not met.

However, being too honest or giving patients more information than necessary for their decision-making purposes can also frustrate the project of attending to their needs. Clinical judgment is required for us to determine acceptable levels of information for a given patient; that is, what will permit the patient's participation in decision making. For example, to the family nurse practitioner (FNP) for Ms. Jones, a 60-year-old patient in a rural family practice clinic, it has become obvious that Ms. Jones needs to add an anti-hypertensive drug to her care plan. Although for several years Ms. Jones has with the FNP's help managed to control her blood pressure by increasing her exercise regimen, reducing stress, and being careful with her diet—her blood pressure is starting to show a pattern of persistent elevation above recommended levels. She does not want to start taking blood pressure pills, but the FNP has done a good job of educating her about long-term effects of poorly controlled hypertension, so she is willing to start taking them. What drug the FNP tries initially and how much information she gives her depends on what the FNP knows about Ms. Jones. Discussion of the side effects she is most likely to experience and how these match her lifestyle and preferences will facilitate a first choice. Explanation of likely side effects will also be tailored to her needs. However, transparency about the extensiveness of what is known related to the drug and the amount of information the FNP gives are also important. These are all clinical judgments based on knowledge of the patient, and like many clinical judgments, they have some element of uncertainty. So, with Ms. Jones, in my judgment, I would discuss major side effects with her, whether these effects are acceptable to her, and what she should report to me. Additionally, I would acknowledge that there are possible side effects that she may not experience and that the best way to deal with this is to remain accessible for questions she may have should she experience unexpected changes.

In palliative care or EOL care settings, problems of veracity can occur when relatives pressure nurses and others to withhold the truth about a condition from patients. Veracity has some implications in the care of patients from cultures where the patient is traditionally protected from knowledge of the criticality of the condition. "Decision making about whether to honor (the demands) of veracity in such cases must take into consideration what is known about the culture, the particular patient, the strength of his or her personal and cultural beliefs, and whether there is evidence about what sort of things the patient would like to know" (Grace, 2004b, p. 316). If the patient is asking questions about his condition, then we need to respond accordingly. We need to draw on what is known or has been discovered (evidence) related to a person's needs to come to terms with his or her condition and nearness to death. But we also may need to assist the family with their needs to fulfill cultural responsibilities. Resources may be found within the cultural community.

In pediatric settings, the issue of veracity is also complicated. Questions arise about how to communicate information in age- or developmentally appropriate ways. How do we interact with parents or guardians who seem overly protective or are working in ways that seem at odds with what is known about the child? This issue is discussed further in Chapter 8.

PRIVACY AND CONFIDENTIALITY

The healthcare principles of privacy and confidentiality are also derivations of the ethical principle of autonomy. The terms *privacy* and *confidentiality* are often lumped together as if they mean the same thing. Privacy, however, is "the broader concept and includes the right to be free from the interference of others" (Grace, 2004a, p. 33) and freedom to grant or withhold access to information about oneself. Justifications for the right to privacy, as noted by Beauchamp and Childress (2001), "flow(s) from fundamental rights to life, liberty, and property" (p. 295). Confidentiality is related more specifically to the protection of a person's information, particularly the person's healthcare information. Beauchamp and Childress (2001) note that in healthcare settings, the right to privacy is most often a control right of sorts: it is the right to control both access to and distribution of information.

For Beauchamp and Childress (2001), a helpful distinction can be made between privacy and confidentiality in terms of the status of violations of these. For confidentiality to be violated, one person discloses information about another person, whereas for privacy to be violated, one person gains access to another person's personal data. Rights to privacy and confidentiality in healthcare settings are contemporary recognitions. The reason for recognition of these rights is that a person's healthcare information can be used in negative ways that can harm that person. In nonhealthcare situations, the status of confidentiality is considered so important that it is protected by privilege and is "shielded from exposure by the legal system" (Grace, 2005, p. 114). For example, the clergy–supplicant privilege prevents courts from forcing clergy to reveal confidential information entrusted to them by congregants.

Limitations on the Right to Privacy

For healthcare providers, honoring privacy, which includes the maintenance of patient confidentiality, is important but does not supersede all other considerations. There may be occasions when an APN should break confidentiality to prevent serious harm to another person. The difficulty, however, lies in making the assessment of dangerousness, how imminent it is, and how severe the likely consequences.

The well-known *Tarasoff* case set a precedent in the United States related to limitations in provider–patient privilege. In October 1969, Prosenjit Poddar killed Tatiana Tarasoff. Poddar had been seeing a psychiatrist and told the therapist he was going to kill a woman, who was easily identifiable as Tatiana. At the time of Poddar's statement to his therapist, Tatiana was out of the country in Brazil. The therapist sought to have Poddar committed but was unsuccessful because Poddar appeared rational. No one warned Tatiana or her family of the threat, and on her return Poddar killed her. The courts in this case, aligning against the idea that psychiatrist–patient privilege is absolute, concluded that "once a therapist does in fact determine, or under applicable professional standards reasonably should have determined, that a person poses a serious danger of violence to others, he bears a duty to exercise reasonable care to protect the foreseeable victim of that danger" (*Tarasoff v. Regents of University of California*, 1976).

Beauchamp and Childress (2001) note three main areas where limits on privacy might require a "balancing of privacy interests against other interests" (p. 297). These areas are "(1) screening and testing for HIV infection, (2) ensuring effective treatments for patients with active tuberculosis (TB), and (3) human genetics" (p. 297). Contemporary issues of dangerousness to others include the deliberate dissemination to, or careless exposure of, others by someone with a transmissible disease, such as human immunodeficiency virus or TB. For example, recently there was a highly publicized case of a patient with extensively drug resistant TB who traveled across the continent on public airliners.

Meaning of Privacy in Health Care

The concept of privacy is important to the preceding discussion of informed consent, although this wasn't explicitly stated. Essentially, the privacy principle means two things: (1) patients should have a say in who is allowed access to their bodies or, for the purposes of evaluation and treatment, other information, and (2) unless the patient gives explicit permission, there is a proscription against healthcare personnel sharing information gained except for the purposes of helping that patient.

The protection of a patient's privacy has a variety of implications both within institutional settings and in primary care. It requires us to think carefully about our actions related to patients, including what we tell referral sources, how we transfer information, and what the implications of testing are related to privacy and protection. It is a reminder not to take our privileged access to sensitive patient information for granted. So, respecting a patient's right to privacy means that when a student APN interacts with a patient as part of gaining clinical expertise, the student status should be revealed. In patient rounds, the identity of persons in the rounding group should be identified. Patients can waive this right but should be made aware of it.

The principle of privacy has other numerous implications; for the most part, concern for the delivery of good patient care will ensure that a patient's privacy is respected. For example, the privacy principle means that we protect those who are not capable of protecting themselves from the intrusion of others, perhaps because they are not aware of the possibility that sharing personal information can affect such opportunities as job prospects and the ability to have health insurance. All providers should know something about the so-called Privacy Rule and its impact on their practice. This rule is explored in more detail in the following section.

HIPAA and the Privacy Rule: History

According to Beauchamp and Childress (2001), "Privacy received little attention in the law or legal theory until the late 19th century" (p. 294), and then it was concerned with protecting family life, child-rearing practices, and other areas of personal choice. Confidentiality as a subcategory of privacy refers to patient rights to have their healthcare information safeguarded. The irony of confidentiality is that to receive care highly personal information has to be revealed to those who will be providing that care. Those providing direct care may sometimes need to share patient information with others whose expertise is important in meeting patient needs. Thus, illness makes one vulnerable to one's healthcare needs, but in trying to address that vulnerability a person becomes vulnerable to those who have access to that personal information.

Prior to 1996, rights to privacy and confidentiality were protected by state laws, professional ethical codes, and ethical deliberation. The advent of large electronic databases for storing medical records, however, jeopardized providers' ability to protect their patients' records. Most who have been involved in health care have recently become familiar with the Health Insurance Portability and Accountability Act (HIPAA); however, much confusion about this act remains (Anderson, 2007).

In 1996, Congress passed HIPAA. The act was initially designed to ensure, among other things, that people would not lose health insurance when they changed jobs. Prior to HIPAA, people could be, and frequently were, denied health insurance when they moved to a new workplace. Grounds for denial of health insurance were preexisting health conditions. Additionally, "HIPAA was meant to protect the privacy of individually identifiable health information in the face of advances in electronic technology" (Grace, 2005, p. 115), as noted earlier. Suggestions had been made for the development of a mega database that could track almost everyone's health care in the United States from birth to death. So, HIPAA was supposed to accomplish two somewhat contradictory tasks: (1) allow for the flow of information that would enable research and access to patient care records for the purposes of improving care and public health, and (2) act as a brake on covered entities' free use of medical information enabled by such a database. A *covered entity* is a person, practice, clinic, pharmacy, or institution covered by HIPAA. Essentially, a covered entity is anyone providing patient care services or undertaking research on human subjects.

Subsequently, a privacy rule was attached to HIPAA (U.S. Department of Health and Human Services, Office for Civil Rights, 2003). The Privacy Rule specifically covers all individually identifiable information including written, oral, or computerized. This went into effect in 2003. An important point to note is that if state rules about privacy are more stringent than HIPAA, then the more stringent standard applies. That is, state regulations trump HIPAA if they are more rigorous than HIPAA standards.

The problem with the Privacy Rule, as noted earlier, is that it is impossible to delineate all imaginable scenarios related to privacy infringements, so clinical judgment, including ethical reflection, is still needed for its interpretation in specific situations. "A rule of thumb for health care professionals related to sharing information with others is to disclose only as much information as is necessary to permit optimal care and only information that is pertinent to the situation" (Grace, 2005, p. 115). Additionally, prudence and mindfulness are required when other people's healthcare records are in your hands.

Anderson (2007) provides tips for ensuring that patient information is not overheard or overseen. Importantly, care must be taken not to leave information lying around and not to discuss patients in public places, and you must consider whether an outsider could identify the person being discussed if he or she overheard your conversation. In rural settings, maintaining confidentiality can be especially difficult. Providers are often members of the small communities in which they practice. It is not unusual for an APN encountered in a grocery store or other local gathering place to be asked about the status of a family member's or friend's health. Additionally, in rural settings office staff may have access to the records of family members or friends. Part of the APN's responsibilities in such settings is education of staff about the implications of accessing information to which they neither have a need nor a right to access.

In a recent *American Journal of Nursing* article offered for continuing education credit, Anderson (2007), the privacy officer for her institution, provides and answers some questions that may be helpful in understanding the intent of the rule. I recommend this article because it has some very helpful information related to HIPAA and the Privacy Rule. Anderson poses some common questions to highlight confusions and to illustrate commonsense answers.

- Is it permissible to call or write to a community provider when referring a patient? *Yes, if the disclosure is for treatment purposes.*
- Am I allowed to e-mail a diagnostic report to another provider for treatment or consultation purposes? *Yes, but encryption is strongly encouraged.*
- May I videotape or photograph patients for teaching purposes? *Yes, but consent should be obtained or patients should be "de-identified."* (Anderson, 2007, p. 67)

Additional insights into experiences of APNs related to privacy and confidentiality are provided by Deshefy-Longhi and colleagues (2004). They conducted a series of studies aimed at describing the views of APNs and their patients related to the protection of healthcare data. Of nine issues identified in focus group explorations, six were identified by both patients and nurses. One of these mutual concerns was the issue of "breaches in privacy occurring through carelessness" (p. 387). Examples given included phone conversations that could be overheard, conversations about patient information that took place in public spaces, and patient information lying around or viewable on computer screens. Additionally, both groups worried that excessive regulation prevented needed information from being communicated to appropriate resources. Even the need to leave a telephone message for a patient at home posed concerns. Nurses wondered how much, if any, information to leave. Additional concerns of the APN group were abuses of privacy related to the use of computers and problems attending to the privacy concerns of adolescents.

SUMMARY

This chapter discusses characteristics important for good nursing care and good decision making in APN settings. It presents an argument for the APN to engage in ongoing professional and personal development in the interests of good patient care. The possession of certain nursing virtues is necessary both for facilitating patient decision making and protecting patient information.

This discussion provides a basis for the ensuing content related to the ethical nature of all healthcare practice that involves individual human beings. Honoring the ethical principle of autonomy was seen to be the underlying assumption for the topics of this chapter. The idea is that a person has the right to make personal decisions both about what care will or will not be accepted and who may have access to personal information and for what purposes. The APN has responsibilities to help patients safeguard these rights.

Ironically, as hard as we work to secure information, insurance companies that are privy to the private information of their subscribers are not always so scrupulous. Chapter 5 investigates ethical issues specifically related to advanced practice nursing environments and the healthcare system, including environments of managed care. The following topics are explored: partnerships; conflicts of interest, including those created by managed care and the pharmaceutical industry; collaboration; and referral, including referrals for genetic counseling.

DISCUSSION QUESTIONS

1. A case study outlined in the Hastings Center Report (2004) describes the case of a 15-year-old daughter of a Chinese immigrant man who was

admitted with a cardiac problem. Circumstances are such that the physician cannot get a Cantonese translator in the middle of the night, and he wishes the daughter to translate for her father, among other things, the seriousness of the man's condition.

What are the implications of asking an adolescent to interpret for a family member?

What would we need to know to decide appropriateness?

What risks are involved?

How would you resolve this issue for the current situation? For the future?

2. Have you cared for a patient that you would describe as difficult? Explore with classmates or colleagues the situation you encountered. Identify assumptions that you are making about the patient. What is the basis for these assumptions? Do you think the patient is responsible for the characteristic that makes him or her difficult? In what ways is he or she responsible? How would you like the person to act? Have you ever been thought difficult or misunderstood?

3. Joe, a 17-year-old patient, is scheduled for a sports physical at your clinic. After examining him, you decide to draw a complete blood count because he complains of feeling a bit "more than usually tired" after 30 minutes of shooting hoops. Joe asks you to tell his dad what you are doing because "he gets antsy when he has to wait." You bring Joe's dad into your office to talk to him, and he asks you to draw extra blood for drug testing and not to tell Joe what you are doing. He says, "I just know he is taking something."

What is the main issue in this case?

What are the APN's responsibilities?

What are the implications of the Privacy Rule?

Discuss with classmates or peers how this situation should be addressed.

4. What is the relevance of discussing ADs with your population of patients? (Neonatal intensive care unit nurses may have to imagine caring for another population.)

Do you have an AD? Why or why not?

What innovative approaches to educating patients about ADs might be used?

What obstacles would you anticipate?

REFERENCES

American Nurses Association. (2001). *Code of ethics for nurses with interpretive statements.* Washington, DC: Author.

American Nurses Association. (2006). *Risk and responsibility in providing nursing care.* Retrieved August 7, 2007, from http://www.nursingworld.org/readroom/position/ethics/RiskandResponsibility07.pdf.

Anderson, F. (2007). Finding HIPAA in your soup: Decoding the Privacy Rule. *American Journal of Nursing, 107*(2), 66–71.

Angell, M. (2004). *The truth about drug companies: How they deceive us and what to do about it.* New York: Random House.

Anscombe, G. E. M. (1958/1981). Modern moral philosophy. In *Ethics religion and politics: Collected Papers, Vol. 3* (pp. 1–19). Minneapolis: University of Minnesota Press (Reprinted from *Philosophy, 33* (124), 1958.)

Armstrong, A. E. (2006). Towards a strong virtue ethics for nursing practice. *Nursing Philosophy, 7,* 101–124.

Baker, M. (2002). Economic, political and ethnic influences on end-of-life decision-making: A decade in review. *Journal of Health and Social Policy, 14*(3), 27–39.

Beauchamp, T. L., & Childress, J. F. (2001). *Principles of biomedical ethics* (5th ed.). New York: Oxford University Press.

Begley, A. M. (2005). Practising virtue: A challenge to the view that a virtue centered approach to ethics lack practical content. *Nursing Ethics, 12*(6), 622–637.

Benjamin, M. (1990). *Splitting the difference.* Lawrence, KS: Lawrence University Press.

Buchanan, A. E., & Brock, D. W. (1989). *Deciding for others: The ethics of surrogate decision-making.* New York: Cambridge University Press.

Broadstock, M., & Michie, S. (2000). Processes of patient decision making: Theoretical and methodological issues. *Psychology and Health, 15,* 191–204.

Chambliss, D. F. (1996). *Beyond caring: Hospitals, nurses, and the social organization of ethics.* Chicago: University of Chicago Press.

Charles, C., Gafni, A., & Whelan, T. (1999). Shared decision-making in the medical encounter: What does it mean? (or it takes at least two to tango). *Social Science and Medicine, 44,* 681–692.

Charo, R. A. (2005). The celestial fire of conscience—refusing to deliver medical care. *New England Journal of Medicine, 352*(24), 2471–2243.

Clarke, D. B. (1998). The patient self-determination act. In J. F. Monagle & D. C. Thomasma (Eds.), *Health care ethics for the 21st Century* (pp. 92–116). Gaithersburg, MD: Aspen.

Coyle, S. L. (2002). Physician-industry relations. Part I: Individual physicians. *Annals of Internal Medicine, 136*(5), 396–402.

Deshefy-Longhi, T., Dixon, J. K., Olsen, D., & Grey, M. (2004). Privacy and confidentiality issues in primary care: Views of advanced practice nurses and their patients. *Nursing Ethics, 11*(4), 378–393.

Feldman, F. (1978). *Introductory ethics.* Englewood Cliffs, NJ: Prentice Hall.

Fry, S. T., & Grace, P. J. (2007). Ethical dimensions of nursing and healthcare. In J. L. Creasia & B. J. Parker (Eds.), *Conceptual foundations: The bridge to professional practice* (4th ed., pp. 273–299). St. Louis: Mosby Elsevier.

Gafni, C. C., & Whelan, T. (1999). Decision-making in the physician-patient encounter: Revisiting the shared treatment decision-making model. *Social Science and Medicine, 49*(5), 651–661.

Grace, P. J. (2004a). Ethical issues: Patient safety and the limits of confidentiality. *American Journal of Nursing, 104*(11), 33–37.

Grace, P. J. (2004b). Ethics in the clinical encounter. In S. K. Chase (Ed.), *Clinical judgment and communication in nurse practitioner practice* (pp. 295–332). Philadelphia: F. A. Davis..

Grace, P. J. (2005). Ethical issues relevant to health promotion. In C. Edelman & C. L. Mandle (Eds.), *Health promotion throughout the lifespan* (6th ed., chap. 5). St. Louis: Elsevier/Mosby.

Grace, P. J., & McLaughlin, M. (2005). When consent isn't informed enough: What's the nurse's role when a patient has given consent but doesn't fully understand the risks? *American Journal of Nursing, 105*(4), 79–84.

Haggerty, L. A., & Grace, P. J. (In press). Clinical wisdom: Approximating the ends of individual and societal health. *Journal of Professional Nursing.*

Hanson, C. M., & Hamric, A. B. (2003). Reflections on the continuing evolution of advanced practice nursing. *Nursing Outlook, 51*(5), 203–211.

Hastings Center Report. (2004). A fifteen-year-old translator. *Hastings Center Report, 34*(3), 10–13.

Hiltunen, E. F., Medich, C., Chase, C., Peterson, L., & Forrow, L. (1999). Family decision making for end-of life-treatment: The SUPPORT nurse narratives. *Journal of Clinical Ethics, 10*(2), 126–134.

Hutchinson, D. S. (1995). Ethics. In J. Barnes (Ed.), *The Cambridge companion to Aristotle* (pp. 195–232). New York: Cambridge University Press.

Jacobson, J. (2005). When providing care is a moral issue. *American Journal of Nursing, 105*(10), 27–28.

Kassirer, J. P. (2005). *On the take: How medicine's complicity with big business can endanger your health.* New York: Oxford University Press.

Kegley, K. A. (2002). Genetics decision-making: A template for problems with informed consent. *Medicine and Law, 21,* 459–471.

MacIntyre, A. (2007). *After virtue* (3rd ed.). Notre Dame, IN: Notre Dame University Press.

Marshall, P. A. (1995). The SUPPORT study: Who's talking? *Hastings Center Report, 25*(6), S9–S11.

McAliley, L. G., Hudson-Barr, D. C., Gunning, R. S., & Rowbottom, L. A. (2000). The use of advance directives with adolescents. *Pediatric Nursing, 26*(5), 471–482.

Medical College of Georgia. (2000). *Ethics Syllabus Glossary.* Retrieved August 4, 2003, from www.mcg.edu/gpi/ethics/ph1syllabus/bioethic.htm.

Omnibus Budget Reconciliation Act. (1990). PL 100-508, 42 U.S.C. § 4206.

President's Commission for the Study of Ethical Behavior in Medicine and Biomedical and Behavioral Research. (1982). *Making health care decisions.* Washington, DC: U.S. Government Printing Office. PB 83236703.

Sellman, D. (2000). Alasdair MacIntyre and the professional practice of nursing. *Nursing Philosophy, 1*(1), 26–33.

Steinman, M. A., Harper, G. M., Chren, M. M., Landefeld, C. S., & Bero, L. A. (2007). Characteristics and impact of drug detailing for Gabapentin. *PLOS Medicine, 4*(5), e134. Retrieved August 1, 2007, from http://medicine.plosjournals.org/perlserv/?request=index-html&issn=1549-1676&ct=1.

Tarasoff v. Regents of University of California. (1976, July 1). California Supreme Court 131. *California Reporter, 14.*

Teno, J. M., Gruneir, A., Schwartz, Z., Nanda, A., & Wetle, T. (2007). Association between advance directives and quality of end-of-life care: A national study. *Journal of the American Geriatrics Society, 55*(2), 189–194.

U.S. Department of Health and Human Services. Office for Civil Rights. (2003). *HIPAA Fact Sheet.* Retrieved August 2007 from http://www.hhs.gov/ocr/hipaa/privacy.html.

Wazana, A. (2000). Physicians and the pharmaceutical industry: Is a gift ever just a gift? *Journal of the American Medical Association, 283,* 373–380.

Williams, B. (1985). *Ethics and the limits of philosophy.* London: Fontana.

Wolf, S. M., Boyle, P. Callahan, D., Fins, J., Jennings, B., Lindemann Nelson, J., et al. (2001). Sources of concern about the Patient Self-Determination Act. In W. Teays & L. Purdy (Eds.), *Bioethics, justice and health care* (pp. 411–419). Belmont, CA: Wadsworth Thompson Learning. (Reprinted from *New England Journal of Medicine, 325* (23) (December 5, 1991): 1666–1671.)

Wolf, Z. R., & Robinson-Smith, G. (2007). Strategies used by clinical nurse specialists in "difficult" clinician-patient situations. *Clinical Nurse Specialist, 21*(2), 74–84.

CHAPTER 4

Professional Responsibility, Human Rights, and Injustice

Pamela J. Grace

Where justice is denied, where poverty is enforced, where ignorance prevails, and where any one class is made to feel that society is an organized conspiracy to oppress, rob and degrade them, neither persons nor property will be safe.
—*Frederick Douglass (1817–1895)*

As long as justice and injustice have not terminated their ever renewing fight for ascendancy in the affairs of mankind, human beings must be willing, when need is, to do battle for the one against the other.
—*John Stuart Mill, "On Liberty" (1806–1873)*

INTRODUCTION

Most advanced practice nurses (APNs) would agree that the quality of the nurse–patient relationship is central to good nursing practice. However, this is not the same as saying it is the *only* important factor as argued in earlier chapters where the point was made that the APN's ethical responsibilities are not confined to this fiduciary relationship. Indeed, we often cannot fulfill our professional goals, "the prevention of illness, the alleviation of suffering, and the protection, promotion, and restoration of health" (American Nurses Association [ANA], 2001, preface) if we do not consider the antecedents of patients' problems as arising from within the larger community and society of which they are members. Two important assumptions of professional nursing practice are that each patient is equally worthy of our attention and the concerns of patients cannot be effectively addressed without understanding the environment in which they live out their daily lives. That is, patients are inseparable from their contexts—their families, communities, and society.

Based on the preceding assumptions and their relationship to Western ideas of justice, there are two crucial points to keep in mind as you read this chapter. First, the following paradox must be acknowledged: there are inevitable tensions between trying to meet overall societal needs and meeting everyone's individual needs, and yet both endeavors have the same purpose. Arguably, what is important about societies is that they exist because of the interests of the unique

107

individuals within them, who can't personally meet all of their own needs or the needs of their dependents. However, balancing everyone's needs fairly is a difficult and complex task even if an ideal political system for balancing injustices were possible. Therefore, to lose focus on the importance of treating people as equally worthy of concern within the society weakens the idea that societies themselves are important—these ideas might not be acceptable in other parts of the world where respecting the unique nature of persons is not a priority value.

Second, in balancing the needs of each person within the society against the needs of fellow citizens, some constraints on permissible individual actions are necessary. For example, a person cannot be free to cause another person serious harm. Additionally, balancing is needed in relation to the distribution of benefits and harms that is an inevitable part of communal living. Societal values and powerful interests both play a role in the distribution of benefits and harms; for this reason some inequities are difficult to avoid.

In a just society, certain basic goods such as "food, clothing, shelter, protection from unwarranted bodily harm" (Boylan, 2001, p. 197) are valued, and all persons have rights to pursue or claim these. These rights are protected or enforced by implicit (moral) and/or explicit (legal) rules and guidelines. Although, the complexity of societies is such that even when politicians and leaders have the best intentions, maintaining balance is a struggle that the more powerful members of society tend to dominate. As Hume, an 18th-century philosopher and observer of human nature, argued, if society were perfect and everyone had everything they needed, then the idea of justice would never have arisen (Hume, 1777/1967). But we do need justice because, as history and observation have shown, human beings possess a variety of characteristics including altruism, which furthers the good of others, and self-interest, which can at a minimum bias us against the interests of others and at worst exploit the weaknesses of others. Thus, rules or guidelines are needed that apply to all within the society and for which individuals may be held accountable either legally or morally. It is inevitable that in some cases these rules will cause problems for individuals in having their *particular* interests met, especially if these are interests for luxury or power that impinge on the more basic interests of others within the society.

Many commentators have proposed that a just society would maintain a just healthcare system; support for this proposition is given later. However, a large body of literature critiques the U.S. healthcare system as being systematically unjust (Mechanic, 2006). Even within a just healthcare system accessible to all—that is, where all are able to get help with the resources needed for the protection or improvement of their health (within the boundaries determined by the society's political process)—it would be difficult for nurses, singly or collaboratively, to try to mediate among the health needs of an individual who has presented for care, the needs of other individuals within their practice, and the concessions and compromises perceived necessary for overall societal benefit. To try to do this in a healthcare system where there is uneven access to services has proven very problematic and often distressing for nurses.

This chapter presents an argument that APNs, along with other healthcare providers, have responsibilities to address injustices that affect their population of concern, and these may include political action to influence inadequate local or national policies. Such policies are those that negatively influence health, mistake the actual source of the problem, or don't attempt to anticipate a population's health needs. By political action I mean activities—informed by nursing knowledge and clinical judgment (see Table 4-1)—undertaken by the nurse, often in collaboration with others, with the purposes of influencing necessary changes in policy at the institutional, local, or societal levels. At no time has it been more crucial for APNs to grasp the importance of this responsibility than now. Currently, the U.S. healthcare delivery system, among others (although perhaps for different reasons), has shifted its primary focus to economic concerns and away from the design and support of systems that are accountable for *both* the good of persons and the good of society.

In this chapter, the idea of human rights, health disparities, and the relationship of these to contemporary healthcare arrangements is explored. Although I used the convention of calling the provision of health services in the United States a *system* earlier, it should be noted that no *cohesive system* exists. Perhaps instead we should think of U.S. healthcare services as groups of arrangements because one of the criticisms of U.S. healthcare delivery is that it is not systematic in any sense of the word (Kleinke, 2002; Mechanic, 2006). In fact, because it is not embedded in a coherent structure, it results in severely fragmented services that negatively affect the health of many citizens.

The latter part of the chapter provides examples of types of problems stemming from societal injustices and the nature of healthcare economics. APN responsibilities to address these problems at a multitude of different levels are delineated, and strategies are proposed for effective action, including, where necessary, political activism on behalf of the population served. Chapters 3 and 5 as well as the later specialty practice chapters discuss different aspects of the healthcare delivery environment, implications for APNs, and provide strategies and resources pertinent to the particular context of the issue or specialty.

INDIVIDUALS AND SOCIETY: TENSIONS

Importance of Societies

The discussion that follows lays the foundation for, or strengthens, APNs' understanding that the relationship between individuals and the societies of which they are a part is tightly woven and not entirely separable. Societies have formed both historically and contemporarily because no one individual

Table 4-1   Clinical Judgment in Nursing

Definition: *Clinical judgment in nursing* is the nonlinear process of using knowledge, reasoning, tacit (experiential) skills, and interpersonal skills to determine—within the limits of available information—probable best actions given the inevitable existence of uncertainty about the possession of adequate knowledge and outcome of actions.

Components	Categories
Knowledge	The knowledge base of nursing: • Nature of the discipline • Purposes and goals • Nature of persons and environment • Characteristics of good practitioners • Scope and limits of practice Knowledge derived from other disciplines: philosophical (including ethical theory), physical, social, psychological, spiritual, biological Knowledge related to the situation • Primary subject/who is involved • Subject's understanding of the situation, values, beliefs and context • Goals
Experience	Previous experiences • Personal • Professional
Characteristics and skills	Perceptual • Grasp the nature and complexity of issues • Identification of needed/potential resources • Envision resolution • Reflection on practice and self-reflection • Creative, articulate Relational • Interpersonal • Collaborative • Mediation Motivation • Professional responsibility • Emotional engagement

is capable of providing for all of his or her own personal needs. Contemporary Western societies ostensibly exist to facilitate the lives of the individuals within them. Arguably, and as discussed shortly, not all societies have intended to provide for the freedom or well-being of all persons who fall under their canopy. Historically, many societies have had a free class and an enslaved or indentured class. Nevertheless, contemporary democratic societies such as that of the United States and many European and other countries have as a guiding principle the idea that all citizens are equal under the law. That is, everyone is subject to the same freedoms and the same restrictions upon those freedoms that are needed for a fair distribution of the burdens and benefits of societal living.

Shortly, we look at the issue of rights in general and human rights in particular and explore the relationship of these to a society's responsibilities to its citizens. As background, it is helpful first to take a historical look at the idea of a social contract and the idea of a just society to discover where responsibilities for the maintenance of just practices and institutions might be located.

Social Contract: Hobbes

The mechanisms of many contemporary societies are based in some form of the idea of a social contract. This "is the view that persons' moral and/or political obligations are dependent upon a contract or agreement between them to form society" (Friend, 2006). Although traces of social contract theorizing are visible as far back as the time of the ancient Greeks, contemporary theorizing about the structure of a good society, arguably, begins with the writings and thoughts of Thomas Hobbes (1588–1679). Hobbes is well known in philosophical and other circles both for his assertion that a social contract is necessary for an orderly and mutually beneficial society and for grounding this in a graphic description of what life would be like for human beings without such a contract.

Like all philosophers, Hobbes is influenced by his context. He lived in the turbulent times of the English civil war, a war fought between Royalists (supporters of the monarch) and Oliver Cromwell's supporters who wanted parliamentary rule. His theory is based on a rather pessimistic view of human nature that does not take into account the possibility of human capacity for altruistic actions (action that is either not primarily or not wholly self-interested). Thus, Hobbes felt that an overall ruler, such as a monarch, was necessary to impose order. However, he did not believe that royalty derived its power directly from a supreme being. That is, he did not believe in the divine right of kings. Individuals comprising the potential society would elect a leader they felt could provide the most impartial leadership. Once elected, the ruler would be entrusted with maintaining social order.

Hobbes's particular view of the social contract has been criticized on many levels. Most contemporary critics do not find his characterization of human beings accurate and neither do they agree with the structure he proposes. Nevertheless, his graphic description of life in a state of nature captures some of our worst fears about how human life could be for us in the absence of some sort of societal structure and is exemplified currently by the terrible conditions that exist in certain parts of the world where no identifiable or coherent social infrastructure seems to exist (for example Haiti, Sudan). Hobbes (1651/1967) writes that without a structured society man would be in "continual fear and danger of violent death . . . [and his life would be] solitary, poor, nasty, brutish and short" (p. 223). Some have argued that in fact even within so-called civilized societies, the conditions of certain marginalized groups of people are not so terribly far from Hobbes's conception of life without a social contract (Iceland, 2006; Papadimos, 2006; Rank, 2005).

Social Contract After Hobbes

The structure and functioning of many modern societies are based on some conception of a social contract. Ideas about human nature and the social contract, however, have gone through several evolutions since the time of Hobbes. Contemporarily, many scholarly writers in bioethics and justice have relied on John Rawls's (1971) ideas detailed in *A Theory of Justice* to explore and/or critique the notion that justice is fairness in the distribution of the benefits and burdens of living within a socially contracted society. The idea of justice as fairness is discussed in Chapter 1 and throughout the book.

Criticisms of the social contract as a way to design just societies exist. Feminists worry that the voices of women, the weak, and the vulnerable are muffled or muted by more powerful societal members, and thus their concerns are left out of the contract (metaphorically speaking). Additionally, the person at the center of the contract is generally conceived to be a self-sufficient, rational individual, who is able to reason objectively. However, contemporary philosophers, feminists, and others have pointed out that in fact we live in a web of relationships that inevitably influence us in complex ways not fully understood; therefore, the ideal of a rational person who can be divorced both from emotions and his or her relationships with others for the purposes of objective decision making is a myth. In view of this problem, the existence of a stable, just society is not possible. What is a more reasonable idea is that there is an ongoing struggle to achieve justice within society. This struggle entails, among other things, a concerted effort to bring out and magnify the perspectives of the disempowered by those who are in a position to recognize the nature and origins of perceived injustices. It includes efforts to rein in the influence of the powerful or redirect such influences toward a just cause.

One other conception of justice that is sometimes used especially as a basis for discussions related to the allocation of scarce resources concerns the view that people should receive benefits in proportion to the contributions they have made or according to what they deserve (Pojman, 1999). Whether a person is considered deserving of special consideration or not depends on societal, community, or religious values and these will be discernible from the supporting rationale. The problem for healthcare providers in relying on conceptions of justice as merit is that our knowledge base includes theoretical and empirical evidence that those who are privileged by supportive backgrounds and environments are often those who will appear more meritorious. It is easier to be meritorious if one is not caught up in the struggle of just surviving, for instance.

For present purposes, then, ideas about justice as fairness best capture problems in current healthcare environments that APNs most often encounter. The argument is made later that understanding the inevitability of structured injustices (unfairness) within any society, and thus within healthcare delivery systems, gives us a basis for understanding that responsibilities exist for nurses to recognize and address inequities that lead to poor health. The next section provides a very abbreviated and simplified account of the evolution of contemporary democratic societies and the relationships of individuals to the societies of which they are members by virtue of location or abode. The purpose of this section is to highlight the nature and source of tensions that exist between individuals and society and, thus, implications for advanced practice in negotiating the levels of responsibility that exist.

Individuals and Society

There are, of course, many different types of societies. The idea of a social contract is implied in some societies and not in others. Not all societies either historically or currently have held respect for individuals (see Chapter 1) as a crucial value. In many societies, the interests of the group, or some other value, is considered by the society's rulers or traditions to be more important than respect for the individual. And, as noted earlier, even when consideration for the equal moral worth of each person is valued, some individuals are more powerful than others and thus more capable of ensuring that they are accorded respect.

A scene from the film *Titanic* provides a striking example of this point. The *Titanic* was a new type of oceangoing ship, touted as being indestructible. However, after a catastrophic encounter with an iceberg, many of the lower-class passengers traveling in steerage class were trapped below decks by gates meant to separate the classes. This meant that they could not easily reach the lifeboats (of which there were too few to accommodate everyone) as the ship was sinking. It was obvious that the lower classes were not treated as equally worthy of moral concern as the upper classes—their very lives were obviously deemed less important than those who had paid more for their passage. Although that event took place almost a century ago, disparities based on class and race continue.

For the purposes of this chapter, though, and because this book is written primarily for APNs in contemporary democratic societies such as the United States, my discussion assumes the existence of a society that (1) takes itself to be democratic, (2) values each citizen as being of equal consideration in the distribution of the benefits and burdens of community living, and (3) has developed implicit and explicit (moral and legal) rules for the conduct of its daily business. Another way of saying this is that within the society each citizen is considered to count as the equal of any other citizen in influencing policy, that is, in saying what goods and services are important and what restrictions on personal freedoms are necessary to achieve the desired ends. These assumptions, which represent values espoused in the Constitution of the United States of America and are evident in the constitutions of other democratic countries, allow us to critique contemporary healthcare arrangements that unfairly disadvantage people.

Democratic Societies, Cooperation, and Legal Protection

Democratic societies are to a certain extent cooperative, meaning that such things as goods and services are gained that would not otherwise be accessible to the person, and such things as materials, time, labor, and money are given in exchange for needed goods and services. Cooperation permits efficiency in the production of goods and the delivery of services, but it also means that the actions of individuals within society necessarily have an impact on the lives of others with whom they interact or, even more broadly, on others in society. The impact may be positive in that mutual benefit occurs or negative in that someone's freedom is restricted or the expected or contracted service is not provided.

Tensions between the needs, desires, and freedom of individuals and what is perceived to be the good of the larger society are inevitable and often lead to political unrest. Not surprisingly it is frequently those who are the most powerful or who have the most resources, natural and/or material, whose interests prevail. For societies to be successful (I am using this term loosely) in balancing individual interests with the interests of the larger group, effective rules and guidelines are needed to deal with inevitable tensions.

Each democratic society, supposedly, develops its own system of justice based on the values of the society. "The provision of goods, when these are deemed by the society as vital for the well-being of individuals in the society . . . are safeguarded" (Grace, 1998, p. 98) by a system of laws. "The legislative system [of the society] determines in what manner, and to what extent, people will be legally protected from having their rights to these crucial goods violated" (Grace, 1998, p. 99). These, then, are the legal rights that a person within a society can claim as his or her due. Legal rights, however, are only one type of right. Moral rights also exist. The basis for moral rights may be the same as or different from those of legal rights depending on the underlying value systems of the society, that is, what sorts of belief systems are accorded legitimacy within the system and which values are deemed important enough to protect via formal sanctions.

MORAL RIGHTS

General Moral Rights

Besides legal rights that are conceived within the society, and in democratic societies with the input of citizens, and for which impingements warrant formal sanctions of some kind, other conceptions of rights exist. So-called moral rights, Feinberg (1973) asserts, "exist prior to, or independently of, any legal or institutional rules" (p. 84). Moral rights may or may not be protected by laws. But we might ask what the term *moral rights* means, and just how these differ from legal rights. As usual, in philosophy there is a variety of answers that can be given to these questions—as many answers as the different perspectives or theories that exist. Some of the important aspects of moral rights are sketched in the following paragraphs.

The idea that an individual has certain moral rights is centered on conceptions that some human goods are critically important and should be protected, preserved, or promoted. The actions of protecting, preserving, or promoting human good imply interactions taken by others on behalf of the subject. An evaluation of the proposed or actual actions is made on the basis of whether the action can actually or does serve its purpose. Moreover, some actions may be forbidden if they are likely to cause more harm than good.

In moral philosophy, the appraisal of actions usually falls into one of three categories. The action by the agent is required (obligatory), permissible (neutral), or forbidden. Although here the discussion is about action framed in positive terms, refraining from acting when action is needed to prevent harm or further a person's good is also subject to moral appraisal. The moral status of actions is generally linked to values espoused within the society—such as freedom of speech, equality of opportunity. These values may be based on a variety of moral theories (deontology, utilitarianism, virtue, and so on) or on a belief in divine rules. For example, say that a patient (an individual within society) is conceived as having a right to make his or her own decisions by virtue of societal values; then, not I nor any other provider may interfere with that decision, all things being equal (in the absence of some reason to suppose that the person is incapable of acting independently). Admission to the hospital does not remove that right. This may seem rather obvious, but it is not always honored in fact, and patient rights were often not respected historically—physicians were often considered to know what was best for a patient whether or not the physician had a sense of the patient's own values. Moral rights are not always subject to legal enforcement, although they may be.

Although it is beyond the scope of this chapter to engage in, or even present, some of the many philosophical debates related to rights and obligations, it is perhaps helpful to note one differentiation that is sometimes made between a positive moral right—where a claim may be made against someone or some institution for assistance or for the provision of goods and services (often requires more government regulations)—and negative moral rights—or the right to be left alone and to be free from the interference of others or from the state (often implies limits on government interference or regulations). To make a claim that one has a right to health care is a positive right in this sense. Positive rights mean that a claim may be made against some entity to ensure one's right—in this case the government of one's society. Claims about a right to health care are often made on the basis of human rights. Human rights are one type of important moral right that are said to belong to humans regardless of the values held by their particular society. If we believe that a right to health care is a human right, this has implications for healthcare providers. The implications stem from the supposition that human beings all have the right to at least a minimally good life (Nickel, 2005).

Human Rights

Human Rights as a Category of Moral Rights: History

Human rights are a specific type of moral right that are no less important in healthcare settings than they are in wider contexts. But what are they? Where do they come from? And what is their force? Contemporarily in the United States, many of us talk about human rights in the same way that we talk about having legs or lungs: we do not question their existence, we believe that they are ours to claim. We object to murder and torture whenever they occur and consider these acts as violations of human rights. To take away a person's life puts an end to all of that person's potential future choices, aspirations, and actions. It ends his or her humanity.

Modern ideas about human rights trace their origins as far back as the Magna Carta of 11th-century England. Under pressure from his noblemen, King John was swayed to institute what was essentially a contract between the king and his subjects. It limited the power of the state to control its populace and delineated what individuals could lay claim to in the courts (British Bill of Rights, 1994). In essence, it served as the foundation for contemporary rules of law. This was an important development because prior to the Magna Carta the citizens of many societies were subject to the whims and desires of their leaders, often kings. Individual freedom was limited by the dictates of these rulers. The Magna Carta was pivotal for certain political changes but did not extend to all subjects, only to those who already had some power.

It was several centuries later during the Enlightenment when the issues of moral rights and human rights were taken seriously. The Enlightenment represents a period in American and European philosophy when the use of reasoning or analytic thought became valued as the main route to knowledge and was viewed as an essentially and uniquely human characteristic. Locke (1690/2003), for example, claimed that rights naturally flowed from the nature of humans as free and rational beings. Kant's (see Chapter 1) ideas about the innate dignity of human beings serve as his justification for the existence of human rights. According to Kant (1785/1967), human beings by virtue of their capacity for rational thought and for making moral rules are, and thus should be allowed to be, self-governing. For this reason, they should never be used purely as a means of serving someone else's advantage. Kant has a complicated argument for this but basically proposes that it is irrational to use an individual purely or primarily as a means to someone else's advantage. For example, if a person assented to this, that person would essentially be saying, "Everyone can treat anyone else as a means to an end" (this is Kant's Categorical Imperative roughly stated). But we would not want to be treated purely as a means to someone else's end; thus, it is irrational to treat someone else as a means to one's own end.

Moral rights, then, include such things as being free to make one's own choices and being free from the interference of the state in personal affairs. Human rights are a more fundamental category of rights. Whereas particular moral rights are based in particular theories of moral philosophy and may or may not hold depending on the values of a society, human rights are asserted to apply to every human by virtue of their humanity. Therefore, human rights apply to everyone regardless of the society to which they belong. Some human rights are considered to be inalienable, that is, they cannot be given away by the person. A classic example of an inalienable right is the right to be free. This means that I cannot agree to be enslaved even if this would benefit my family in some way because it is the nature of humans to be free. It is important to note that there is no agreement about exactly what is the set of rights that we can call human rights, although certain rights are generally agreed to be included, as you shall see.

Human Rights: Contemporary Understandings

Following the Enlightenment period, attention paid to the issue of human rights waned temporarily. However, renewed interest emerged partly as a result of human abuses during World War II (1939–1945) (see Chapter 6 on research ethics for a fuller discussion). This prompted a revisiting of the issue of human rights and attempts to further define what they are and why they should be honored. Fagan (2006) notes that contemporarily, "human rights have been defined as basic moral guarantees that people in all countries and cultures allegedly have simply because they are people." According to Nickel (2005), human rights "are concerned with ensuring the conditions . . . of a minimally good life" (p. 386). Fagan (2006) in his thoughtful discussion of human rights notes that this idea of a minimally good life "has been enshrined in various declarations and legal conventions issued during the past fifty years, initiated by the Universal Declaration of Human Rights (1948) and perpetuated by, most importantly, the European Convention on Human Rights (1954) and the International Covenant on Civil and Economic Rights (1966)." Conceptions of a minimally good life are necessarily different depending on the society and its resources.

The idea behind an assertion that all human beings have rights simply by virtue of being human derives from the "philosophical claim: that there exists a rationally identifiable moral order, an order whose legitimacy precedes contingent social and historical conditions and applies to all human beings everywhere and at all times" (Fagan, 2006). We could state this a little differently by saying either each human is equally worthy of moral consideration (viewed as important in his or her own right) or no one is. If no one is to be accorded moral consideration, then any one of us at any time might find our interests discarded on someone else's whim. Indeed, using Rawls's ideas about people in the original position deliberating behind "a veil of ignorance" (Rawls, 1971), we can imagine that no one would feel secure about abolishing human rights for fear their position in society, and their assets might make them particularly vulnerable to the absence of such rights.

Human rights, however, are not bound to a particular society but are taken to apply across societal and national borders and political contexts. The declarations cited earlier allude to human rights as supporting such goods as a basic standard of living that includes education, provisions for health care, and protection from the effects of destitution. They prohibit torture, slavery, and exploitation. Unfortunately, the interpretation of these rights and how they should be applied in actual situations is a more difficult undertaking than asserting that they exist—as is enforcing them. Currently, in moral philosophy and bioethics circles there is debate about whether human rights imply the right to a certain basic level of health care that is consistent with the status of healthcare knowledge and societal resources. Complicating things further is the absence of a definition of health that everyone can agree upon.

Is There a Right to Health Care?

This question has been raised by many scholars in the United States and elsewhere. It is an important problem to explore within the context of this book because nurses assert via the policies and position statements of their professional bodies (ANA, 2003; International Council of Nurses, 2000) and the writings of scholars that they exist to attend to the health needs of individuals and society in a nondiscriminatory manner (Ballou, 2000; Gaylord & Grace, 1995; Grace, 1998, 2001; Raphael, 1997; Spenceley, Reutter, & Allen, 2006). Thus, clarity about the influence of all of the following on health is important: universal human rights and their demands on societies, societal values implied (what people would tell you) versus actual (how societal institutions are set up), a person's social and/or economic standing, and the nature and accessibility of healthcare services. These are fundamental for understanding what actions are required to meet the health needs of an APN's population (where the definition of health depends both upon the patient's conception of this and insights from nursing knowledge development and the APN's specialty knowledge base).

Nurses, as Curtin (1979) and many other commentators have pointed out, are often the ones who "attend patients when distress is immediate . . . for sustained periods of time" (p. 4) and thus have the opportunity to experience patients in all of their humanity (a philosophical ideal of nursing—see Chapter 2), including the struggle of the poor and otherwise disadvantaged for survival in an inequitable environment. Certain living conditions have been shown to contribute to or exacerbate health problems perhaps even more than a lack of access alone, although often persons living in substandard conditions also lack easy or adequate access to healthcare services. Thus, there are inextricable links among living conditions, social standing, economic status, and health (Danziger & Haveman, 2001; Iceland, 2006; Powers & Faden, 2006; Rank, 2005). For this reason, even if we agree that there is a right to a basic level of health care, this will not ensure good health because even more fundamental justice problems arise within society that also require attention, such as needs for adequate nutrition, housing, and security, as discussed shortly.

Human Rights Arguments for Justice in Health Care

Before discussing professional advocacy for individual and societal health—which means comprehending the effects of poverty and socioeconomic standing on persons' lives and their functioning and flourishing—it is important to gain an understanding of the relationship between human rights and rights to health care. Dernier (2005) notes that when we assert that a right to health care exists, we are essentially making several related claims. A right to health care means that everyone encompassed by the society (regardless of status and perhaps even including illegal immigrants), by virtue of being human, is entitled to a certain level of access to health care and society has a collective responsibility to ensure this. It is a strong societal obligation. This obligation should be reflected in policy debates, and failure to meet this obligation can be said to constitute an injustice.

As a profession, nursing takes the stance that providing basic healthcare services, including those that facilitate the prevention of illness, and the promotion and preservation of health for all members of society are a moral responsibility and should be treated as a human right (ICN, 2000). This is a starting place. A further question that is beyond the scope of this book to explore in detail is to ask, "What are the scope and limits of this right?" Buchanan (1984) noted in the 1980s that there was a growing belief in the idea that "the right to a decent minimum of health care" exists; indeed this is the title of his book. However, d'Oronzio (2001), along with many other philosophers, ethicists, healthcare professionals, and citizens, is concerned that viewing as a human right a basic minimum of health care is not compatible with the current U.S. healthcare financing arrangements. Although efforts to change the U.S. health-care delivery system are in process, certain professional healthcare groups, notably the ANA (2005), have affirmed their belief that there is a right to health care and that this means the system must change. "The ANA endorses a single payer system as a way to integrate services and facilitate accessibility. ANA believes that health care is a basic human right. . . . Thus, ANA reaffirms its support for a restructured health care system that assures universal access to a standard package of essential health care services for all citizens and residents" (ANA, 2005, p. 2).

The following section explores the scope and limits of an APN's responsibilities to patients and society. Role responsibilities are described as both narrow and broad. An argument is presented for understanding responsibilities in three areas: to individual patients, to influence societal conditions that affect groups of patients in terms of access to care or other influences on health, and to overcome obstacles to good care caused by the environment of practice.

ADVANCED PRACTICE NURSING AND PROFESSIONAL ADVOCACY

Professional Advocacy: A Broad Conception of Role Responsibilities

The term *advocacy* is commonly used in nursing circles as an ideal of practice. However, efforts are ongoing to define what this means in nursing contexts (Bu & Jezewski, 2007; Chafey, Rhea, Shannon, & Spencer, 1998; Grace, 1998, 2001; Mallik, 1997; Snoball, 1996; Spenceley et al., 2006). Consequently, the boundaries of nursing responsibilities related to advocacy are often unclearly understood and shift depending on the definition of advocacy assumed. The term has various meanings to various people. I know this to be true both from available literature and from informal surveys of the many graduate and undergraduate students I have encountered over the years. Some say advocacy means defending a patient's rights (Abrams, 1978; Curtin, 1982; Gadow, 1990; Jezewski, 1993; Miller, Mansen, & Lee, 1983; Pagana, 1987; Shirley, 2007; Zussman, 1982); some say that it means ensuring that a patient gets his or her immediate needs met; still others might say that it is a role-related responsibility of nursing, meaning that any action taken by the nurse while acting in the role of a nurse is advocacy. Indeed, all of these definitions appear in the nursing and allied literature (ANA, 2001; Annas, 1974/1990; Bernal, 1992; Chafey et al., 1998; Gaylord & Grace, 1995; Grace, 2001; Hewitt, 2002; MacDonald, 2007; Mallik, 1997; O'Connor & Kelly, 2005; Snoball, 1996; Spenceley et al., 2006).

Elsewhere, I have examined the concept of advocacy in great detail (Grace, 1998, 2001); indeed, it was the topic of my doctoral dissertation. A colleague and I were initially stimulated to explore this topic by an article that appeared in the *Hastings Center Report* in 1992 by nonnurse ethicist Ellen Bernal. In the article, she chastised nursing for taking the stance that we are patient advocates. She argued that nursing uses advocacy to advance its autonomy as a discipline and thus improve its professional status. On closer reading, we realized she was using an interpretation of advocacy as meaning only a defense of patient rights and were moved to explore in more depth what nursing means by *advocacy* (Gaylord & Grace, 1995). This problem of ambiguity of meaning and thus expectations of the nurse became the impetus for a whole program of study related to professional responsibility.

Perhaps the most interesting insight gained during this investigation of advocacy concerned the roots of the term in legal settings. Advocacy as a practice ideal has its origins in the field of law. In law, it means the verbal act of arguing for a person's cause against the cause of an adversary. Lawyers, while advocating, have responsibilities only for that client (or group of clients) and his or her cause. If there are system injustices, these are dealt with outside of the immediate lawyer–client situation.

Nurses, however, do not have such limited responsibilities. In advocating for one patient to have his or her needs met, we may well cause disadvantage to another. For example, a primary care nurse practitioner (NP) in a busy clinic is told by one of her patients that she is being physically abused by her boyfriend. This is an urgent matter and the patient needs time and attention. But the nurse is in a practice with two physicians, who in response to economic pressures have limited the time allocated for nurse visits. The APN is the sole available provider this afternoon, and she has three other patients also waiting to be seen. She must make a decision that will affect somebody's care: an immediate decision must be made that balances the risk to the other patients against the likely benefit to the abused patient of spending more time with her. The APN has simultaneous responsibilities to more than one patient; thus, advocating for one to receive extra attention may well disadvantage others. So, her responsibilities cannot end with the immediate decision and ensuing action. The problem of inadequate visit time is recurring and results in part from a misunderstanding about the APN role, deliberate or inadvertent, on the part of the collaborating/ supervising physicians.

Therefore, a different way of looking at the advocacy role of the APN is to view it as *any action taken to further professional goals* (ultimately related to promoting patient good). This permits us to see that our advocacy actions may be directed at different levels. "Professional advocacy, then, may be conceived both as actions taken to further nursing's purposes on behalf of individual patients and actions taken to expose and redress underlying problems that are inherent in the larger contexts of institutions, policymaking, and the health care delivery system" (Grace, 2001, p. 161). Many so-called advocacy situations "have their fundamental roots in such things as national health policy decisions, economic conflicts of interests, miscommunication, institutional barriers or a host of other grounds" (Grace, 2001, p. 152).

To provide some coherent structure to the exploration of advocacy viewed as professional responsibility to further nursing goals (responsibilities of the nursing role), the next section is divided into three parts. The first part describes advocacy viewed as the APN's professional responsibilities to individual patients encountered in practice settings. Second, advocacy is viewed as the responsibilities to address the environment in which the APN practices is discussed. Finally, the APN's role in influencing social policy is discussed. However, this is an artificial categorization because in many cases all three levels of responsibility may coexist. When the APN is faced with a tension between trying to provide what is needed for a particular patient and the needs of others within the practice, clinical judgment is needed to prioritize action. Clinical judgment in this sense is synonymous with ethical or moral reasoning (see Table 4-1).

Case: An Example of Common Issues

This case appeared in the *Louisville Courier-Journal* (Coomes, 2007) recently. It exemplifies the various levels of advocacy needed to ensure good care for this patient. Additionally, Ms. Henley's predicament is familiar, one to which many nurses at all levels of practice can relate. "Portia Henley, a 50-year-old [African American] grandmother from Louisville [is] unable to keep a steady job. She has diabetes and struggles to pay for the better food and special drugs her condition requires; asthma inhibits her ability to exercise. 'I'm fighting a real battle,' said Henley. 'It's hard to stay on the straight and narrow in terms of what you eat when you don't have the income to handle the price of medicine, the price of going to doctors and the price of keeping a roof over your head, plus the cost of buying food for this one specific health problem.'"

Professional Advocacy for Individual Patients

Nurse–Patient Relationship

As noted in Chapter 1, the essence of nursing care is the individual nurse–patient relationship. This is a fiduciary relationship based on trust. Whether patients do or do not actually trust us, in the sense of knowing who we are and having confidence in our abilities, nevertheless, they are forced to trust that we do in fact have their individual best interests in mind, know what we are doing, understand the limits of our knowledge and skills, and will steer them in the right direction or put them in touch with needed resources when we have reached the limits of our expertise. For this reason, transparency of purpose and affiliation is important. In some cases, especially in advanced practice settings, our work is not directly aimed at patient benefit. Here, I mean such activities as performing preemployment wellness screenings or serving in the role of research nurse coordinator. In such cases, we have responsibilities to reveal our purpose and any existing conflicts of interest, to address misunderstandings, and to direct the involved person to a source of help as needed.

However, mostly our role is to further patient good related to individual persons' actual or potential health needs. To further this good we use clinical judgment to determine appropriate actions. A definition of clinical judgment that was synthesized from extant literature in nursing, medicine, and the cognitive sciences appears in Table 4-1. Clinical judgment is needed to identify patients' needs, anticipate future needs, and facilitate care that is most likely to meet these needs. Because the goals of care involve understanding what is best for the patient whose life is necessarily contextual and nuanced, we need to engage with the patient (and with family members when this is indicated) to discover the patient's beliefs, values, and preferences so that our actions are tailored to that person's needs. Additionally, because we too are human and have our own beliefs, values, and biases, we must be careful to understand what these biases are and how such prejudices (prejudgments about the nature or attributes of a person) are likely to affect our clinical judgment in particular situations.

Biases

Ms. Henley's case serves as an example of a possible bias that providers may exhibit and relates to poverty. Many people do not have a good understanding of the nature of poverty and its antecedents. Coryn (2002), in his literature review, notes that there are three distinct categories of attitudes people have related to poverty: these are "individualistic/internal, structural/external, and fatalistic." In the United States, the predominant attitude of the middle class is individualistic/internal, meaning the poor person is blamed for possessing a character flaw such as laziness or lack of ambition that has led him or her to the present condition. Perhaps not surprisingly, among the poor themselves the predominant attitude is structural/external, meaning they attribute poverty to external circumstances (Coryn, 2002). Because, as has been noted, most healthcare professionals are middle class, a bias against the poor can be anticipated (Crandall, 1990).

One way to avoid the effects of bias that arises from inexperience or ignorance is to try to understand what the person's life is like for him or her. What are the daily experiences and struggles like? Other biases or prejudices may exist because of negative past experiences with someone. For example, a nurse whose parent suffered from alcohol abuse has a negative attitude toward patients she views as alcoholic. Advocacy, viewed as professional responsibility to further the goals of the profession for good care, obligates us to understand who the patient is, what is needed for the patient's care, and what obstacles exist to getting the patient the care he or she needs.

Identifying and Addressing Obstacles

Obstacles to providing what the APN determines to be necessary for the good of an individual patient may take many shapes and forms. Table 4-2 lays out the different levels at which obstacles may present and provides a synopsis

Table 4-2   Categories of Obstacles to Ethical Nursing/Health Care

Category	Obstacles
Individual patient	1. Patient not viewed as unique • Standardized patient care • Provider lacks understanding of important contextual details' influence 2. Prejudgment of patient (bias/prejudice) 3. Patient or family needs for knowledge not fully addressed (related to above) 4. Interpersonal conflict • Provider–patient • Patient–family • Provider–provider 5. Poor communication • Provider–patient/family • Provider–provider 6. Power imbalances—coercion/silencing 7. Inadequate time—resources to evaluate and address needs (also a practice environment problem)
Practice environment	1. Lack of primary focus on patient good • Economic conflicts of interest • Practice philosophy is to meet economic goals 2. Autonomous practice constrained • Senior colleagues • Institutional mission • Managed care mandates 3. Unsupportive environment
Social injustices	1. Unjust aspects of the healthcare system • Access • Financing • Priorities • Failure to attend to the real origins of certain health problems (below) 2. Socioeconomic disparities • Education • Poverty • Discrimination 3. Profit motive or business emphasis 4. Fragmented services

of common problems. Strategies to address obstacles are presented shortly. The later chapters of this book, which cover issues in specialty APN practice, feature specific types of problems and methods to identify and overcome obstacles that are prevalent within or associated with the particular settings. However, the types of problems Portia Henley encounters daily, like many of the examples given in Chapter 3, cut across settings. We can see that many obstacles exist to her achieving optimal health even within the limits of her complex issues. Because some of these issues arise as a result of social inequities, addressing these requires influencing social policies, as addressed shortly.

In caring for Ms. Henley at the nurse–patient relationship level, our immediate concern is to assist with her current problems. Professional advocacy at this level means using an approach that is based in nursing's philosophy of care and goals of practice (discussed in Chapter 1). Although priority goals are to meet her immediate needs, we still need to have an idea of who Portia is as a person. In the absence of a life-threatening emergency that would require immediate measures, we cannot adequately help Portia meet her health needs if we don't know more about her. We need to know, for example, how her maladies are affecting her, what she views as the priority issue, what she knows about her physical conditions, what resources are available to her, and what her priorities are. Advocacy at the level of nurse–patient relationship, then, means professional responsibility to ensure good patient care. This entails understanding what good actions are likely to be for this patient, working with Portia to determine what are good avenues of action from her point of view, and recognizing and accounting for potential and actual obstacles to good action.

Advocacy viewed as professional role responsibilities for good care presents the same obligations regardless of setting and is based in nursing's philosophy of care and disciplinary goals. So, Ms. Henley could have presented for care at any number of different specialty practices—primary care adult health, family practice, women's health primary care, emergency room, as a preanesthesia workup, in a diabetes or asthma clinic, and so on. The time required to address all of her issues may be different in different settings because some aspects of her care may well be beyond the knowledge and skills of the clinician, who will then need to refer Portia to others for care of those aspects. Nevertheless, the APN's responsibilities include evaluating the quality and appropriateness of the referral made (as discussed in Chapter 5).

One could object that advocacy, as described earlier, is an onerous and unrealistic responsibility given current environments of practice with their inevitable time constraints and pressures. This objection is not uncommon and may be true in many settings. Nevertheless, our role responsibilities include understanding and influencing the context of care so that nursing goals can be met. In those situations where the APN finds intractable differences between his or her philosophy of care and those of her practice colleagues, it is the nurse's responsibility to consider whether a different type of setting might be more fitting. (See Chapter 5 for APN role issues.)

Nurses see firsthand the effects of unaddressed or poorly addressed problems upon their population of patients. They may be the first or only ones to understand both what those effects are and what changes are needed. Therefore, our responsibilities do not end when the presenting patient's priority needs are met, especially when it is recognized that the practice environment may actually be working against nursing goals of providing care for the patient as a person.

Professional Advocacy and Practice Environments

The varied environments in which APNs work and care for patients also give rise to problems that can interfere with optimal care for a given patient (see Table 4-2). Role responsibilities exist so that nurses can understand in what ways the particular setting and its values are impinging on ethical patient care. The problem may involve a particular patient or may be seen as recurrent. In the case of Portia Henley, a practice focus of constricted time slots or on managing only the acute presentation would lead to fragmented care, is at odds with nursing goals that include anticipation and prevention of future problems, and would affect many of the patients within the practice. As another example, in correctional settings the facility's goal of prisoner behavior control may interfere with a nursing emphasis on providing for the prisoner's well-being. In yet other settings, unit, institutional, or practice policies, conventions, or expediencies may raise barriers to good patient care. Like other healthcare providers in primary care settings especially, constraints related to financing arrangements, reimbursement issues, and managed care practices pose some of the most troubling, difficult, and time-consuming problems for nurse practitioners (Johnson, 2005; Ulrich et al., 2006; Ulrich & Soeken, 2005). Issues associated with managed care organizations and financing are discussed in more detail in Chapter 5.

Professional Advocacy and Social Injustices

At the broadest level, APNs in concert with other nurses, physicians, and allied health professionals have a collective interest in addressing social injustice. This is because the goals of almost all healthcare professions have to do with improving the health of individuals. Improving the health of individuals often requires addressing injustice that is deeply rooted in a society. It is not expected that most APNs will be capable of single-handedly tackling an issue; however, their knowledge and experiences place them in the ideal situation to join with colleagues or collaborate with other professionals to inform policy debates.

Nurses, both because they provide direct care and have a perspective and approach that permits hearing patients' health and illness stories within the contexts of patients' daily lives, may be the first or only ones to recognize existing and developing patterns of injustice or disparity. Nurses, along with other healthcare providers, see firsthand the end results of poor access to health care or poor health maintenance. Thus, viewing advocacy as a broader responsibility to further professional goals at both the individual and societal level highlights the range of knowledge, skills, and actions that may be needed. Besides the fact that taking a broad view of nursing responsibilities is needed for meeting nursing goals, positive action at a level different from the immediate situation is also a way of mitigating the moral distress or unease felt when we are unable to provide the care needed for a particular patient because of environmental or other obstacles (Arthur, 1995; Corley, 1995; Corley, Minick, Elswick, & Jacobs, 2005; Erlen & Sereika, 1997; Fowler, 1989).

Health Disparities and Poverty

Although health disparities are by no means the only nursing care issues that require professional advocacy at the societal level, the issue of poverty in the United States and its influence on health provides an important exemplar and argument for APNs to take seriously their ethical responsibilities to advocate for health policy changes. Poverty affects people in a variety of ways that are not always easily discernible but that have been well documented in the literature and supported by empirical studies (Danziger & Haveman, 2001; Iceland, 2006; Rank, 2005). Patients like Portia Henley, for whom daily life is an ongoing struggle to make ends meet, may delay seeking care until their problems are out of control. They may have inadequate insurance, transportation difficulties, lack of family support, be the primary caretaker for others whose needs they put first, or have any number of other obstacles to getting the assistance they need. As a diabetes clinical nurse specialist (CNS) or APN, my immediate goal would be to assess Ms. Henley's priority needs for knowledge, self-care, nursing, and other necessary therapeutics, which would include understanding her values and priorities. Next steps would be to help her obtain the resources and supports she needs to achieve a level of health that she desires and that is realistic in the context of her life. Finally, what is really needed is an exploration of the environmental and economic conditions that resulted in her current status.

Strategies for recognizing and addressing ethical issues arising in direct patient care settings were given in Chapter 2 and are discussed throughout this book. The next section briefly presents some ideas for influencing change in the broader healthcare environment. Nursing has a rich history of activism to improve health care, starting with the efforts of Florence Nightingale (1820–1910). Nightingale used evidence and influence to change the way wounded soldiers were treated during the Crimean War, and she used her knowledge, skills, and influence to ensure that a patient's environment would be conducive to his or her healing.

Professional Advocacy: Influential Strategies

As APNs, we are uniquely positioned to research and articulate the likely consequences of problematic practices to those in charge of policy decisions, whether this is at the institutional, local, and/or societal levels. The current healthcare climate necessitates the political action of nurses individually, collectively, and in collaboration with others and is exceptionally open to the input of nurses because "physicians have lost much of their influence and control to corporate medicine in recent years" (Mechanic & Reinhard, 2002, p. 7). Although not all nurses can, as Malone (2005) notes, "become policy experts . . . in addition to providing direct patient care . . . all nurses can assess, identify, and articulate for [or on behalf of] patients" on certain problematic issues and "provide information to patients on options for impacting policy; and work to effect policy change through professional and advocacy organizations" (p. 136).

One can (*should*) include in one's nursing assessment possible "policy factors that may have preventive, etiological, or therapeutic significance" (Malone, 2005, p. 136). This may sound complicated but is actually elementary. For example, it means asking why certain poor patients with diabetes are not managing their diet and medicines well. Is it because they are unaware of resources (the system is not allowing for adequate patient education), they can't afford the medicines (health insurance problems), have access problems, or some other issue? One effective strategy is to join forces with other nurses, physicians, and allied professionals whose concerns mirror yours. Publicize the problem, provide convincing rationale, and outline probable consequences. Providing a submission to the op-ed page of a newspaper or a letter to the editor often gets public attention and raises questions for discussion in a more public forum. Membership on pertinent, institutional, or local committees is another good strategy and can open an important forum for educating other committee members about nursing concerns. For example, acute care CNSs or NPs can provide a valuable voice for patients on hospital ethics committees and patient care committees.

APNs can be instrumental in educating and providing information for grassroots patient organizations. Recognize that the information you have about patient situations is valuable and can be articulated in a variety of arenas and forums to inform needed changes. For example, family nurse practitioner students joined with their mentors and a specialty organization to change the practice of one managed care company related to antihistamine prescriptions. The formulary allowed only diphenhydramine for seasonal allergy treatments, but this was making many of the children drowsy. A letter-writing and publicity campaign managed to change the practice and make better options available to these children. Another example of effective nursing political activity is given by Murphy and colleagues (2005) and is related to improved pain control. "Through regulatory policy advocated for by nurses and many others in the political arena, optimal pain control is now part of standard practice" (p. 22). Join with colleagues and/or collaborate with allied professionals to publicize a problem. This can also be done via letters to the editor of local papers, or by e-mailing, calling, or writing to one's local or state representative.

Conclusion

Professional advocacy is synonymous with the idea that all nursing actions have ethical implications. This is because all nursing actions have the ultimate purpose of furthering the goals of nursing related to patient well-being. The goals of nursing involve providing this good of health and well-being for individuals who are inextricably a part of the larger society in which they reside. Consequently, patients are susceptible to inequities occurring as a result of societal arrangements. Good patient care, then, often requires attention to the underlying circumstances that have given rise to the need for nursing's services, including poverty and other disparities that leave patients especially vulnerable to their healthcare needs.

SUMMARY

This chapter provides an essential background for understanding the breadth of APN responsibilities to attend to the health needs of both individuals and society. An argument is provided for the importance of balancing the needs of individuals with societal needs related to health and health care. To fulfill professional goals APNs need to engage with individual patients, taking into account the patients' unique needs and addressing obstacles that prevent meeting these needs. Additionally, APNs may need to engage in political activity at a variety of levels, either singly or in collaboration with others.

DISCUSSION QUESTIONS AND EXERCISES

1. We all have patients or types of patients that we find ourselves avoiding—this is human nature. The person reminds us of someone in the past, perhaps, who treated us badly or at whose hands we suffered, or the person may just be difficult to please. In light of the previous discussion of advocacy, explore ways in which you might make a connection with a difficult patient.
2. In your practice or from your nursing experience, identify the common barriers/obstacles that make it difficult for you to give the care that in your clinical judgment is required. How should such problems be addressed?
3. You are one of the two APNs in a group practice. You and your colleague are being pressured to assume the same approach to practice as your physician colleagues and the physician assistant. Your colleagues are receptive to your input and you have a collegial relationship. How would you explain to them that your nursing perspective requires a different approach?
4. What does it mean to be self-reflective? How does one know when one has been genuinely self-reflective versus justifying the values one has?
5. Do you think that everyone should have access to the same basic level of health care? What would this include?

REFERENCES

Abrams, N. (1978). A contrary view of the nurse as patient advocate. *Nursing Forum, 17*, 258–267.

American Nurses Association. (2001). *Code of ethics for nurses with interpretive statements.* Washington, DC: Author.

American Nurses Association. (2003). *Social policy statement.* Washington, DC: Author.

American Nurses Association. (2005). *Health Care Agenda.* Retrieved July 9, 2007, from http://www.nursingworld.org/readroom/anahca05.pdf.

Annas, G. J. (1974/1990). The patient rights advocate: Can nurses effectively fill the role? In T. Pence & J. Cantrall (Eds.), *Ethics in nursing: An anthology* (pp. 83–86). New York, NY: National League for Nursing Publication.

Arthur, E. (1995). Coping with moral distress. *Minnesota Nursing Accent, 67*(3), 5.

Ballou, K. A. (2000). A historical-philosophical analysis of the professional nurse obligation to participate in sociopolitical activities. *Policy, Politics, & Nursing Practice, 1*(3), 172–184.

Bernal, E. W. (1992). The nurse as patient advocate. *Hastings Center Report, 22*(4), 18–23.

Boylan, M. (2001). A universal right to healthcare. *International Journal of Policy and Ethics, 1*(3), 197–211.

British Bill of Rights. (1994). *The Magna Carta.* Retrieved June 30, 2007, from http://www.hrweb.org/legal/otherdoc.html.

Bu, X., & Jezewski, M. A. (2007). Developing a mid-range theory of advocacy through concept analysis. *Journal of Advanced Nursing, 57*(1), 101–110.

Buchanan, A. (1984). The right to a decent minimum of health care. *Philosophy and Public Affairs, 13*(1), 55–78.

Chafey, K., Rhea, M., Shannon, A. M., & Spencer, S. (1998). Characterizations of advocacy by practicing nurses. *Journal of Professional Nursing, 14*(1), 43–52.

Coomes, M. (2007). Kentucky's health: Critical condition. *Louisville Courier-Journal,* May 11. Retrieved June 24, 2007, from http://www.kctcs.edu/todaysnews/index.cfm?tn_date=2007-05-11#10533.

Corley, M. C. (1995). Moral distress of critical care nurses. *American Journal of Critical Care, 4,* 280–285.

Corley, M. C., Minick, P., Elswick, R. K., & Jacobs, M. S. O. (2005). Nurse moral distress and ethical work environment. *Nursing Ethics, 12*(4), 381–390.

Coryn, C. (2002). Antecedents of attitudes towards the poor. Unpublished paper. Retrieved June 24, 2007, from http://www.iusb.edu/~journal/2002/coryn/coryn.html.

Crandall, L. A. (1990). Advocacy of just health policies as professional duty: Cultural biases and ethical responsibility. *Business and Professional Ethics Journal, 9*(3&4), 41–53.

Curtin, L. (1979). The nurse as advocate: A philosophical foundation for nursing. *Advances in Nursing Science, 1*(3), 1–10.

Curtin, L. L. (1982). What are human rights? In L. L. Curtin & M. J. Flaherty (Eds.), *Nursing ethics: Theories and pragmatics* (pp. 3–16). Bowie, MD: Brady Communications.

Danziger, S. H., & Haveman, R. H. (2001). *Understanding poverty.* Cambridge, MA: Harvard University Press.

Dernier, Y. (2005). On personal responsibility and the human right to healthcare. *Cambridge Quarterly of Healthcare Ethics, 14,* 224–234.

d'Oronzio, J. C. (2001). A human right to health care access: Returning to the origins of the patients rights movement. *Cambridge Quarterly of Healthcare Ethics, 10,* 285–298.

Douglass, F. (1982). U.S. abolitionist. In J. W. Blassingame (Ed.), *The Frederick Douglass Papers.* New Haven, CT: Yale University Press. (Original speech April 1886, Washington, DC.)

Erlen, J. A., & Sereika, S. M. (1997). Critical care nurses, ethical decision-making and stress. *Journal of Advanced Nursing, 26,* 953–961.

Fagan, A. (2006). Human rights. *The Internet Encyclopedia of Philosophy.* Retrieved July 7, 2007, from http://www.iep.utm.edu/s/soc-cont.htm#H6.

Feinberg, J. (1973). *Social philosophy.* Englewood Cliffs, NJ: Prentice Hall.

Fowler, M. D. M. (1989). Moral distress and the shortage of critical care nurses. *Heart and Lung, 18,* 314–315.

Friend, C. (2006). Social contract theory. *The Internet Encyclopedia of Philosophy.* Retrieved July 7, 2007, from http://www.iep.utm.edu/s/soc-cont.htm#H6.

Gadow, S. (1990). Existential advocacy: Philosophical foundations of nursing. In T. Pence & J. Cantrall (Eds.), *Ethics in nursing: An anthology* (pp. 40–51). New York: National League for Nursing. (Reprinted from *Nursing Images and Ideals,* 1980, pp. 79–101.)

Gaylord, N., & Grace, P. (1995). Nursing advocacy: A ethic of practice. *Nursing Ethics, 2*(1), 11–18.

Grace, P. J. (1998). *A philosophical analysis of the concept "advocacy": Implications for professional–patient relationships.* Unpublished Dissertation. University of Tennessee Knoxville.

Available at http://proquest.umi.com. Publication No. .AAT9923287, Proquest Document ID No. 734421751.

Grace, P. J. (2001). Professional advocacy: Widening the scope of accountability. *Nursing Philosophy, 2*(2), 151–162.

Hewitt, J. (2002). A critical review of the arguments debating the role of the nurse advocate. *Journal of Advanced Nursing, 37*(5), 439–445.

Hobbes, T. (1967). Leviathon. In A. I. Melden (Ed.), *Ethical theories: A book of readings* (2nd ed., pp. 218– 231). Englewood Cliffs, NJ: Prentice Hall. (Original work published in 1651.)

Hume, D. (1967). An enquiry concerning the principles of morals. In A. I. Melden (Ed.), *Ethical theories: A book of readings* (2nd ed., pp. 273–316). Englewood Cliffs, NJ: Prentice Hall. (Original work published in 1777.)

Iceland, J. (2006). *Poverty in America* (2nd ed.). Berkeley: University of California.

International Council of Nurses (with the assistance of J. Robinson). (2000). ICN on nursing and development: Policy background paper. Retrieved July 8, 2007, from http://www.icn.ch/policy_ paper1.htm#wealth.

Jezewski, M. A. (1993). Culture brokering as a model for advocacy. *Nursing and Health Care, 14*, 78–85.

Johnson, R. (2005). Shifting patterns of practice: Nurse practitioners in a managed care environment. *Research and Theory for Nursing Practice, 19*(4), 323–340.

Kant, I. (1967). Foundations of the metaphysics of morals. In A. I. Melden (Ed.), *Ethical theories: A book of readings* (pp. 317–366). Englewood Cliffs, NJ: Prentice Hall. (Original work published in 1785.)

Kleinke, J D. (2002). *Oxymorons: The myth of a US health care system.* Hoboken, NJ: Jossey-Bass.

Locke, J. (2003). *Two treatises of government and a letter concerning toleration* (ed. I. Shapiro). Binghamton, NY: Vail-Ballou Press. (Original work published in 1690.)

MacDonald, H. (2007). Relational ethics and advocacy in nursing: Literature review. *Journal of Advanced Nursing, 57*(2), 119–126.

Mallik, M. (1997). Advocacy in nursing—a review of the literature. *Journal of Advanced Nursing, 25*, 130–138.

Malone, R. E. (2005). Assessing the policy environment. *Policy, Politics and Nursing Practice, 6*(2), 135–143.

Mechanic, D. (2006). *The truth about health care: Why reform is not working in America.* Piscataway, NJ: Rutgers University Press.

Mechanic, D., & Reinhard, S. C. (2002). Contributions of nurses to health policy: Challenges and opportunities. *Nursing and Health Policy Review, 1*(1), 7–15.

Mill, J. S. (1862). The contest in America. *Harper's New Monthly Magazine, 24*(143), 683–684.

Miller, B. K., Mansen, T. J., & Lee, H. (1983). Patient advocacy: Do nurses have the power and authority to act as patient advocates? *Nursing Leadership, 6*(6), 56–60.

Murphy, N., Canales, M. K., Norton, S. A., & DeFilippis, J. (2005). Striving for congruence: The interconnection between values, practice, and political action. *Politics, Policy and Nursing Practice, 6*(1), 20–29.

Nickel, J. (2005). Poverty and rights. *Philosophical Quarterly, 55*, 385–402.

O'Connor, T., & Kelly, B. (2005). Bridging the gap: A study of general nurses' perceptions of patient advocacy in Ireland. *Nursing Ethics, 12*(5), 53–67.

Pagana, K. D. (1987). Let's stop calling ourselves "patient advocates." *Nursing, 17*, 51.

Papadimos, T. J. (2006). Charles Dickens hard times and the academic health center: A tale of the urban working poor and the violation of a covert covenant, an American perspective. *Online Journal of Health Ethics, 1*(2). Retrieved July 2, 2007, from http://ethicsjournal.umc.edu/ojs2/index.php/ojhe/article/view/56/64.

Pojman, L. (1999). Merit: Why do we value it? *Journal of Social Philosophy, 30*(1), 83–102.

Powers, M., & Faden, R. (2006). *Social justice.* New York: Oxford University Press.

Rank, M. R. (2005). *One nation underprivileged: Why American poverty affects us all.* New York: Oxford University Press.

Raphael, A. R. (1997). Advocacy oral history: A research methodology for social activism in nursing. *Advances in Nursing Science, 20*(2), 32–43.

Rawls, J. (1971). *A theory of justice.* Cambridge, MA: Belknap/Harvard University Press.

Shirley, J. L. (2007). The limits of autonomy in nursing's moral discourse. *Advances in Nursing Science, 30*(1), 14–25.

Snoball, J. (1996). Asking nurses about advocating for patients: Reactive and proactive accounts. *Journal of Advanced Nursing, 24*, 67–75.

Spenceley, S. N., Reutter, L., & Allen, M. N. (2006). The road less traveled: Nursing advocacy at the policy level. *Policy Politics and Nursing Practice, 7*(3), 180–194.

Ulrich, C. M., Danis, M., Ratcliffe, S. J., Garrett-Mayer, E., Koziol, D., Soeken, K. L., et al. (2006). Ethical conflict in nurse practitioners and physician assistants in managed care. *Nursing Research, 55*(6), 391–401.

Ulrich, C., & Soeken, K. L. (2005). A path analytic model of ethical conflict in practice and autonomy in a sample of nurse practitioners. *Nursing Ethics, 12*(3), 305–316.

Zussman, J. (1982). Want some good advice? Think twice about being a patient advocate. *Nursing Life, 2*(6), 46–50.

CHAPTER 5

Collaborative Relationships—Promoting Patient Good

Deborah Giambarco

Great discoveries and improvements invariably involve the cooperation of many minds. I may be given credit for having blazed the trail but when I look at the subsequent developments I feel the credit is due to others rather than to myself.
—*Alexander Graham Bell (1847–1922)*

INTRODUCTION

The purpose of this chapter is to provide advanced practice nurses (APNs) with an understanding of their professional responsibilities to collaborate with peers and other professionals in the interests of good patient care and also to present strategies for effective collaboration. The chapter explores the foundation for the APN scope of practice including ethical and legal obligations to collaborate with others. The need for collaboration in APN practice, regardless of specialty setting, requires discernment both in the choice of collaborators and the nature of information shared. Effective collaboration also requires understanding common barriers to inter- and intradisciplinary communication and useful strategies to overcome or circumvent such obstacles.

Although the scope of practice guidelines developed within the nursing profession delineates the minimum standards for APN competency when addressing issues of patient care, it is understood that ethical practice requires ongoing personal and professional development that goes beyond achieving minimum competencies. The chapter provides a brief discussion about collaboration in APN settings, its historical development, controversies over definitions, and associated responsibilities to clarify the current status of collaborative activities and provide direction for future collaboration.

APNs face many issues and dilemmas in patient care today. Any obstruction to what is seen, in the clinical judgment of the APN, as needed care for a patient is an ethical issue. Sometimes the problem is very complex and no good solution is easily available. These more complex issues where the right action is difficult to determine are *dilemmas*. APNs encounter issues surrounding informed consent, care at the edge of viability, resuscitation against parental wishes, a patient's right to refuse treatment, quality of life, and length of life. APNs may even be asked by patients to assist them in ending their suffering, that is, to assist them in achieving suicide. Additionally, APNs may be involved in providing information about stem cell use for scientific research, withdrawal of care, and interpreting the requirements of the Health Insurance Portability and Accountability Act of 1996 (HIPAA) for maintaining patient privacy and confidentiality.

The complexity of the healthcare environment and the nature of knowledge needed to provide good care in the face of such complexity mean that all health providers have responsibilities to confer with colleagues from within their own profession, from other professions, and/or from other specialty areas. The question remains how to do this judiciously and effectively so that good practice is enabled. Many of the issues facing APNs are well documented in other parts of this book—this chapter provides a more in-depth look at the problems associated with collaboration and ways to address these.

The ability of the APN to collaborate with patients, families, and multiple members of the healthcare team is necessary for optimal patient care. Care is becoming more and more complex as scientific advances are made, and care is also affected by the economic arrangements associated with the provision of health care (at least in the United States). The concept of APN collaboration has been studied for several decades. Research findings support the benefits of collaboration and point to improved patient outcomes (Knaus, Draper, Wagner, & Zimmerman, 1986), increased nursing job satisfaction and retention (Baggs & Ryan, 1990), improved teamwork (Abramson & Mizrahi, 1996), reduced length of stay (Rubenstein, Josephson, & Wieland, 1984), and cost savings (Barker, Williams, & Zimmer, 1985). It would appear that collaboration is beneficial. This is not surprising in that no one person can possibly hold all the answers when problems are complex or out of one's area of expertise. But how do we know when we have enough information to make a decision or to act and when to seek further assistance? How do we know who the best person to consult is, or who or what are sound sources of information? The answer lies in part in knowing oneself, as discussed in Chapter 2, and in understanding the boundaries of one's knowledge and experience.

What, then, is collaboration and why do we need it? The following definition of collaboration provides some guidance. However, additional information is necessary to understand how this definition applies to, or must be modified related to, APN efforts on behalf of patients.

COLLABORATION DEFINED

Formal Definitions of Collaboration

Government Guidelines

Although state laws vary in the degree of leeway granted to APNs to practice independently from supervising physicians, thus sometimes directing that formal collaborative arrangements exist and otherwise leaving collaboration arrangements to the discretion of the APN, the U.S. federal government has continued to uphold the idea of supervisory collaborative arrangements for the purpose of reimbursement for services provided under government funding agencies such as Medicare, Medicaid, and the Veterans Administration system. It has not, however, succeeded in being so clear about what it takes collaboration to be. A brief review of how these formal definitions of collaboration might affect our practice is reflected in the following. The federal government defines collaboration related to APN and Medicare reimbursement as follows:

> (i) . . . a process in which a nurse practitioner works with one or more physicians to deliver health care services within the scope of the practitioner's expertise, with medical direction and appropriate supervision as provided for in jointly developed guidelines or other mechanisms as provided by the law of the State in which the services are performed. (ii) In the absence of State law governing collaboration, collaboration is a process in which a nurse practitioner has a relationship with one or more physicians to deliver health care services. Such collaboration is to be evidenced by nurse practitioners documenting the nurse practitioners' scope of practice and indicating the relationships that they have with physicians to deal with issues outside their scope of practice. Nurse practitioners must document this collaborative process with physicians. (U.S. Department of Health and Human Services, 2001, §410.75)

Another definition, which has applied since 1990 to APNs practicing in rural areas who seek Medicare reimbursement as a result of the 1990 Omnibus Budget Reconciliation Act of 1990 (OBRA '90), notes that billing of professional services (under Medicare Part B) should be done "in collaboration with a physician" to be eligible for payment. Section 1866 states the following related to collaboration. Collaboration is

> a process in which a nurse practitioner [or clinical nurse specialist] works with a physician to deliver health care services within the scope of the nurse practitioner's [or clinical nurse specialist's] professional expertise, with medical direction and

appropriate supervision as provided for in jointly developed guidelines or other mechanisms as defined by the law of the State in which services are performed.

Like the previous definition, what this means is not clear and differs from state to state. Thus, APNs need to understand their state rules related to independent practice (Boards of Nursing in the United States). Rules that do not serve the population well may need to be addressed via APN practice organizations. (See Chapter 4 for political action strategies.) Additionally, these definitions talk only about supervisory or directive types of collaborative roles. A hierarchy is implied that does not take into account the fact that nursing has it own perspective on care, practice goals, knowledge, and skills. Thus, the definitions of collaboration given earlier are not informative about other collaborative needs related to everyday issues and where a more egalitarian relationship involving trust and respect might better allow for the meeting of patient needs. In any case, for APNs, as it should be for any provider, the need for collaboration may take a variety of forms and will depend on the nature of the setting and the nature of the problem.

Collaboration: ANA Code of Ethics for Nurses with Interpretative Statements

The American Nurses Association (ANA) has remained interested in the idea of collaboration, nurse responsibilities related to it, and what collaboration entails. It further developed the concept of collaboration in the process of the latest code of ethics project. The project was initiated by the ANA Board of Directors and the Congress on Nursing Practice in 1995 in response to perceived changes in environments of practice. A need to update the previous code of ethics to better capture current environments of nursing practice was viewed as important. By June of 2001, the ANA House of Delegates voted to accept the nine major provisions of the revised *Code of Ethics* sending it then to the Congress of Nursing Practice and Economics. In July 2001, the new language of the interpretive statements was approved, resulting in a completely revised *Code of Ethics for Nurses with Interpretive Statements* (the Code). The Code provides guidance in evaluating collaborative skills utilized in nursing practice. The Code also provides the "nonnegotiable ethical standard" (ANA, 2001, p. 5) that calls for each nurse to act ethically, including acts of collaboration. "Collaboration is not just communication but is the concerted effort of individuals and groups to attain a shared goal" (ANA, 2001, Interpretive Statement 2.3).

Balanced Budget Act

Since the Balanced Budget Act of 1997, APNs in all geographic locations are eligible for Medicare Part B reimbursement when providing Medicare-eligible services. The Health Care Financing Administration (HCFA) has not provided any specific guidance in interpreting the definition of collaboration as it applies to Medicare reimbursement. HCFA's instructions to Medicare carriers and intermediaries (private contractors administering Medicare in each state) regarding APN reimbursement under OBRA repeat the statutory language used by the Balanced Budget Act of 1997.

Physician Payment Review Commission

During the meeting of the Physician Payment Review Commission in 1993, the ANA expressed its concerns about statutory requirements for "collaboration" (ANA, 1993):

> Advanced practice nurses are, as are all registered nurses, independently licensed and accountable for their actions, able to deliver services independent of their relationship with physicians or other health care providers. Collaborating with and referring to other health providers is a matter of standard professional practice. Regardless of practice setting or supervision requirements, advanced practice nurses, like most health professionals, generally maintain a network of specialists and colleagues for referral and collaboration to achieve optimal patient care. (ANA, 1998b)

In 1992, national discussion on healthcare reform began. With the differing views on the definition of collaboration, the increasing popularity of the APN to provide affordable and accessible health care resulted in the President's Health Security Act, which included expansion of reimbursement for APN services and, more important, preempted state laws that previously restricted the practice of APNs.

Although this was a huge accomplishment for nursing, it did not go unnoticed by the American Medical Association (AMA), which continued to assert opposition to direct reimbursement for advanced practice nursing services. Its continued message was that APNs must act only under physician "supervision." With continued debate between the ANA and the AMA, leaders of both groups met during 1993 and 1994 with the goal of further defining the nurse–physician relationship and establishing a mutually agreeable definition of collaboration. The following definition of collaboration was developed during these talks:

> Collaboration is the process whereby physicians and nurses plan and practice together as colleagues, working interdependently within the boundaries of their scopes of practice with shared values and mutual acknowledgment and respect for each other's contribution to care for individuals, their families, and their communities. (ANA, 1998a)

The ANA Board of Directors adopted this definition in 1994. The AMA has still yet to adopt the definition. There have been no further formal discussions regarding the definition or issue of physician–nurse collaboration since this meeting. The definition refers to the APN scope of practice. To more fully understand what collaboration requires, a good understanding of the APN's scope of practice and ethical responsibilities related to this scope of practice is important.

SCOPE OF PRACTICE

An APN's scope of practice is the range of care, therapeutics, and interventions that he or she may ethically and legally deliver and is based on his or her experience, education, knowledge, and skills. The boundaries of practice are also determined by the legal requirements of the state in which the person practices. Guidance about one's scope of practice can be obtained from one's specialty organization and the board of nursing for the state in which one practices.

The scope of practice also guides the care the APN is able to give by providing limits through licensure and certification. Thus, the legitimate scope of an APN's practice is determined by several sources and is dependent in part upon area of specialty. The foundational scope of practice in the United States is the same for all nurses, and guidelines for this are published in the ANA's (2004) *Scope and Standards of Practice*. However, at the level of advanced practice the scope of practice is expanded related to the advanced education, knowledge, and skills possessed. APNs should have a good understanding of their scope of practice to understand when collaboration is necessary and what sorts of collaborative arrangements are both necessary and ethical, that is, those that will be most likely to facilitate the good of the patient in question or of the population served.

Billing services in the United States are based on scope of practice, so falling outside one's scope of practice is not only a legal and ethical issue, but also a financial issue. Treatments, medications, and tests must be prescribed within the scope of practice of one's specialty.

This necessarily brief overview gives an idea of how widely the nurse practice acts can vary from state to state. It remains crucial to check the nursing practice of each state for the most current regulations. Keeping current is an ongoing responsibility of advanced practice. At the time of this chapter's writing, and according to the American Academy of Nurse Practitioners, APNs are regulated by nursing boards in all 50 states and jointly by medical boards in 7 states. In addition, 48 states have some form of statute or regulation specifically addressing nurse prescriptive authority. In some states, collaboration is not clearly delineated or defined but is implied by the physician–nurse relationship described in the practice acts. The assumption that collaboration is necessary is often buried within some practice acts and is visible in directions to develop practice guidelines, collaborative agreements, and/or protocols.

According to the most recent Pearson Report (Pearson, 2007), 23 states require no physician involvement for the licensed nurse practitioner (NP) to diagnose and treat, while "the remainder of states require some degree of written or formal physician involvement in NP practice." Some states define collaboration in such a way that it is in reality synonymous with physician supervision, which is not an element of collaboration in any definition, implying a power differential rather than an equal relationship where each party is understood to have a different knowledge base and set of skills that they bring to bear on behalf of the patient.

State regulations vary with level of collaboration for APNs versus collaboration required for a prescriber of medications and/or medical devices (Pearson, 2007). Some states have provisions for different levels of supervision necessary in various practice settings. It's not possible to discuss every state's legislative regulatory structure and governing body, but it is imperative that APNs are knowledgeable about the state regulations in which they practice.

An example of the variety of regulatory functions is provided by Alabama and Mississippi regulations. They are examples of states with joint regulation of advanced practice. Alabama defines collaboration in its regulations and does require "the collaborating physician to be present in a practice site with the CRNP a minimum of 10% of the CRNP's collaboration time" with a few exceptions noted such as acute care facilities. Mississippi's joint regulatory committee is responsible for writing regulations based upon medical diagnoses, prescriptive privileges, or other corrective measures. Mississippi defines the role of the APN as a "collaborative, consultative relationship" with a physician whose practice is compatible with the NP (Pearson, 2007).

Standing in contrast to Alabama and Mississippi is Alaska, which has one of the most liberal regulatory boards for APNs. It does not include a definition of collaboration in its statute but does have a state law requiring APNs to construct a consultation and referral plan that outlines procedures for consultation with other healthcare professionals in appropriate circumstances (Pearson, 2007). According to the most recent Pearson Report (2007), all practice models require that the provider know, be accountable for, and function within the provider's scope of practice. The care administered through supervision, collaboration, or delegation cannot be used to replace scope of practice and individual provider responsibility.

According to Pearson (2007), some states have separate levels of required collaboration for APNs with prescriptive authority. Some APNs can practice independently without prescriptive privileges, but if the APN prescribes, a collaborative practice agreement with protocols must be utilized for prescription. The disparity and incongruence for regulatory guidelines continue from state to state, making it tricky for APNs to stay current with regulatory trends, but staying current is a necessary part of the APN's professional role. So, now that I have established what scope of practice is and what we are mandated by law to follow, where does collaboration fit in?

Many people discuss the use of collaboration in practice, but few practice the actual art. Before deciding whether or not we collaborate, we first need to define collaboration in a way that is useful for APNs. A variety of sources can aid in the defining of collaboration, but in application to the APN role, the boundaries become gray. APNs are involved in the care of the whole person. In that sense, they do many different things and tend to many aspects of a person's health and well-being.

Although, as we have established, federal law defines *collaboration* as "a process in which a NP works with a physician to deliver health care services within the scope of the practitioner's professional expertise, with medical direction and appropriate supervision as provided for in jointly developed guidelines or other mechanism as defined by the law of the State in which the services are performed" (Pearson, 2007). This is too simplistic a definition and does not provide guidance for practice. A history of the evolution of the idea of collaboration in health care and related to APN practice is informative.

HISTORY OF COLLABORATION

During the 1960s, the issue of collaboration began to develop as the role of the APN began to grow. APNs were initially trained for independent practice, diagnosing and treating patients using medications, medical therapies, and treatments. However, the role as noted earlier was nevertheless rooted in nursing goals and nursing perspectives on their practice. Many of the nurse practice acts of the time restricted the independent role in practice. In states where the practice act did allow for a more independent scope of nursing practice, regulators feared the development of an autonomous APN. The Boards of Registration in Medicine responded to any attempts of nursing groups to become more autonomous by using inflammatory language to describe what these groups were proposing. Terms such as *medical diagnosis* or *delegated medical acts* became common in the arguments. The inference was that APNs would be practicing medicine without a medical license.

Lack of agreement about what exactly the APN could and could not do led to confusion, which was evidenced in the various nurse practice acts. This gave rise to the acceptance of widely varied definitions of collaboration as part of the scope of practice among states. Practicing outside one's scope of practice presents a legal liability for all involved. According to Nurses Service Organization's (NSO) malpractice claims data from 2004, APNs practicing beyond scope accounted for 6% of all claims filed. The scope of practice determines the "minimum standard" of competency for a healthcare provider. According to NSO, 32% of claims in the same data report from 2004 were related to "failure to meet minimum standards." Without a defined specialty and in turn a defined body of knowledge inherent to your education, board certification, or other credentialing mechanism to measure APNs in their specialties, the standard of practice you are held accountable for could vary considerably.

The Federation of State Medical Boards (2004) confirms that the "American Medical Association does not have an official definition of collaboration." In 1994, the American Nurses Association endorsed the statement that collaboration involves physicians and nurses working "together as colleagues, working interdependently within the boundaries of their scope of practice." According to the Federation of State Medical Boards, collaboration is regulated as a relationship between two healthcare providers, usually a physician and an APN, though the structure of this relationship has wide variation from state to state.

According to the Federation of State Medical Boards, delegation is still used to define APN practice in a few states. In some cases, delegation allows a licensed provider who practices independently to permit certain functions to be performed under supervision by another person who does not have these functions expressively provided for in his or her own practice act. According to the Federation of State Medical Boards: "Delegated services must be ones that a reasonable and prudent physician using sound medical judgment would find appropriate to delegate and *must be within the defined scope of practice both of the physician and the non-physician practitioner.*" According to the IOM report (Institute of Medicine, Committee on Quality of Health Care in America, 2001) *Crossing the Quality Chasm: A New Health System for the 21st Century*, all health professionals should be educated to deliver patient-centered care as members of an interdisciplinary team, emphasizing evidence-based practice, quality improvement approaches, and informatics. As health care continues to evolve with rapidly changing technology and increasing needs for nursing services, the APN should be an integral part of the changing dynamics. APNs are uniquely positioned both to care for persons and to value the knowledge and skills that others can add.

HOW TO COLLABORATE

Collaborative relationships are notoriously difficult to build and/or maintain. This is true for many reasons, including the fact that history has shown us that it is human nature to want to construct and maintain hierarchies. Additionally, other psychosocial and institutional influences such as time pressures, access to the appropriate experts, and lack of institutional or office support for collaboration can get in the way of effective relationships. Finally, APNs and others need to be self-reflective about their personal inhibitions or worries related to collaboration. It takes self-confidence and confidence in one's particular knowledge base and skills to convincingly articulate the nursing perspective to others who may be skeptical that APNs have a knowledge base and a perspective on patient care that are both valid and valuable.

Knowing the limits of one's own practice and admitting to them can be a daunting endeavor. It is difficult to admit that we cannot provide all the services necessary to treat our patients and to let go of some of the control. However, only by knowing our limits are we able to allow our patients to get the best possible health care. A few simple legal guidelines derived from the previous readings about deciding whether it is necessary to collaborate about a patient are as follows:

> Do I have the knowledge base to treat this patient?
> Do I have the appropriate licensing, education, and credentialing to treat this patient?
> Do I have subspecialization if necessary for this case?
> Am I following professional standards of care?

If the answer is no to any of these questions, collaboration and/or referral is required by law or state legislation. If the answer is yes, but there are remaining questions or problems that the APN is not equipped to address, then a referral to a subspecialist or colleague with the appropriate expertise may be in order or a consultation may provide the appropriate assistance. The unanswered questions do not go away and may mean that optimal care for the patient will not be facilitated. APNs have fought hard for the independence they have earned. Some may well worry that collaborating with others will be seen as a weakness and mean that the nurse's knowledge base is inadequate. The reality is that the more we learn about our area of practice, the more questions we develop. With knowledge comes insight, and insight permits us to recognize when what is needed for a patient's good may be beyond our singular ability to provide.

Barriers to Collaboration

Clarin (2007) provides some simple strategies for understanding and overcoming barriers to collaboration. Barriers to collaboration, according to Clarin, are the following:

- Lack of knowledge about the APN role
- Lack of knowledge about the APN scope of practice

- Poor physician attitude toward APN
- Lack of respect
- Poor communication
- Patient and family reluctance to accept APN care

These are easily addressed by the individual APN. Taking a proactive role in educating the physician as well as the patient in what the APN brings to the healthcare arena can sometimes be all it takes to change to a collaborative environment.

How to Improve Collaboration

Clarin (2007) suggests the following as strategies to improve collaboration:

- Educate and provide formal orientation to physicians and other health-care professionals on the nothing-by-mouth scope of practice and role.
- Expose medical students to graduate nursing students early in the educational process.
- Continue efforts to create uniform NP education and certification.
- Use integrated collaboration models in the development of APN positions.
- Hold all team members accountable for improved communication.
- Hold interdisciplinary rounds with the APN to visibly show the patient and family that the APN is involved in the medical management of the patient.

Physicians and other healthcare providers often do not have formal education about what an APN can and cannot do in practice. APNs are well equipped to educate the others in the practice as to their role in their specific setting.

Consult Services and Networking

When addressing health concerns that fall outside your area of expertise, consult services should be utilized. Over time, a network of health professionals that consult and collaborate in cases can be developed. For example, if you are an APN in a geriatric clinic specializing in Alzheimer's care, but you see many patients with spouses exhibiting symptoms of depression, you can help put a network in place to assist the spouses of your patients. A clinical nurse specialist with specialization in geriatric psychiatric illness may be helpful to your group. Of course, one must diligently evaluate the quality and philosophy of care of those with whom one consults.

APNs have a legal obligation to remain within their scope of practice and know when and how to access appropriate services for their patients. If there is no inside consult service set up, then perhaps phone consultation can be utilized for the desired specialty or subspecialty. Ethics consults should also be considered when especially difficult problems arise. This is especially important for those cases where the team is unable to remain united about care or to maintain a focus on facilitating goals of the patient where these are knowable. Ethics consults can be particularly helpful with end-of-life questions but can also be helpful in assisting the team to provide the care they wish to provide within the legal confines of the law. For example, in the case of end-of-life care in the neonatal intensive care unit, the decision to forgo intravenous fluid and/or enteral feedings can be difficult and a legal gray area. An ethics consult may be of assistance in this case. If there is not a formal ethics consult team in your institution, contact your national credentialing body for further assistance.

Gardner (2005) provides what she defines as 10 essential competencies for collaborative partnerships:

> *Lesson 1: Know thyself.* Know your own strengths, weaknesses, and biases, and accept them, knowing that they affect the way your viewpoint is developed.

> *Lesson 2: Learn to value and manage diversity.* Individual differences are the foundation of multidisciplinary care. Welcome diversity.

> *Lesson 3: Develop constructive conflict resolution skills.* Conflict is a natural part of collaboration. If everyone agreed on everything, we wouldn't need collaboration.

> *Lesson 4: Use your power to create win-win situations.* Use of your power and the sharing of power is an important balance to achieve.

> *Lesson 5: Master interpersonal and process skills.* Clinical competence, cooperation, and flexibility are the most frequently identified attributes important to effective collaborative practice.

> *Lesson 6: Recognize that collaboration is a journey.* It won't happen overnight. Some of the skills needed for effective collaboration such as conflict resolution, clinical excellence, appreciative inquiry, and knowledge of group process are all continually evolving and developing as practice develops.

> *Lesson 7: Leverage all multidisciplinary forums.* Active participation in multidisciplinary team meetings, rounds, conferences, and other forums can provide an opportunity to nurture collaborative partnerships.

Lesson 8: Appreciate that collaboration can occur spontaneously. If the circumstances are right, sometimes collaboration requires no additional effort.

Lesson 9: Balance autonomy and unity in collaborative relationships. Being part of a team does not mean your own point of view is always the correct course of action. Be willing to see others' viewpoints and accept constructive feedback on your own plan of care.

Lesson 10: Remember that collaboration is not required for all decisions. Collaboration is not a universal solution and is not needed in every situation, but knowing when it is needed is a necessary skill to develop as an APN.

Following are a few case studies to illustrate points covered in this chapter. These cases are purely fictitious and for the purposes of further discussion.

CASE STUDIES

A pediatric nurse practitioner (PNP) in a primary care setting has been treating a child with a complex congenital heart disease for a number of years. The patient is now 24 years old and is beginning to exhibit clinical symptoms of gastro-esophageal reflux. The PNP prescribes routine gastroesophageal medications used in her practice to treat pediatric patients with similar symptoms. The first round of medications fails to control the symptoms; a second multimedication trial is undertaken. The patient has now been experiencing symptoms for a little longer than 2 months. The medications fail to achieve control of the symptoms, and the patient presents with hematemesis to a local emergency department.

Did this patient receive optimal care?

Would the patient have benefited from collaboration with an adult NP or gastrointestinal specialist?

Does the APN have a legal obligation to collaborate in this case?

Although the condition the APN is treating is a commonly occurring pediatric condition, the symptoms are occurring in an adult. The differential diagnosis is different in the adult patient versus the pediatric patient. This APN should have collaborated with an adult APN or a gastrointestinal specialist before beginning treatment for this patient. There is a legal obligation to collaborate on this case because the patient is not covered in the pediatric APN's scope of practice.

I am a geriatric NP who has expertise in Alzheimer's disease. Many of these patients with significant cardiovascular disease are seeing internists who may not be familiar with their condition. Can I still treat the cardiovascular disease in these patients?

Perhaps. A geriatric NP with an expertise in diagnosis and treatment of a condition that presents in a patient and for which he or she has an established relationship should at least be utilized as a consultant for that patient's continuing medical condition. The patient also needs to be managed in collaboration with a cardiovascular specialist because some of the patient issues to be encountered would not be under the scope of practice of a geriatric APN.

I am a neonatal NP working in a collaborative practice in neurosurgery. The collaborating physician sees children under 13 years of age with neurologic conditions. Can I provide follow-up care or write prescriptions for these children?

No. The expertise for treating these conditions is outside of the specialty of neonatal critical care. The NP has no educational basis that would support seeing patients older than the age of 6 months, regardless of the presence of a collaborating or supervising physician. A physician, as per the Federation of State Medical Boards, also has no foundation to delegate care for a condition that he or she knows is not in the scope of practice for the NP.

I am an adult critical care NP working in the emergency department. Is there a problem if I treat a 14-year-old presenting with a hypertensive crisis because I have expertise in treating this condition?

The etiology of hypertension in a 14-year-old versus and in an adult varies considerably, leading to a very different differential diagnosis. The etiology, therapies, and treatments for these two groups, pediatrics and adults, can be entirely different. Without specialized training in pediatric critical care, the clinical and didactic training in this population are lacking. An APN with adult critical care expertise would not be able to demonstrate validated education, competency, and skill in effectively diagnosing and treating the underlying cause of this life-threatening symptom. A pediatric critical care/cardiovascular APN should be consulted for collaboration in this patient's care.

You have been caring for a patient in a long-term skilled nursing facility for 5 years. The patient has periods of lucidity but also periods of confusion consistent with dementia. The patient's son is assigned as the healthcare proxy. The patient has expressed a desire to you on more than one occasion that she does not wish to be aggressively resuscitated should a life-threatening event occur. The son is always present at the visits and is able to talk the patient out of her desire for a do-not-resuscitate (DNR) order. You have discussed this case extensively on monthly rounds and with a covering physician who has never met the patient or the family. The physician and other care team members do not see any reason to pursue a DNR if the patient won't take a stand against her son. Are you, as the APN, obligated to collaborate further in this case?

Yes. The patient has expressed a desire for a DNR order but seems not to be able to take a forceful stand with her child in the room. Whether this is because of indecision or an inability to advocate for herself, you don't know. There are other support systems available to explore this question. An ethics consult or palliative care team consult can be considered. Collaborating outside the practice, keeping HIPAA guidelines in place, can also provide a source of additional information.

You are an APN in an health maintenance organization obstetrical outpatient clinic. You are reviewing ultrasound reports prior to patient visits. One patient is described as having a complete placenta previa at 23 weeks gestation. You have not had time to discuss these findings with your supervising physician prior to the patient's visit. During the visit, the physician instructs the patient to limit heavy lifting, but no other restrictions are placed on activity. You wait to discuss the conversation with the physician until after the patient leaves the room. At that time, you ask why the patient was not placed on bed rest and told of the previa. The physician tells you that she has seen this in many cases and most of the time it turns out to be nothing to worry about. You attempt to continue the conversation, but the physician states that it is her decision, not yours. Are you legally obligated to inform the patient of the potentially life-threatening condition?

Yes. It is within your scope of practice and within your nurse practice acts.

How do you approach the physician who is not willing to discuss the case any further?

One course of action is to do your own research on the findings and treatments of a complete previa at that given edge-of-viability gestation and ask to speak with the physician again with the goal of education. Ask the physician to educate you and see if the material is congruent with your own research findings; maybe one of you is unaware of recent research findings. Is there a piece of information you may be missing? You could discuss the case with another colleague in the practice in a nonjudgmental manner as seeking more information regarding findings of a complete previa and the criteria of high-risk referrals. Another course of action is to check referral guidelines for a referral to a high-risk obstetrician. If all else fails, as the APN your allegiance is to your patient and you can educate your patient to advocate for herself. This patient would meet qualifications for a high-risk pregnancy and deserves a referral on both legal and moral obligations.

CONCLUSION

As the complexity of care increases and the need for multidisciplinary input for optimal patient outcomes becomes more evident, the APN must be prepared to collaborate in patient care. The concept of collaboration is complex and changes depending on the specific situation. But, keeping in mind the limits of the APN scope of practice, nurse practice acts, and state-specific legislation, APNs can effectively advocate for their patients in a collaborative manner.

Collaboration is a very complex undertaking that occurs and develops over time. It requires respecting the knowledge and perspective of the other parties. It requires integration of all the perspectives of the team members, along with that of the patient or the patient's proxy. Some conflict is natural and to be expected. Working through conflict can build a more collaborative environment because it is by listening to others that we really begin to open the doors to collaborative communication. Realize that you will not always be "right" nor do you have to be right is every situation, but realize that your contribution is going to improve your patients' outcomes. By allowing team communication to develop, collaboration will also develop, leading to an enhanced understanding of what each team member has to offer. If we can keep the focus of collaborative efforts on mutual goals of patient good, then collaborative relationships are likely to be effective in achieving these goals.

DISCUSSION QUESTIONS

1. Think about a situation involving collaboration that you have experienced (within or outside of your professional practice). Was the collaboration egalitarian in nature? If yes, what evidence can you present to argue that the relationship among the parties was egalitarian? If not, what were the relationships and how did they play out?
2. Are all effective collaborative endeavors egalitarian in nature? Give rationale for your negative or positive answer to this question.
3. What responsibilities do APNs have to ensure that the quality of the referrals they make, the consultations they seek, or the collaborative relationships in which they engage are appropriate. Can you give examples of situations where you think that the collaborative relationship was less than optimal? What was going on? Could the situation have been addressed? What strategies might be helpful?

I not only use all of the brains I have, but all I can borrow.
—Woodrow Wilson, 28th President of the United States (1856–1924)

REFERENCES

Abramson, J. S., & Mizrahi, T. (1996). When social worker and physicians collaborate: Positive and negative experiences. *Social Work, 41*(3), 270–281.

American Nurses Association. (1993). Testimony to the Physician Practice Review Commission, November 1993. Retrieved from http://www.hhs.gov/asl/testify/t980310b.html.

American Nurses Association. (1998a). Executive summary. Collaboration and independent practice: Ongoing issues for nursing. *Nursing Trends and Issues, 3*(5). Retrieved February 14, 2008, from http://nursingworld.org/DocumentVault/NTI/Vol3No5May1998.aspx.

American Nurses Association. (1998b, March 16). Statement on physician supervision of allied health professionals before the Practicing Physicians Advisory Council, Health Care Financing Administration. Retrieved from http://www.medpac.gov/publications/congressional_reports/jun02_NonPhysPay.pdf.

American Nurses Association. (2001). *Code of ethics for nurses with interpretive statements.* Washington, DC: Author.

American Nurses Association. (2004). *Scope and standards of practice.* Washington, DC: Author.

Baggs, J. G., & Ryan, S. A. (1990). Intensive care unit nurse-physician collaboration and nurse satisfaction. *Nursing Economics, 8*, 386–392.

Balanced Budget Act of 1997, 42 USC section 1395x(s)(2)(K) (1997).

Balanced Budget Act of 1997, 42 USC section 1395x(aa)(6) (1997).

Barker, W. H., Williams, T. F., & Zimmer, J. G. (1985). Geriatric consultation teams in acute hospitals: Impact on back-up of elderly patients. *Journal of American Geriatrics Society, 33*, 422–428.

Bell, A. G. Quote from the Collaboration page. Learning to Give website. Retrieved March 20, 2008, from http://www.learningtogive.org/search/quotes/Display_Quotes.asp?subject_id=51&search_type=subject.

Boards of Nursing in the United States. State-by-state Web links. Retrieved from http://www.medscape.com/viewarticle/482270.

Clarin, O. (2007). Strategies to overcome barriers to effective nurse practitioner and physician collaboration. Medscape. Retrieved November 30, 2007, from http://www.medscape.com/viewarticle/564327.

Federation of State Medical Boards. (2004, February). Increasing scope of practice: Critical questions in assuring public access and safety. Draft report presented at Annual Meeting of FSMB in Dallas, Texas.

Gardner, D. (2005). Essential competencies for collaborative partnerships: Ten lessons. *Online Journal of Issues in Nursing* (10)1. Retrieved from http://www.medscape.com/viewarticle/499266_3.

Institute of Medicine, Committee on Quality of Health Care in America. (2001). *Crossing the quality chasm: A new health system for the 21st century.* Washington, DC: National Academy Press.

Knaus, W. A., Draper, E. A., Wagner, D. P., & Zimmerman, J. E. (1986). An evaluation of outcomes from intensive care in major medical centers. *Annals of Internal Medicine, 104*, 410–418.

Nurses Service Organization. (2004). NP practice continues to evolve. *NSO Risk Advisor, 12*, 1–2.

Omnibus Budget Reconciliation Act of 1990, Pub.L. 101–508, 104 Stat. 1388, enacted 1990-11-05.

Pearson, L. (2007). Pearson report 2007. Annual update of how each state stands on legislative issues affecting advanced nursing practice. *American Journal for Nurse Practitioners, 11*(11/12). Retrieved March 20, 2008, from http://www.webnp.net/images/ajnp_feb07.pdf.

Rubenstein, L. S., Josephson, K. R., & Wieland, G. D. (1984). Effectiveness of a geriatric evaluation unit: A randomized clinical trial. *North Eastern Journal of Medicine, 311*, 1664–1670.

U.S. Department of Health and Human Services Office of the Inspector General. (2001, June). *Medicare coverage of non-physician practitioner services.* Retrieved November 3, 2007, from http://oig.hhs.gov/oei/reports/oei-02-00-00290.pdf.

CHAPTER 6

Research Ethics: Advanced Practice Roles and Responsibilities

Pamela J. Grace

Science has given to this generation the means of unlimited disaster or of unlimited progress. There will remain the greater task of directing knowledge lastingly toward the purpose of peace and human good.
—*Sir Winston Churchill, speech, New Delhi, January 3, 1944*

Man who lives in a world of hazards is compelled to seek for security.
—*John Dewey, The Quest for Certainty*

INTRODUCTION

Aims of Research

The preceding quote is from Dewey's (1929/1980) lectures entitled *The Quest for Certainty*. Dewey, a philosopher of the American Pragmatist School, observed that it is characteristic of human nature to seek control over, and thus stability in, the experienced world. This inherent drive has produced philosophers and empirical scientists. *Empirical* means planned and structured observations of experiences and nature. Philosophers try to make logical sense of the world and discover meaning via reasoning (thought), and scientists have tried both to make sense of the world through formal methods of study and experimentation (action) and more recently to control aspects of the world using their discoveries. The distinction between science and philosophy is somewhat artificial because many philosophers have also engaged in practical experiments, and philosophically derived theories often provide the foundation for empirical studies. As Dewey (1929/1980) noted, "The problem of philosophy concerns the *interaction* of our judgments about ends to be sought with knowledge of the means for achieving them. Just as in science the question of the advance of knowledge is the question of *what to do*, what experiments to perform, what apparatus to invent and use. . . . (T)he problem of practice is what do we need to *know*, how shall we obtain that knowledge and how shall we apply it?" (p. 37, italics as in original), and these are philosophical questions.

We know from records that the human quest for knowledge of both kinds—theoretical and practical—has been ongoing since as early as the era of the Presocratic Greek philosophers, that is, from roughly the sixth and fifth centuries B.C. (Wheelwright, 1988). Our ability to satisfy this drive has been developing in sophistication over the past two and a half millennia. Over the past few centuries, our ability to study the natural world has accelerated rapidly as a result of technological and biological knowledge development. Often innovations occur so rapidly that they outpace our ability to come to terms with the philosophical and ethical implications of them.

Philosophical inquiry historically involves asking questions about observed events, phenomena, and human characteristics. It attempts to analyze the elements of them to discover relationships and causes. Wheelwright (1988) argues that we can discern three fundamental human drives underlying philosophical inquiries. He concludes this from a review and synthesis of historical philosophical writings. One of the drives is the religious drive to discover what is "greater and more excellent" (p. 2) than man. Explorations and questions that result from this drive constitute the study of metaphysics or attempts to understand what, if anything, underlies or transcends the physical world. For example, questions about whether there is a creator or overseer of the universe are metaphysical questions not directly observable in nature. The second drive is the scientific quest to understand physical matter, measurement (for example, how to divide property and how to quantify things), and the relationship of the stars and solar system to earth. Thus, philosophy and research are intimately related and can be seen as different faces of the same coin. A third drive can also be identified in historical as well as contemporary literature and that is the attempt to understand self.

Contemporary researchers have built upon previous knowledge developments and/or used their imaginations, undoubtedly fed by prior experiences, to derive new questions and ideas that can then be tested for soundness or validity. They have used increasingly sophisticated tools to carry out in-depth explorations of the nature of the world and of human beings. The results of these explorations include innovations that although they have the capacity to do much good also possess the power to harm when these are used without deliberative forethought or mindfulness of their possible impact on individuals, society, and in some cases the world. This is the status of research, generally, and human subjects research, particularly. The results of research endeavors have greatly improved the human potential for living a good life, but unethical research has caused immeasurable suffering.

Aims of Research Involving Human Subjects

In human subjects research, the temptation and tendency of researchers to lose sight of the ultimate goals of research—the promotion of human good—has been well documented, and illustrative examples are given later. Research aimed at developing knowledge about human beings logically derives its focus from the idea that facilitating the human good is a worthy goal. The research community, professionals who design studies or use research findings, and society—via its philosophers, activists, and citizens—all bear responsibility for ensuring that the focus on human good is maintained. Vigilance and mindfulness of the ease with which such a goal can become perverted are needed to prevent the true aims of human subject research from fading in the course of the research process. Additionally, it does not make sense to ignore or discount a given individual participant's needs so that a greater societal good can be achieved because individual human beings make up the greater society, and without individuals society would not exist. If an individual is not of strong concern, what are the grounds for asserting that the ends of research are best aimed at a societal good?

Ironically perhaps, research completed in the cognitive, psychological, and social sciences has supported the idea that the motivation and disposition of human beings to good action can be influenced both by internal factors and situational aspects (Zimbardo, 2005), as discussed in more detail later. Knowledge developments in the preceding areas, stimulated in part by the long history of the abuse of human beings by others in their species, support the idea that it is easy for human beings either not to recognize the moral components of human interaction or to stray from the moral path related to treatment of their fellow human beings. The most difficult task for those in human services professions or engaged in human subjects research is that of staying true to the purpose of the work.

Research-Related Roles of the APN

As healthcare professionals, advanced practice nurses (APNs) may be involved in all aspects of human subjects research, from study design to the use of the knowledge gained in practice settings. We may contribute unanswered questions that arise from practice experiences. We may assist in research studies or oversee the clinical aspects of them. Our patients may be subjects of research or request our advice about whether enrolling in a given study is prudent in light of their health concerns. We may even be the designers and principal investigators for a study. As APNs working in nursing roles, however, our profession's goals provide the foundation for all of our actions and take priority over all other concerns when conflicts occur. They give us a point of view from which to advocate for the patient/subject's or healthy subject's safety and ongoing informed consent to participate. APNs who work in clinical research settings are not subject to different rules or responsibilities. Responsibilities relate to individual good as well as societal good and are not to be subverted by the goals of scientists and other professionals, whether serving as researchers or otherwise (ANA, 1994).

This next section explores the history of human subjects research, highlighting the source and nature of benefits and abuses. It traces regulatory efforts to overcome the ethical issues inherent in human subjects research settings. Finally, the chapter uses cases and examples to illustrate issues that APNs may face in their various roles related to the conception and conduct of research and the use of research findings in practice. The cases serve as a springboard for discussion and clarification. Some strategies for dealing with unethical conduct in the context of human subject research are proposed.

BACKGROUND: HUMAN SUBJECTS RESEARCH

Definition of Research

Although most of us in healthcare settings probably feel that we have a good grasp of the meaning of human subjects research based on our experiences with research protocols and from reading research findings, what constitutes human subjects research is not always clear-cut. Some studies that don't seem to involve a risk to persons, perhaps because they don't involve a direct interaction with a human being, may nevertheless present some danger—perhaps the data gathered can be misused and add to a person's vulnerability. For example, revealing genetic information or the probability of developing a disease may jeopardize a person's ability to obtain health or life insurance. Genetic information gained about one person also may carry implications for another person's privacy. Our professional goals, as discussed throughout this book, have to do with providing a good for individuals, and in so doing we must also be careful to minimize the possible harms that could come from our actions. So, our interests in research endeavors are necessarily focused on the impact, negative or positive, of the given research on the well-being of persons. This requires diligence, vigilance, and rigor in uncovering the hidden implications—long term and short term—of innovations on the lives of individual human beings and on society. The next section provides information about the history of human research and its abuses as a foundation for developing confidence in decision making when research issues are an aspect of the practice environment.

In the United States, research is defined by the federal government in the Code of Federal Regulations (CFR) as a "systematic investigation, including research development, testing and evaluation, designed to develop or contribute to generalizable knowledge" (National Institutes of Health, Office for Human Research Protections, 2004). This definition is broad and not confined to human subjects research. A more particular definition given in the CFR demarcates a human subject as "a living individual about whom an investigator (whether professional or student) conducting research obtains (1) Data through intervention or interaction with the individual, or (2) Identifiable private information" (National Institutes of Health, Office for Human Research Protection, 2004).

Intervention includes both physical procedures by which data are gathered (for example, venipuncture) and manipulations of the subject or the subject's environment that are performed for research purposes. Interaction includes communication or interpersonal contact between investigator and subject. *Private information* includes information about behavior that occurs in a context in which an individual can reasonably expect that no observation or recording is taking place, and information which has been provided for specific purposes by an individual and which the individual can reasonably expect will not be made public (for example, a medical record). Private information must be individually identifiable (i.e., the identity of the subject is or may readily be ascertained by the investigator or associated with the information) in order for obtaining the information to constitute research involving human subjects. (National Institutes of Health, Office for Human Research Protections, 2004)

Together these two definitions delineate what is meant by human subjects research. The ensuing discussion uses this description along with the APN's professional responsibilities as discussed in earlier chapters to explore the history of human subjects research, its uses and abuses, as well as contemporary implications for advanced nursing practice.

HISTORICAL DEVELOPMENT OF RESEARCH ETHICS

Human Subject Research: Researcher Motivations

Evidence suggests that human vivisection took place in ancient Rome with the possible aim of understanding more about the human body. Vivisection is the dissection or cutting up of live beings. The literature extensively supports the idea that since ancient times research efforts have been viewed as important, and the development of research methods and tools has continued through the ages. There is, however, also a long history of what we currently refer to as human subject abuses. These abuses are indicative of several attitudes: (1) the predisposition on the part of researchers toward furthering the social good even when this may be risky for individual participants; (2) a disposition to gain knowledge by whatever means necessary (human subjects are not a significant moral concern); (3) certain classes of persons (slaves, minorities, lower classes) are not viewed as equally worthy of concern as are others; (4) the perspective that some groups of persons are disposable and thus expedient objects of research (e.g., the Nazi experiments); or (5) a desire to fulfill personal/professional ambition. Because there are areas of overlap among these, the following examples may evince more than one of them. However, grasping this point is important for APNs in considering the source of problems with research integrity.

1. *Society versus individuals.* Public health or societal interests in healthy people have often provided the impetus for research endeavors that involve populations. These studies try to understand how to prevent, attenuate, or cure diseases that are either serious and pervasive in the population (for example, cardiovascular diseases) or affect large numbers of people (for example, infectious diseases). History has shown that sometimes in the urgency to resolve pressing societal problems, the interests of individuals have been trampled. Katz (1992) documents the comments of a Swedish investigator who used young children as subjects in a variola vaccine experiment: "(P)erhaps I should have first experimented upon animals, but calves—most suitable for these purposes—were difficult to obtain because of their cost and their keep" (p. 230). This attitude signifies a fairly common theme in research aimed at stopping the ravages or spread of communicable diseases; vaccines were often developed and tested on healthy persons, frequently children. Testing has not always involved knowledgeable consent. Indeed, many of these studies involved healthy children who were not of an age where they could be considered developmentally capable of processing the information necessary for understanding. These efforts have been termed "challenge studies" (Hope & McMillan, 2004). Perhaps the most well known of these studies is Jenner's inoculation with cowpox (a mild form of smallpox discovered in cows) of an 8-year-old boy, James Phipps. This took place in 1796. When Phipps recovered from the cowpox, he was then inoculated with smallpox without ill effect. It had been noted that

milkmaids who had had cowpox didn't seem to succumb to smallpox—a much deadlier disease.

2. *Knowledge for its own sake.* Some scientists have been interested in seeing if their theories are right regardless of, or perhaps despite, their ability to further human good or cause harm. Although most scientists involved in human subjects research would probably deny that they have any but the most altruistic motives for their research, historically knowledge developments related to the human psyche point to the possibility of other motives, whether these are conscious and/or subconscious. The most infamous examples of research carried out without any intention of benefit to subjects were the Nazi experiments on concentration camp inmates. Experiments included grafting bone and muscle tissue from one person to another to study nerve regeneration, immersion in freezing water to track the limits of human endurance, the effects of poison, and so on (Jewish Virtual Library, 2008). In fact, many such studies were aimed at helping the war effort by understanding the effects of adverse conditions upon the armed forces.

3. *Inequality of moral concern, and*

4. *Perceived disposability.* Some segments of society have historically been more susceptible to research abuses related to their subservient status in a society or vulnerability to the whims or design of others. Savitt (2001) notes that especially in the Old South slaves "were considered more available and more accessible (for experimentation purposes) . . . they were rendered physically visible by their skin color but were legally invisible because of their slave status" (p. 215). Axelsen (2001) describes Dr. Marion Sims (1813–1883) the "father of gynecology" as having shown a "shocking disregard for the personhood of African-American women" (p. 225) on whom he practiced experimental surgeries. The infamous Tuskegee study, which lasted several decades (until 1972), studied untreated syphilis in African American men. Even when treatment did become available, it was withheld from them. At the Willowbrook State School for retarded children, a study was conducted ostensibly to see the effects of gammaglobulin inoculation. However, children were deliberately infected with hepatitis and treatment was often withheld (Ramsey, 2001). In 1966, Beecher published an article in the *New England Journal of Medicine* detailing 22 cases of ethically suspect research that had appeared in the medical literature, including the Willowbrook study.

5. *Personal/professional ambition.* It is widely recognized that humans are susceptible to favoring personal gain, material or psychological, over

benevolent actions toward others when they perceive that providing for someone else's needs would disadvantage them in some way. This susceptibility is stronger for some than for others and depends for its strength on a variety of factors related to an individual's background, experiences, and the current circumstances. The susceptibility may be consciously experienced and result in "cognitive dissonance" (Festinger, 1957) or is subconscious and not noted by the agent. This is not to discount the idea that we are also capable of altruism (Nagel, 1991) but rather to make the point that no matter how objective we think we are being, we can never be completely free from a variety of influences. Research and theoretical work in cognitive, motivational, and social psychology, and moral development has increased our understanding of the influence of bias, prejudice, and self-interest on action. The human predisposition to rationalize behavior is extensively documented (Bandura, 1986, 1999; Tavris & Aronson, 2007; Weiner, 1992; Weston, 2005). Rationalizing behavior means that we use our reasoning ability to justify the action we prefer over an alternative that is just as reasonable or even more so or that we offer justification as an explanation for behavior that has occurred. Rationalizations do not usually hold up under objective scrutiny. So, for example, a nurse who was complicit in the Nazi euthanasia experiments might claim that she had no option but to follow orders. Yet we know from other nurses who objected that this choice existed (Benedict & Kuhla, 1999).

Human Malleability

One further problem associated with ethical research, and associated with the problems noted earlier, has to do with the human predisposition to act in accord with situational conditions. One can see oneself as powerless to affect a bad situation and become numb or immune to the problem and/or continue to participate in the bad situation, thus perpetuating the unethical practice. Additionally, a subtle shift in perspective can occur, causing one to believe what others are saying (Bandura, 1999; Chambliss, 1996; Mohr & Mahon, 1996). The possibility of situationally influenced perspective shifts is illustrated by the Stanford Prison Experiment conceived and executed in 1971 by Zimbardo, a psychologist (although it was terminated before completion). The experiment's aim was to explore the effects of prison on individuals. It used college student volunteers and a simulated prison environment to study the ways in which people react or behave under those types of conditions. The experiment was to have lasted 2 weeks but was terminated after 6 days (in response to criticism from a person of importance to the researcher). There was no disinterested oversight of the research, and the researchers themselves admit to failing to notice the seriousness of the psychological impact of the study upon the participants, both prisoners and guards. Although the experiment has been criticized as unethical, findings from the study support the idea that human beings can be influenced by situational factors to behave badly toward one another. As Zimbardo (2005) states of the study, the "power of social situations to distort personal identities and long cherished values and morality as students internalized situated identities in their roles as prisoners and guards" was striking. The experiment *randomly* assigned volunteers to one of two groups, prisoners and guards. The prisoners were subjected to dehumanizing and demoralizing routines, and the guards were reminded of the inferior nature of the prisoners. Both groups came to assume the characteristics of the roles assigned to them. "Within a few days the role dominated the person," Zimbardo noted (Alexander, 2001).

Development of Human Subjects Research Regulations

In the United States and in many other countries, contemporarily it has been recognized that there must be independent oversight of research processes to lessen the likelihood that participants of biological or behavioral research will be wittingly or unwittingly abused. There is wide recognition that certain ethical principles should underlie all aspects of the research process, from the conceptualization of a question to be studied to the use of findings. The Nuremberg Code (1949), which was formulated as a result of the Nazi Doctors Trial after World War II, stresses the importance of voluntary participation of subjects. It provides support for the "judgment of the Nuremberg Tribunal that the Nazi physician-scientists had been guilty of perpetrating deeds of agony, torture, degradation and death on human beings in the name of medical science" (Katz, 1992, p. 228).

Katz writes that, interestingly, the only antecedent to the Nuremberg Code was promulgated in 1931 in Germany. This document, entitled "Regulations on New Therapy and Human Experimentation," was issued by the Reichsminister of the Interior and in many ways mirrored the eventual prescriptions for ethical research laid out in the Nuremberg Code, including the need for voluntary informed consent of the participant. Vollman and Winau (1996) note that the need for ethical rules to guide research had been discussed in Prussia for several decades before the edict from the Reichsminister. The 1931 document also makes a distinction between "therapeutic . . . and nontherapeutic research . . . and set out strict precautions" (p. 1446) to be followed.

Therapeutic research involves testing potential new treatments or therapies for their ability to provide benefit. Nontherapeutic research is experimentation on healthy subjects or without the aim of possible subject benefit. The significance of this distinction is discussed in more detail later. The prescriptions of the Nuremberg Code were soon realized by the international medical community to be too stringent and in some cases involved injustice. Requiring voluntary informed consent left several groups of people out of consideration for studies that might have led to benefit for them or their cohort. This realization led to the formulation of the Declaration of Helsinki with its ongoing revisions. Subsequent to the Declaration of Helsinki and in response to ongoing research abuses, the Belmont Report was issued in the United States. All of these documents and their implications are discussed briefly in the following sections.

The Nuremberg Code

The Nuremberg Code (U.S. Department of Health and Human Services, 1949) was conceptualized and formulated as an attempt to protect human rights. It is best viewed in the context of its development over the course of the Nazi Doctors Trial and subsequent deliberations about the atrocities perpetuated on the captive populations of the Nazi concentration camps. Its priority tenet, a reaction to the involuntary nature of the manipulation of human subjects that occurred, states that "(T)he voluntary consent of the human subject is absolutely essential" (cited in Katz, 1992, p. 227) in research endeavors. Although many of its other guidelines have been incorporated into contemporary documents on the protection of human subjects, the first principle of the code was soon realized to be problematic. If only voluntary participation is allowed, those who might benefit from research, such as the cognitively challenged and children, would be left out of research endeavors, yet such studies might be necessary to address their particular types of health problems. As Munson affirms, "(F)ew people [actually] doubt the need for research involving human subjects" (2008, p. 7). The results of research studies have provided significant improvements in the human life experience. Thus, to leave out of research endeavors those who might benefit or whose cohort might eventually benefit is a justice issue, as discussed shortly.

Additionally, many researchers outside of the Nazi context saw the Nuremberg Code as not pertinent to them and their research efforts. The Nazi's actions were seen as aberrations. Such blatant disregard by researchers and physicians of their obligations to do no harm was generally and naively taken to be unlikely in the research and medical communities. Yet, innumerable cases in which human rights were discounted and subjects of research misused have subsequently been documented.

The Declaration of Helsinki—1964 and Later Revisions

The World Medical Association (WMA) is an international body representing physicians. It was founded in 1947 in response to the events of WWII that resulted in the Nuremberg Tribunals. Initially, 27 countries had representatives in the WMA. The purpose of the WMA was "to ensure the independence of physicians, and to work for the highest possible standards of ethical behavior and care by physicians, at all times" (WMA, 2003). The Declaration, which has been revised several times since first adopted (most recently in 2000), introduced the idea of proxy consent. As noted earlier, the Nuremberg Code's proscription of any but voluntary participation gave rise to another set of ethical issues related to justice. (This topic is discussed later under ethical principles.) Proxy consent permits a responsible person, chosen in light of certain criteria, to enroll in a research study an individual who does not have decision-making capacity. The criteria and considerations for enrollment are discussed in a later section. Additionally, the distinction between therapeutic and nontherapeutic research was articulated more clearly with rationale provided.

Events Leading to the National Research Act of 1974

During this same time frame in the United States (1945–1960s), no independent oversight of research endeavors existed. Physicians and other researchers continued to be responsible for policing themselves. Rothman (1991) describes the tremendous upsurge, however, in research endeavors that followed World War II and resulting in part from the availability of federal funding. The existence of funding changed the nature of research endeavors from small independent initiatives to, in many cases, much larger enterprises. Although the importance of informed consent was acknowledged, many studies nevertheless proceeded without the participants or participant proxies being informed of important aspects of the study or in the absence of careful scrutiny of the possible deleterious effects on individual subjects. This occurred despite the fact that the Nuremberg Tribunal had codified these as crucial considerations. Important safeguards and guidelines from the Nuremberg Code related to research design, conduct, and human subject protections included the advice that research results should be likely to benefit humanity in some way, influence or coercion of subjects to participate is forbidden, in certain cases prior research on animals should be completed, likely results should justify any risks, and risks should be minimized including mental or physical suffering, which are not permissible.

In 1966, Henry Beecher, a Boston physician, published an article in the *New England Journal of Medicine* detailing problems in the ethical conduct of research. Although he had gathered from the medical literature many more than the 22 examples he described in his article, what he presented was a "devastating indictment of research ethics" (Rothman, 1991, p. 15). The research studies had taken place in a wide variety of settings, so they could not be ignored as aberrances—the problem was apparently widespread. Even Beecher's exposé, however, was not enough to radically change the status quo in the United States.

On July 26, 1972, a journalist brought to attention a study that had been carried out on black men to explore the effects of untreated syphilis. The study had been ongoing over a period of 40 years, and many publications had been issued from it—thus, the study was not carried out in secret. The informed consent of the men not only was not sought; deceptive practices were used to keep them from seeking effective treatment even after it became available. The widespread exposure of the Tuskegee Experiment, as it was called after the location of its study population, finally mobilized a change in the oversight, regulation, and ethical conduct of research and led to the National Research Act of 1974. It is important to know that although most unethical research involved or involves biomedical research, research in the social sciences also came under fire. The Stanford Prison Experiment described earlier and the Milgram (1974) experiment, which was designed to understand obedience to authority and involved subject deception and psychological distress, provide just two of many possible examples.

The National Research Act of 1974

In 1974, the National Research Act was passed. This act led to the creation of the National Commission for the Protection of Human Subjects of Biomedical and Behavioral Research.

> One of the charges to the Commission was to identify the basic ethical principles that should underlie the conduct of biomedical and behavioral research involving human subjects and to develop guidelines which should be followed to assure that such research is conducted in accordance with those principles. In carrying out the above, the Commission was directed to consider: (i) the boundaries between biomedical and behavioral research and the accepted and routine practice of medicine, (ii) the role of assessment of risk-benefit criteria in the determination of the appropriateness of research involving human subjects, (iii) appropriate guidelines for the selection of human subjects for participation

in such research and (iv) the nature and definition of informed consent in various research settings. (National Institutes of Health, Office of Human Subjects Research, 1979)

The *Belmont Report* identified three crucial ethical principles that should frame the research process as it applies to researchers in the United States and U.S. government–funded research studies conducted abroad. These principles are respect for persons, beneficence, and justice. Although these principles were explored in earlier chapters, a more specific discussion of them as they relate to the human subjects research process occurs later in this chapter. The Belmont Report led to 1981 regulations entered into the CFR under Title 45 (Public Welfare), Part 46 (Protection of Human Subjects). A further development from the *Belmont Report* was the inception of institutional review boards (IRBs), also sometimes called human subjects review boards or committees and discussed later. In 1991, 17 different federal departments and agencies agreed to be governed by these regulations, and the regulations became known as the Common Rule relating to research or the use of innovative techniques and technology on human subjects (Dunn & Chadwick, 2001).

Institutional review boards are committees based within institutions where research is conducted and funded either directly or indirectly by the U.S. government. IRBs function in accord with the CFR to ensure the ethical conduct of research within the given institution. The purpose of IRBs is to discern unethical aspects of a research project including the rigor, soundness, and integrity of the design; ability to answer the question posed; the safety of participants; and the voluntariness of subject participation. All federally supported research projects at an institution, academic or healthcare delivery, must be approved by an IRB prior to commencing. Additionally, ongoing protocols are reviewed annually. Any amendments made by the research team after initial approval are also reviewed either by individual committee members or full board review, depending on the nature of the amendment. Initial protocol reviews may be one of three types: full review, expedited, or exempt. Expedited reviews undertaken by one or more IRB members may be carried out for research involving minimal risk. Protocols that are exempt from review fit in one of six categories (U.S. Department of Health and Human Services, 2005). The makeup of IRBs varies by institution. Box 6-1 explains the minimum criteria set by the Office for Human Research Protections (OHRP). Some studies that might be considered under an expedited review when conducted on adults might nevertheless require full board review when conducted on children.

Box 6-1

Makeup of Institutional Review Boards: Minimum Membership

- A minimum of five members with varied backgrounds, some with expertise in the types of protocols typically reviewed
- Professional members are experienced and qualified and include persons from more than one profession
- Inclusion of at least one member whose concern is primarily scientific and one whose concern is not scientific
- At least one member who is not affiliated with the institution—citizen members represent the population served or have specialist expertise
- For protocols involving vulnerable groups, a member of that group or someone knowledgeable about them is advisable
- When protocols involve information that is beyond the expertise of the committee, an expert can be invited to assist but will not have voting privileges unless accepted to ongoing membership

Source: Data adapted from U.S. Department of Health and Human Services. (2005). DHHS, 2005 Title 45, Part 46, Subpart D, Section 46.402. *Additional protections for children involved as subjects in research.* Retrieved January 10, 2008, from http://www.hhs.gov/ohrp/humansubjects/guidance/45cfr46.htm#subpartd.

RESEARCH ETHICS: GUIDING PRINCIPLES

Chapter 1 provides an in-depth discussion of ethical principles used in healthcare decision making. The philosophical origins and implications of those principles are pertinent in research settings and should be reviewed if necessary. The implications of the Belmont Report principles for APNs in a variety of practice settings where they may be required to advise patients about research protocols or may serve in a research-related role are exemplified here. External oversight and regulation of research are necessary to protect human subjects, even though such rules and direction may be limiting for researchers and in some cases may defeat the purpose of the research. Nevertheless, participants or potential participants of research are not necessarily aware of the complexity of the research process. Additionally, and it is easy for participants to forget or discount this idea, the motives behind a research endeavor are not primarily to promote the given individual's well-being; research is different from a purely clinical setting. Potential subjects may need assistance in the decision-making process and require an advocate or interpreter to help them understand what participation in the research means for them and how it is, or is not, likely to further their particular goals.

The meaning and implications of each of the research ethics principles set out by the *Belmont Report* (National Institutes of Health, Office of Human Subjects Research, 1979) are discussed separately in the following paragraphs; in many ways the principles are related or overlapping. They all have their basis in the idea that human beings are equally worthy of moral consideration and concern and should not be used as a means to achieve another person's or society's goals. For such reasons, Miller and Wertheimer (2007) have argued that it is important to understand that although paternalism (beneficence) is pervasive in contemporary human research endeavors, it is not necessarily incompatible with respect for persons. That is, there is a need and an obligation on the part of researchers and others to *protect* subjects from study harms that would be impossible for them to anticipate.

Paternalism, as discussed in an earlier chapter, means acting in the patient's best interest and preventing the patient from coming to harm. Paternalism may or may not be in accord with a given patient's autonomous choice—that is, a person's *right* to make his or her own decisions—however, when we grasp that someone is not in possession of appropriate information to make a decision in his or her own interests, paternalism may well be justified and respectful of the individual as a person.

For example, Mrs. Jones may wish to be involved in a trial where the principle investigator Dr. Green is a physician she knows and trusts. The study is aimed at testing the safety and efficacy of a new anti-hypertensive drug. Her blood pressure is well controlled with the drug she is currently taking, which has minimal side effects. Mrs. Jones is sure that Dr. Green would not offer to enroll her if the doctor did not think the research would benefit her, so she is willing to follow Dr. Green's advice. This willingness hints at Mrs. Jones's misunderstanding of the goals of research and calls into question how informed she is. To respect Mrs. Jones as a person is to understand what is required for her autonomous decision making and to facilitate this. In line with the discussions in Chapters 1 and 3, this problem demonstrates a failure of the informed consent process. Dr. Green's responsibility is to ensure that Mrs. Jones understands the distinction between the primary goals of the healthcare provider and of the researcher. Without being assured of this, Mrs. Jones should not be permitted to enroll. Moreover, if Mrs. Jones eventually enrolls because she becomes more fully informed, her best interests would be served by having a separate primary care provider.

Besides the regulatory aspects guiding human research in the United States, clinical judgment (Chapter 4, Table 4-1) is required to ascertain what the patient needs to know to make an informed decision about what is acceptable. As Miller and Wertheimer (2007) have pointed out, "(T)he question arises . . . whether standard protections for research subjects are inherently paternalistic" (p. 24) and how this paternalism coexists with the "primacy of informed consent."

An additional question is, when is paternalism justified and when is it not? IRBs, for example, do not approve protocols when the language is not clear or the description of the study is not well articulated because a subject entering is unlikely to be adequately informed, and a subject cannot enroll until the study is approved. So, although this is warranted paternalistically to protect the subject, it also shows respect for persons.

Respect for Persons

Autonomy and Its Limits

The principle of respect for persons has its philosophical roots in the ethical principle of autonomy. As noted in the *Belmont Report* (National Institutes of Health, Office of Human Subjects Research, 1979), "(R)espect for persons incorporates at least two ethical convictions: first, that individuals should be treated as autonomous agents, and second, that persons with diminished autonomy are entitled to protection" (Principle 1). As in general healthcare practice, this principle serves both as the foundation for obtaining informed consent from those with decision-making capacity and places responsibilities on the researcher or patient advocate, including APNs, to ensure that a proxy decision maker is appropriate and able to make an informed and uncoerced decision for the person with diminished autonomy. It also means understanding under what other circumstances a person's autonomy might be constrained.

Vulnerability

Vulnerability to coercion or persuasion limits a person's capacity for autonomous decision making. For example, a prisoner may be influenced to enter a research trial through fear of retribution from prison officials or in the hopes that this will facilitate an early release. Thus, the principle of respect for persons also takes into account inordinate vulnerability. Another way of looking at this principle is to see that the particularities of a person, including context and influences, are important aspects of respecting that person.

All of the following groups have been viewed as vulnerable: those with impaired cognition (congenital, developmental, or organic), prisoners, pregnant women (because of the implications for both the woman and her fetus), and children.

The fact of vulnerability does not mean that these groups cannot be enrolled as subjects. Indeed, as discussed later, justice requires that they are not left out of studies that might benefit them and that special consideration be given to the study of their particular issues. "The particular needs of the economically and medically disadvantaged must be recognized" (World Medical Association

Declaration of Helsinki, 2004, Section A8). Rather, the issue of vulnerability means that special precautions must be taken to ensure that consent is informed, that the research does not pose inordinate risks, that the potential benefits of the research outweigh the risks to the subject, and where benefit to the subject is not possible that any likely benefits will accrue to the subject's cohort. So, for example, in the case of prisoner research, the results of the research are aimed at benefiting other prisoners in similar circumstances. Research on prisoners remains controversial (Parascandola, 2007). APNs working with especially vulnerable populations need to familiarize themselves with the literature about ethical issues and research implications for their populations and area of practice.

Another example of vulnerability concerns the situation of immigrant communities and populations. In such cases, the persons may not be proficient in the English language and/or the U.S. culture. In such cases, researchers must first consider whether it is just (discussed later) to leave such populations out of consideration as potential subjects. If it is decided that immigrant populations should be offered the opportunity to participate, the question of what special accommodations are needed must be addressed. Knowledge of the culture, language, and other aspects of their situation is crucial. For nurses, there is the additional question of whether there is a professional responsibility to ensure that we learn what the particular needs of such groups are to best serve these needs. Many studies initiated by doctorally prepared nurses or predoctoral nursing scholars have been focused on understanding the very nature of a population's vulnerability with the aim of designing interventions; thus, being aware of ethical issues involved in studying such populations is a professional responsibility.

Altruism

One further implication of respect for persons viewed as the right to make one's own choices is that one has the right to participate in research for altruistic purposes even if that choice is highly risky. For example, Ms. Brown has a genetic form of a chronic lung disease that is in its advanced stages. She has two sons and a daughter. A research study aimed at preventing the progress of this disease has been approved by the IRB at the institution where Ms. Brown is an outpatient. It is under way and enrolling participants. She meets the criteria for participation. As the clinical nurse specialist (CNS) in the pulmonary clinic, Ms. Darrowby is asked by Ms. Brown about the study. Her son read about it on the Internet. Ms. Darrowby is familiar with the study, although not involved directly in it. Because several of her patients have asked for more information about the study, she talked with the researcher about it and has familiarized herself with the protocol. She discusses what she knows with Ms. Brown and helps her to understand that because of her advanced disease, personal benefit is either extremely unlikely or not possible and that there are serious risks involved, including the risk of death. Ms. Brown is insistent that she would like to participate. She is able to articulate her understanding of the purposes of the study and its implications for her. She views her participation as a legacy for her children and others like them. It is a meaningful and considered request. So, Ms. Darrowby refers Ms. Brown to the principal investigator for further information, assuring Ms. Brown that she will continue to provide her care and help her process information about the study as necessary. If all other aspects of the study are sound, and ongoing protections are in place, Ms. Brown would be permitted to enroll. Ms. Darrowby's professional responsibilities would be to monitor her, provide care that is in line with the protocol criteria, and ensure that Ms. Brown knows she can withdraw later if she wishes and still receive appropriate care.

Adequately Informed

In the case of Ms. Brown, we have made a determination after much exploration and discussion that she is making an informed, uncoerced, and voluntary decision to participate. Although we may not agree with her choice—it is hers to make and we can continue to support her. However, in many cases the individual's decision-making process and influences upon it are not so transparent. In such cases, determining what is needed for informed consent is more difficult. What does it mean when we say that a person who is deemed to have decision-making capacity and who is not more than usually vulnerable (we are all somewhat vulnerable to the unpredictable nature of daily life) can give or has given informed consent?

There is no one reliable answer to this question even after a great deal of attention has been paid to it in the bioethics literature. How we come to terms with the difficulty of understanding what constitutes informed consent—given knowledge about human nature and the complexities of information processing—remains problematic and is the subject of ongoing debates. Although the issue of uncertainty related to informed consent cannot be resolved here, understanding the difficulties involved permits thoughtful and careful decision making on the part of the APN, along with the recognition that collaboration or the marshalling of other resources on the patient/subject's behalf may be warranted.

Informed Consent and Its Limits

For current purposes, then, although it is important to note that the difficulties inherent in protecting human research subjects have not been resolved, the results of research endeavors have often greatly improved human quality of life and lifespan. For such reasons, we as a society continue to appreciate the ongoing need for human subject experiments and explorations. For many people, participating in a research study holds out the potential of direct benefit, especially for those whose mental or physical condition cannot be relieved by any available treatment. In addition to the potential positive effects of biomedical research, some qualitative research endeavors have been shown to provide therapeutic effects, too. "Qualitative research is a form of social inquiry that focuses on the way people interpret and make sense of their experiences" (Holloway & Wheeler, 2002, p. 1). Qualitative research endeavors, those designed to understand experienced phenomenon such as postpartum depression, victimization, grief, sadness, and moral distress, often provide a therapeutic effect (Shamai, 2003).

With this in mind, our goals as healthcare professionals must include helping people decide whether they wish to participate in research endeavors, for what purposes, and under what circumstances. These are examples of what is meant by respect for persons in research settings. Respect for persons in health care or the healthcare research setting means taking responsibility for understanding who the patient is as an individual with particular needs and concerns and what information that person likely needs to meet his or her own goals. This is true whether a choice is being made about whether to accept treatment or whether to become a subject of research. Respecting persons, then, means facilitating informed decision making and assisting in making an authentic choice. An authentic choice is one that is based on an understanding of what is being proposed and the ways in which the decision once made may affect the person, including the impact it is likely to have on personal lifestyle and goals. As noted earlier, it also means recognizing when persons are not capable of informed decision making and assisting proxy decision makers as they strive to fulfill their responsibilities.

Requirements of Informed Decision Making

All of the following are ethical and legal requirements of informed decision making:

- The provision of knowledge and information appropriate to a person's situation and capacities
- The individual's ability to process and comprehend information and show how it is likely to affect him or her
- Freedom from unduly coercive influences (psychological, physical, or environmental)

These represent the criteria of "disclosure . . . comprehension . . . (and) voluntary agreement" spelled out in more detail in the *Belmont Report* (National Institutes of Health, Office of Human Subjects Research, 1979). In the *Belmont Report* and subsequent discussions, it is recognized that obtaining adequately informed consent under the best of conditions and even with the purest of researcher motivations is difficult. Knowledge development in this area is ongoing. Scholars from various disciplines have been concerned to learn more and have undertaken to study what subjects understand as a result of the consent process and whether this matches the intent of the process. In several research studies, this was shown not to be the case (Hutchison, 1998; Kenyon, Dixon-Woods, Jackson, Windridge, & Pitchforth, 2006; Lynöe, Sandlund, Dalqvist, & Jacobsson, 1991); however, more research is needed to discover which strategies are facilitative of quality informed consent processes.

Table 6-1 lists the basic and essential elements of informed consent that, with much thought and discussion, have been deemed by regulatory bodies to be necessary but perhaps not always sufficient for a quality informed consent process to occur. Certain circumstances require additional elements to be included. For example, some populations are considered vulnerable for a variety of reasons and require special protections.

Table 6-1   Essential Aspects of Research Subject Informed Consent

Interpretation of NIH OHSR Elements	APN Applications in Clinical Research Settings and Advisory Role to a Patient or Family
- Acknowledgment that what is being proposed is a research study and that any questions will be answered by the researcher or designee - The purpose of the study - How long the study will take - Which procedures are experimental and which established	Explain the difference between treatment goals and research goals and how this applies in the particular person's case and relates to the person's goals. Help potential participants to explore in what ways participating might or might not serve their purposes. Explore whether they are feeling any pressure to agree. What are their concerns? Discuss with them what sorts of questions they might want to pose to the researcher or person obtaining consent. If the study cannot benefit the potential participant directly, what would be good reasons for participating (help others later)?

Interpretation of NIH OHSR Elements	APN Applications in Clinical Research Settings and Advisory Role to a Patient or Family
- The important details of the study: tests, procedures, extra visits, possible risks, and expected benefits - What alternative treatments are available if the person decides not to participate	Map it out. Help potential participants understand what this would mean in terms of their lives, time frame, and commitment. Do the potential benefits make it worth the effort? What is the likelihood or magnitude of the risks and benefits? Have any treatments or interventions been used before on other populations? What other treatments exist and what has the experience of these been? Explain that they will continue to receive good care whether or not they agree to participate. People are sometimes fearful that if they don't agree, they will be abandoned by their healthcare provider.
- Voluntariness of participation is maintained throughout. Possibility of withdrawal at any time without penalty - They may be withdrawn by their provider or the researcher physician if conditions (theirs or adverse events associated with the study) warrant it - What they can expect if withdrawn - How unforeseen expenses or problems will be addressed	Subjects/patients have the right to withdraw at any time—they do not always understand this. The research team will not necessarily remind them. Some persons may need to be empowered to withdraw when the study becomes too burdensome for them. Primary care providers, not involved in the research, may be the best advocates for the patient. Sometimes the researcher or provider may decide that the person should be withdrawn from the study—they may need help understanding the reason for this and finding appropriate alternative care including hospice or palliative care when warranted.
- How confidentiality will be maintained	Help the person think about how his or her confidentiality will be protected. What might the implications be for the person if personal information got into the hands of the insurance company or an employer?

continue

Table 6-1   Essential Aspects of Research Subject Informed Consent (*continued*)

Interpretation of NIH OHSR Elements	APN Applications in Clinical Research Settings and Advisory Role to a Patient or Family
- Contact information for researcher or resource person	Help subjects/patients think through how to get information in an emergency—who to call and who to inform. If hospitalized, the receiving institution needs to know what protocol is in effect related to interventions they are planning.

Source: National Institutes of Health (NIH), Office of Human Subjects Research (OHSR). (2006). Sheet 6— Guidelines for writing informed consent documents. Retrieved January 7, 2008, from http://ohsr.od.nih.gov/info/ sheet6.html.

A crucial point for the APN is that regardless of whether a person is a subject of research or a patient in need of nursing care, the goals of nursing services are unchanged. Nurses acting in a nursing capacity (i.e., relying upon their professional status as registered nurses) continue to be accountable for practicing in accord with their professional Code of Ethics (ANA, 1994). Anecdotally, on several different occasions over my years of teaching nursing ethics, I have been told by nurses who practice in clinical research settings that they are pressured to ignore nursing concerns related to the individual in favor of maintaining the integrity of the research protocol. I believe this is a mistaken understanding both of the nursing role in research settings and researcher responsibilities. Indeed, the Declaration of Helsinki affirms, "(I)n medical research on human subjects, considerations related to the well-being of the human subject should take precedence over the interests of science and society" (World Medical Association, 2004, Section A5). The complex and uncertain nature of most research requires that "the responsibility for the human subject must always rest with a medically qualified person and never rest on the subject of the research, even though the subject has given consent" (World Medical Association, 2004, Section B15).

Children and Assent

As Munson (2008) notes, "one of the most controversial areas of all medical research has been that involving children as subjects" (p. 14). Children are especially vulnerable to abuse for obvious reasons but most particularly because they are dependent on adults to meet their everyday needs and to make decisions on their behalf. Research in the biological, social, cognitive, and psychological sciences has revealed that capacity for reasoning and decision making is developmental and varies related to biological factors, the age of the child, the type of environment in which the child is raised, and the types of experiences the child has had or to which he or she has been exposed. Consequently, in the case of children, ability to meet the criteria for informed consent, which requires decision-making capacity, must be viewed as occurring along a continuum. It requires understanding the child in context, just as it does for adults. Because it is often difficult to determine just how capable a child is to make informed decisions, legal regulations apply. However, legal regulations alone do not make for ethical practices.

We might ask why enroll children in research at all? Munson (2008) answers this question by reminding us that children are not just small adults. There are differences in biology, metabolism, and biochemistry such that we need to tailor treatments and interventions to their specific needs. Additionally, many illnesses are seen only in childhood either because the illness is so severe the child dies or, in the case of infectious diseases, most adults are immune to the disease, having experienced the illness as a child. "To gain the kind of knowledge and understanding required for effective medical treatment for children, it is often impossible to limit research solely to adults" (Munson, 2008, p.15). The same is true of research studies conceived in the social sciences and designed to understand more about how children relate to the world. Addressing the mental health of children requires understanding more about positive and negative influences on their health and ability to adapt to changing conditions.

Legal Requirements

The protection of children and information related to informed participation are laid out in the CFR (U.S. Department of Health and Human Services, 2005, Title 45, Part 46, Subpart D). Before looking at these in more detail, it might be helpful to understand the definitions that the Department of Health and Human Services relies upon. Additionally, it is important to know that the age at which a person may legitimately make personal decisions related to health care varies from state to state. Rules about the conditions of obtaining emancipated minor status also vary by state. An emancipated minor is a person younger than 18 years of age who is granted the legal right to make his or her own decisions. It is important that APNs understand their state's rules about emancipated minors.

The fact that rules about appropriate age vary from state to state lend logical strength to the idea that no agreement exists about who is a child and thus not capable of decision making and who is an adult and presumed, all things being equal, capable of personal decision making. CFR definitions are as follows:

> (a) *Children* are persons who have not attained the legal age for consent to treatments or procedures involved in the research, under the applicable law of the jurisdiction in which the research will be conducted.
>
> (b) *Assent* means a child's affirmative agreement to participate in research. Mere failure to object should not, absent affirmative agreement, be construed as assent.
>
> (c) *Permission* means the agreement of parent(s) or guardian to the participation of their child or ward in research.
>
> (d) *Parent* means a child's biological or adoptive parent.
>
> (e) *Guardian* means an individual who is authorized under applicable State or local law to consent on behalf of a child to general medical care. (U.S. Department of Health and Human Services, 2005 Title 45, Part 46, Subpart D, Section 46.402)

For the purposes of discussing assent and its requirements, I assume that the child in question is a nonemancipated minor. Generally, children under the age of 6 years are not considered capable of assent. However, recent research has shown that children with a chronic illness may demonstrate an advanced ability to understand how their illness affects them and are able to manage aspects of it (Alderson, Sutcliffe, & Curtis, 2006).

What, then, are the considerations? The guidelines for IRBs are instructive (U.S. Department of Health and Human Services, 2005). IRBs will grant approval for studies involving children when it is felt that the study is well designed and likely to produce results and that every effort is being made to safeguard the child's interests. From my experience on two different IRBs over the past 8 years, I can say that such committees take this charge extremely seriously. Protocols are read very carefully by committee members, the principal investigator (PI) is charged with answering clarification questions, and the protocol is approved only when all are satisfied that the child subject's well-being is a priority.

For research endeavors that have the probability of no greater than a minimal risk to the child, a child may be enrolled with the permission of one parent and the assent of the child. For children to assent, they need to be given information and allowed to process it in developmentally and circumstantially appropriate ways. This necessitates understanding who the child is in terms of his or her capacities and skills. What constitutes minimal risk has not been well defined and is the subject of ongoing debate in the ethics literature. But for our purposes, it can be thought of as equivalent to those perils that the child would be likely to encounter in the course of daily life. For example, a child with diabetes would be likely to encounter hypodermic needles more often than other children, so research involving injections would not be considered more than minimally risky.

For research that involves the possibility of more than minimal risk, a child may be enrolled if there is the prospect of direct and likely benefit, no treatment exists that is comparable, and the child's current status is such that the potential benefit is substantial in terms of quality of life. In such cases, the assent of the child is necessary along with the permission of one parent. Where there is greater than minimal risk and no prospect of direct benefit to the child, the assent of the child and the permission of both parents is needed (where both parents are available). Such situations may be when the child has an incurable disease for which generalizable knowledge is needed to develop ways of preventing or ameliorating the disease in the future for other children.

APNs and Conditions of Assent

Parents or guardians may seek the professional opinions of APNs about whether to enroll their child in a study. Additionally, pediatric nurse practitioners (NPs) may be asked to identify children from their patient populations who are potential subjects for a study. Therefore, it is important to keep in mind possible factors that could endanger a child's welfare either from being inappropriately enrolled in a study or not being enrolled in a study that could potentially provide a benefit.

Besides understanding the nuances of the research project and ensuring that it is scientifically and ethically sound, as discussed elsewhere, APNs have other responsibilities. In the course of informing and supporting parents or guardians interested in a research study and helping them to determine its appropriateness, the APN should be alert to other factors that could harm the child such as being persuaded to assent when it is obvious that the child does not wish to participate. Possible factors that would provoke further exploration of a given situation or raise concerns include when parents who are financially burdened talk about the financial or in-kind incentives to participate (perhaps there will be free care or medications); they may need help getting resources from other avenues. On rare occasions, parents may be abusive or influenced by the possibility of secondary gains (e.g., extra attention). Children without a parent or caregiver (for example, wards of the state) should have an advocate appointed who will look after their interests.

Beneficence

The ideal overall purpose of research on human beings is one of beneficence; that is, the results of empirical endeavors are expected to contribute positively to society and its constituents. In the process of making positive contributions, harms to individuals must be minimized. Researchers are responsible for the physical, mental, and social well-being of subjects. They cannot fulfill this responsibility if they are not willing to understand individual subjects within their contexts, beliefs, values, and plans. Unfortunately, as noted and exemplified earlier, a host of factors can interfere with researcher interest in the good of an individual subject. A variety of conflicts of interest can weaken researcher willingness to adhere to the goal of beneficence. There may also be financial inducements related to the funding source. It is beyond the purposes of this chapter to detail the commercialization of the biomedical research enterprise that has occurred over the past several decades in the United States; however, this development has raised further possibilities for researcher conflicts and is an important consideration for APNs and others who are concerned about protecting subjects from harm.

Human subjects protection regulations stipulate that conflicts of interests be disclosed in the informed consent process in such a way that the potential subjects understand the implications for them. However, the possible effects of conflicts of interests are not always easy to identify or sort out. This is evident from the expanding body of literature on this topic. Implications of this for advanced practice is that nurses who frequently find themselves involved in the recruitment or informing stages of the research process have responsibilities to understand the issues involved so that they can assist their patients or subjects in the decision-making process.

The Two Branches of Beneficence

In the Chapter 1 discussion of ethical principles, the principles of nonmaleficence (do no harm) and beneficence (promote the good) were discussed separately. Philosophically, they are related, but there is disagreement about whether nonmaleficence should be subsumed under the umbrella term of *beneficence*. In research ethics discussions, this is the convention. Beneficence, as noted earlier, is closely related in purpose to the principle of respect for persons.

Beneficence is an obligation both of healthcare professionals and those engaging in research endeavors that involve human beings. For the purposes of undertaking research, "Two general rules have been formulated as complementary expressions of beneficent actions in this sense: (1) do not harm and (2) maximize possible benefits and minimize possible harms" (National Institutes of Health, Office of Human Subjects Research, 1979). Although this seems like a relatively straightforward principle, it is very "complex and ambiguous in application" (Smith, 2000, p. 7). The very nature of most research means that there are unforeseeable risks and potential benefits. Estimating the likelihood, quantity, or quality of the benefits and balancing them against the possibility and likelihood of risk is a very tricky task. Additionally, although the hoped-for benefits may be either to an individual subject or to society, the risks are usually to the well-being of a particular subject.

Therapeutic versus Nontherapeutic Research

In the Declaration of Helsinki, the distinction between therapeutic and nontherapeutic research was made. Therapeutic research is that which holds out the hope of treatment for a malady or condition experienced by the subject and takes place as part of patient care. It is sometimes also called clinical research. Nontherapeutic research is that which aims to contribute more generally to the knowledge base for benefit of others rather than of the subject. Subjects of nontherapeutic research may of course benefit in a variety of ways, for example, feeling good about contributions they are making to health improvements in the future. Capron (1998) and others have called into question the importance of the distinction because it implies that research combined with clinical care is therapeutic. Such research nevertheless involves experimental aspects, and the danger is that the physician, when he or she doubles as researcher, may be lulled into "treating the project as inherently more justified" (p. 143) than nonclinical research. Additionally, for APN purposes, both beneficence and respect for persons require attention to the experimental nature of clinical research with its inherent risks.

APNs employed in research settings may be exposed to nontherapeutic research protocols. Nontherapeutic trials often but not always involve healthy volunteers. Some have noted that phase 1 drug trials involving seriously ill persons should be considered nontherapeutic because they are not expected to benefit participants, although participants often do not grasp this fact despite the informed consent process. (Box 6-2 explains what types of subjects participate in phased trials.) Regardless of whether or how this controversy is resolved, the important point to take away is that research has uncertain aspects as does clinical care—beneficence requires that harm to individual patient subjects is reduced and that the individual patient/subject good is considered paramount.

Box 6-2

Phases of Drug Trials

Research that involves the development and testing of new drugs generally takes place in four phases. Each phase is distinct and involves different groups of subjects. Following is my synthesis of the pertinent literature over time including the National Institutes of Health (NIH).

Phase 1	Occurs after testing in animals when feasible. Uses a small group of people. The aim is to see both what is a safe dose and what dose is effective for the purpose designed. May use healthy subjects or subjects with a disease process. Is not designed to benefit the subject, although it sometimes provides a placebo effect (Grace, 2006) and in some cases has an effect on a patient's disease process. Often called safety and efficacy trials. Escalating doses of a drug are given to successive patients or patient groups.
Phase 2	Uses larger groups of people, usually those who have the condition targeted, to further test for safety, side effects, and effectiveness.
Phase 3	Uses a large group of subjects who have the condition the drug is designed to treat. Further tests safety and effectiveness, generally over a longer time frame. The number needed for the study is based on statistical estimates of what is needed to validate findings. Subjects are usually monitored by their physicians and the study PI.
Phase 4	After Food and Drug Administration (FDA) approval of the drug for general use, these studies monitor for adverse findings over a period of time.

Justice

The third important principle in research ethics is that of justice. For healthcare purposes, the two salient questions related to knowledge development for human good are (1) what constitutes an ethically sound study, and

(2) "(W)ho ought to receive the benefits of research and bear its burdens?" (National Institutes of Health, Office of Human Subjects Research, 1979). In Chapter 1, I noted that the favored conception of justice in healthcare situations is that of justice as fairness. That is, justice means that we try to ensure that all individuals and groups have the opportunity to benefit from societal provisions. Meanwhile, we recognize that it is more difficult for the disadvantaged and the impoverished to have their needs met.

However, another problem that was discussed previously related to vulnerability is that historically some persons have been studied because they were convenient, unlikely to object, or easily deceived. So, there are three main aspects of justice that are important, as discussed in the following subsections.

Failure to Study an Important Issue Affecting a Vulnerable Group

Justice as fairness requires that healthcare professionals and scientists study issues, psychosocial and biological, that especially affect certain groups of vulnerable people or to which these persons are especially susceptible. For example, to avoid studying factors associated with Alzheimer's disease for the reason that in the later stages of the disease people are not capable of informed consent represents an injustice. Likewise, to avoid investigating problems associated with certain immigrant populations because it requires translating documents and information also fails to meet justice criteria.

Minimizing Harms and Maximizing Benefits

This is a very difficult task in view of the complexity and uncertainty associated with much medical research—it requires paying scrupulous attention to all aspects of the project from conception through study termination and publication of findings. It involves understanding the particular risks to both individuals and the group based on the type of vulnerability present.

Fair Selection of Subjects

Subject selection cannot be based on mere expediency. The history of research ethics provides vivid examples of studies that were carried out upon people who were easily deceived or who could not object. One rule of thumb is that research using subjects from vulnerable or disadvantaged groups should be aimed at benefiting those people or their cohort group. The Belmont Report proposes the following:

> Justice is relevant to the selection of subjects of research at two levels: the social and the individual. Individual justice in the selection of subjects would require

that researchers exhibit fairness: thus, they should not offer potentially beneficial research only to some patients who are in their favor or select only "undesirable" persons for risky research. Social justice requires that distinction be drawn between classes of subjects that ought, and ought not, to participate in any particular kind of research, based on the ability of members of that class to bear burdens and on the appropriateness of placing further burdens on already burdened persons. Thus, it can be considered a matter of social justice that there is an order of preference in the selection of classes of subjects (e.g., adults before children) and that some classes of potential subjects (e.g., the institutionalized mentally infirm or prisoners) may be involved as research subjects, if at all, only on certain conditions. (National Institutes of Health, Office of Human Subjects Research, 1979)

PROBLEMS FACING NURSES IN RESEARCH ROLES AND SETTINGS

APNs may function in one of several roles related to research. As primary care providers they may be caring for patients who are on a protocol of some sort. They may be asked to select and recruit patients from their population who would be good subjects for a particular research study. As specialists, they may be asked to be consultants for a research study. The identification of unanswered practice questions may spur the conception of a study where APNs serve as investigators or co-investigators. Many NPs and CNSs serve as study coordinators and are responsible for oversight of study integrity and subject safety and well-being. Another role is that of an IRB member. This is an excellent way for nurses to develop a more in-depth knowledge of the ethical and regulatory issues surrounding healthcare research. All of these roles require different skills and expertise. There is always a period of intense learning for any new role undertaken, and the issues associated with each role cannot be detailed here.

Some of the problems most commonly faced are discussed in the following list. I do not attempt to propose a course of action for all of these because solutions depend upon more detailed data gathering and what constitutes good action varies depending on the data. Chapter 5 discusses collaboration, which is helpful in certain cases. For more troubling issues, enlist the assistance of the principal investigator. If you feel that serious breaches of ethics are occurring, and the PI seems uninterested in the problem, then it might be helpful to speak to a member or the chair of the IRB that approved the study.

1. Patients who don't seem to understand the goals of the research. For example, a patient thinks a study is to benefit him when in fact he may

be selected to the group receiving a placebo or alternative treatment. For a more in-depth discussion of placebos and randomized control trials (RCTs), see Michels and Rothman (2003). Another example is when the patient thinks the drug is designed to cure when in fact at best it is to prolong life.

2. Patients who have expressed a desire to withdraw from the study but are being pressured to continue. First, it must be ascertained why the patient wants to withdraw, and then a way must be found to support that person in his or her wishes.

3. A patient seems to be experiencing a lot of suffering and isn't aware of alternatives to the protocol such as hospice or palliative care. A discussion should be initiated that seeks to discover under what conditions he or she would wish to continue, what the patient's goals are, and what is most likely to meet these.

4. A person enters the trial with decision-making capacity but has become cognitively unable to agree to continue or request withdrawal.

5. A researcher, colleague, or surrogate decision maker appears to be acting unethically. For example, Ms. Jacques, a 75-year-old woman, is about to be discharged after suffering an acute coronary event with subsequent congestive heart failure (CHF). Ms. Vitale, the critical care unit (CCU) NP, is completing her discharge summary when Dr. Gould, one of the CCU attending physicians, asks if he can speak to Ms. Jacques about a study he is doing. He tells Ms. Jacques that he thinks she would benefit from being in this study that will look at the effect of exercise on CHF. Ms. Jacques says that would be a lot of traveling for her and asks if there are any alternatives. Dr. Gould says, "There isn't anything available where you would be so closely monitored and so well cared for." Ms. Vitale knows this is not exactly true because the local hospital near to Ms. Jacques's home has a cardiac rehabilitation program for which she is eligible. Attending that program would require a lot less traveling, and the unit has a good reputation. Thus, Ms. Jacques's best interests would probably be served by this option.

6. A surrogate decision maker seems to be making decisions that are not in the subject's interest. For example, Timmy, 10 years old, is being kept in the hospital to complete a drug study. He is experiencing uncomfortable but not life-threatening side effects from the study drug for which there are alternative treatments with fewer side effects. Timmy has been on these alternatives before and with less problems. Timmy tells you he wants to go home. You overhear Timmy's stepfather say to his wife (Timmy's mother), "But if we kept him in the study one more week, we could get this week's compensation money."

SUMMARY

This chapter has provided an overview of ethical issues associated with research conducted in healthcare settings. Such research is necessarily based on the premise that it will further some sort of good or benefit to individuals and society related to health. This chapter provides a basis for understanding the nature and complexity of the research endeavor and locates the APN's responsibilities related to research subjects firmly in the goals of nursing to promote individual and social good. Nurses working in clinical research settings sometimes find their professional goals seemingly at odds with the apparent goals of a researcher, who seems more interested in preserving the integrity of the study at the expense of an individual participant's needs. The reality is that the goals of both the nurse and the researcher (who may also be a nurse) are really in concert. Both are ethically charged with ensuring that in the process of the research endeavor, the protection of the individual subject's good remains the priority goal.

DISCUSSION QUESTIONS

1. Discuss with peers the ways in which your thinking about APN responsibility related to human subjects research has or has not changed as a result of reading this chapter.
2. You are an APN in a nurse-run inner-city family practice clinic. The clinic practitioners are trying to decide whether to recruit part of their patient population to an obesity control trial (phase III) at the local university hospital, which involves random assignment to receive either a new drug and support plus exercise sessions, or a placebo and support plus exercise sessions. The purpose is to see if the drug is more effective than support and exercise alone in achieving significant weight loss.
   a. What further information about the study would you need to know before deciding whether you will recruit? What are the implications for provider–patient relationships at the clinic?
   b. You decide that this would be a good opportunity for your population. You are the APN who is most knowledgeable about the problems and promises of research and the associated ethical issues and have been charged with sharing your knowledge with your colleagues. How would you prioritize the issues? Why?
   c. Additionally, because many of your teenage patients suffer from obesity, discuss the potential for them to participate. What special considerations are necessary when recruiting children for experimental research studies?

REFERENCES

Alderson, P., Sutcliffe, K., & Curtis, K. (2006). Children's competence to consent to medical treatment. *Hastings Center Report, 36*(6), 25–36.

Alexander, M. (2001, August). Thirty years later Stanford prison experiment lives on. *Stanford Reporter, 22.* Retrieved March 31, 2008, from http://news-service.stanford.edu/news/2001/august22/prison2-822.html.

American Nurses Association. (1994). *Position statement: The nonnegotiable nature of the ANA code for nurses with interpretive statements.* Washington, DC: Author.

Axelsen, D. (2001). Race, gender and medical experimentation: J. Marion Sims' surgery on slave women. In W. Teays & L. Purdy (Eds.), *Bioethics, justice and healthcare* (pp. 224–230). Belmont, CA: Wadsworth/Thompson Learning.

Bandura, A. (1986). *Social foundation of thought and action.* Englewood Cliffs, NJ: Prentice Hall.

Bandura, A. (1999). Moral disengagement in the perpetration of inhumanities. *Personality and Social Psychology Review, 3,* 193–209.

Beecher, H. (1966). Ethics and clinical research. *New England Journal of Medicine, 274,* 1354–1360.

Benedict, S., & Kuhla, J. (1999). Nurses participation in the euthanasia programs of Nazi Germany. *Western Journal of Nursing Research, 21*(2), 246–263.

Capron, A. (1998). Human experimentation. In R. Veatch (Ed.), *Medical ethics* (2nd ed., pp. 135–184). Sudbury, MA: Jones and Bartlett.

Chambliss, D. (1996). *Beyond caring: Hospitals, nurses and the social organization of ethics.* Chicago: University of Chicago Press.

Dewey, J. (1980). *The quest for certainty.* New York: Putnam Publishing—Perigee Books. (Original work published in 1929.)

Dunn, C., & Chadwick, G. (2001). *Protecting study volunteers in research: A manual for investigative sites.* Boston: Center Watch.

Festinger, L. (1957). *A theory of cognitive dissonance.* Stanford, CA: Stanford University Press.

Grace, P. (2006, February). The clinical use of placebos: Is it ethical? Not when it involves deceiving patients. *American Journal of Nursing, 106*(2), 58–61.

Holloway, I., & Wheeler, S. (2002). *Qualitative research in nursing* (2nd ed.). Malden, MA: Blackwell.

Hope, T., & McMillan, J. (2004). Challenge studies of human volunteers: Ethical issues. *Journal of Medical Ethics, 30*(1), 110–117.

Hutchison, C. (1998). Phase I trials in cancer patients: Participants' perceptions. *European Journal of Cancer Care, 7*(1), 12–22.

Jewish Virtual Library. (2008). *Bone, muscle, and nerve regeneration and bone transplantation experiments.* Retrieved April 4, 2008, from http://www.jewishvirtuallibrary.org/jsource/Holocaust/bonexp.html.

Katz, J. (1992). The consent principle of the Nuremberg Code: Its significance then and now. In G. J. Annas & M. A. Grodin (Eds.), *The Nazi doctors and the Nuremberg Code: Human rights in human experimentation* (pp. 227–239). New York: Oxford University Press.

Kenyon, S., Dixon-Woods, M., Jackson, C., Windridge, K., & Pitchforth, E. (2006). Participating in a trial in a critical situation: A qualitative study in pregnancy. *Quality and Safety in HealthCare, 15*(2), 98–101.

Lynöe, N., Sandlund, M., Dahlqvist, G., & Jacobsson, L. (1991). Informed consent: study of quality of information given to participants in a clinical trial. *British Journal of Medicine, 303*(6803), 610–613.

Michels, K., & Rothman, K. (2003). Update on unethical use of placebos in randomised trials. *Bioethics, 17*(2), 188–204.

Milgram, S. (1974). *Obedience to authority.* New York: Harper & Row.

Miller, F., & Wertheimer, A. (2007). Facing up to paternalism in research ethics. *Hastings Center Report, 37*(3), 24–34.

Mohr, W., & Mahon, M. (1996). Dirty hands: The underside of marketplace healthcare. *Advances in Nursing Science, 19*(1), 28–37.

Munson, R. (2008). *Intervention and reflection: Basic issues in medical ethics* (8th ed.). Belmont, CA: Wadsworth/Thomson Learning.

Nagel, T. (1991). *Equality and partiality.* New York: Oxford University.

National Institutes of Health, Office for Human Research Protections. (2004). Title 45 Code of Federal Regulations, part 46, 102(d). Retrieved October 28, 2007, from http://www.hhs.gov/ohrp/humansubjects/guidance/cdebiol.htm.

National Institutes of Health, Office of Human Subjects Research. (1979). *The Belmont report: Ethical principles and guidelines for the protection of human subjects of research.* Retrieved January 6, 2008, from http://ohsr.od.nih.gov/guidelines/belmont.html.

Parascandola, M. (2007). Use of prisoners in research. *Research Practitioner, 8*(1), 12–24.

Ramsey, P. (2001). Judgment on Willowbrook. In W. Teays & L. Purdy (Eds.), *Bioethics, justice and healthcare* (pp. 245–249). Belmont, CA: Wadsworth/Thompson Learning.

Rothman, D. (1991). *Strangers at the bedside.* New York: Harper Collins—Basic Books.

Savitt, T. L. (2001). The use of blacks for medical experimentation and demonstration in the Old South. In W. Teays & L. Purdy (Eds.), *Bioethics, justice and healthcare* (pp. 215–224). Belmont, CA: Wadsworth/Thompson Learning.

Shamai, M. (2003). Therapeutic effects of qualitative research: Reconstructing the experience of treatment as a by-product of qualitative evaluation. *Social Service Review, 77*(3), 455–467.

Smith, M. B. (2000). Moral foundations. In B. Sales & M. Folkman (Eds.), *Ethics in research with human participants* (pp. 3–10). Washington, DC: American Psychological Association.

Tavris, C., & Aronson, E. (2007). *Mistakes were made (but not by me): Why we justify foolish beliefs, bad decisions and hurtful acts.* Orlando, FL: Harcourt.

U.S. Department of Health and Human Services. (1949). *Nuremberg Code. Trials of war criminals before the Nuremberg Military Tribunals under Control Council Law No. 10,* Vol. 2 (pp. 181–182). Washington, DC: U.S. Government Printing Office. Retrieved January 6, 2007, from http://www.hhs.gov/ohrp/references/nurcode.htm.

U.S. Department of Health and Human Services. (2005). DHHS, 2005 Title 45, Part 46, Subpart D, Section 46.402. *Additional protections for children involved as subjects in research.* Retrieved January 10, 2008, from http://www.hhs.gov/ohrp/humansubjects/guidance/45cfr46.htm#subpartd.

Vollman, J., & Winau, R. (1996). Informed consent in human experimentation before the Nuremberg code. *British Medical Journal, 313,* 1445–1447.

Weiner, B. (1992). *Human motivation: Metaphors, theories and research.* Thousand Oaks, CA: Sage.

Weston, A. (2005). *A practical companion to ethics* (3rd ed.). New York: Oxford University Press.

Wheelwright, P. (1988). *The Presocratics.* New York: Macmillan.

World Medical Association. (2003). About the WMA. Retrieved January 6, 2008, from http://www.wma.net/e/about/index.htm.

World Medical Association Declaration of Helsinki (2004). Retrieved April 4, 2008 from http://www.wma.net/e/policy/pdf/17c.pdf.

Zimbardo, P. (2005). Professional profile. Retrieved December 20, 2007, from http://zimbardo.socialpsychology.org/.

Ethical Issues in Advanced Practice Specialty Areas

CHAPTER 7

Nursing Ethics and Advanced Practice: Neonatal Issues

Peggy Doyle Settle

Never give out while there is hope; but hope not beyond reason,
for that shows more desire than judgment.
—*William Penn, Some Fruits of Solitude, 1693*

INTRODUCTION

Good nursing care in the neonatal intensive care unit (NICU) is achieved when nurses are empowered to advocate for infants and their families. As with all patients, the goals of good nursing care in the NICU include the alleviation of suffering and the protection, promotion, and restoration of health in the care of both the infant and family (American Nurses Association [ANA], 2001). Factors influencing good nursing care include the nurse's knowledge and experience, available technology, and an understanding of health policy implications of treatment and supportive environments. Ethical issues and dilemmas arise in the NICU when the goals of good nursing care conflict with the goals of other disciplines and/or family members or when there is uncertainty about what are reasonable goals. This chapter reviews ethical issues that are unique to the neonatal setting. Strategies and tools for exploring or resolving these issues are discussed including the best interest standard, collaborative decision making with healthcare professionals and parents, and understanding medical futility in the newborn period. These issues and many others contribute to the complexity of nursing care in the NICU. Advanced practice neonatal clinical nurse specialists (CNSs), nurse practitioners (NPs), and nurse administrators are in pivotal roles to facilitate discussions with direct care nurses and other health team members when ethical issues arise that jeopardize the delivery of good nursing care.

CONTEXT OF CARE

The care of critically ill newborns is an ethical and emotional challenge for all members of the healthcare team. Uncertainty is often a fact of work in NICU settings. Many critically ill and/or premature infants receive available treatment and recover with no or minimal sequelae (Lantos, Mokalla, & Meadow, 1997; Meadow, Lee, Lin, & Lantos, 2004). However, some NICU infants require prolonged medical treatment, but there may be only a very small chance of recovery (Catlin, 2005). It isn't always easy to know which baby can recover and which will have serious ongoing problems that will impinge on the baby's quality of life (QOL). The rapid pace of technologic developments adds further uncertainty to the decision-making process. What can't be treated very well currently may well have an effective intervention down the road. Moreover, literature suggests that medical treatment decisions and outcomes vary based on geographic location and the technical capability of the institution (Vohr et al., 2004). These variations mean that there may be different treatments applied and different outcomes seen for two infants with similar problems merely as a result of location. Additionally, health policies in different countries influence medical treatment decisions, causing further variations in treatments and outcomes among countries (Rebagliato et al., 2000). These variations also pose ethical issues in the delivery of good nursing care. For example, one family with a critically ill infant may be offered the option of discontinuing treatment based on sociodemographic factors, and another family may not be offered the same option (Orfali & Gordon, 2004; Orfali, 2004).

Before describing the ethical issues encountered with critically ill and premature newborns, a review of the technologic advancements and healthcare regulations affecting treatment decisions is necessary. This will provide you with a more in-depth understanding of the factors influencing care. In addition, the unique role of the direct care NICU nurse is included to fully describe the context of care.

Historical Context of Care

The specialty of neonatology established in 1966 was followed by regionalization of care involving the transport of critically ill and premature newborns in specially equipped vehicles to tertiary care centers. Transport provided to the critically ill or premature infant, from rural or other areas where the sophisticated technology and healthcare professional skills needed to maintain the lives of these infants was not available, improved chances of survival. However, this transport also often resulted in the separation of the infant from his or her parents and placed the infant directly in the healthcare team's control (Pinch, 2002). Treatment decisions for critically ill newborns were made by the healthcare providers directly involved in the infant's care and with little input from parents (Pinch, 2002).

Technology both provided previously nonexistent opportunities but also led to some problematic practices. The public disclosure of certain ethically questionable medical practices regarding critically ill infants who were liable to have a protracted clinical course led to amendments in federal legislation that aimed to provide protections for these infants. As technology became more sophisticated, healthcare providers were able to initiate, sustain, and in some cases prolong the lives of extremely early born infants. And with reported variations in NICU patient outcomes, healthcare providers now wonder, although they can offer treatment to this patient population, should treatment always be offered? And under what circumstances is it permissible or even obligatory to withhold life-prolonging treatment?

Technologic Context of Care

The ongoing fundamental physiologic needs of the critically ill and premature infant are warmth, respiratory and nutritional support, and prevention and treatment of infection (Pinch, 2002). Landmark technologic developments of each decade are listed in Table 7-1.

Despite the technologic advances of each decade, few standardized treatment protocols were developed. Few clinical trials aimed at developing guidelines related to NICU practice were conducted. Healthcare providers initiated treatments for infants with whatever resources were available (Pinch, 2002). The development of biological and technologic innovations that can be applied to the care of high-risk infants continues. These developments enable the NICU team to provide life-sustaining treatment to extremely low birth weight (ELBW) infants born at 22 to 23 weeks gestation, now considered the threshold of viability (Brinchmann & Nortvedt, 2001; Orfali & Gordon, 2004; Pinch, 2002; Sayeed, 2005).

The morbidity and mortality rates related to this "rescue philosophy" (Pinch, 2002, p. 13) of care for ELBW infants is variable. The long-term developmental outcomes related to the application of life-sustaining treatments range from minimal to severe neurodevelopmental complications (Hack et al., 2002; Wilson-Costello, Freidman, Minich, Fanaroff, & Hack, 2005). Few prognostic indicators exist to accurately determine long-term outcomes. This poses decision-making dilemmas regarding whether and

Table 7-1   Landmark Technologic Innovations

1950s	Mechanical ventilator for newborn Phototherapy as a treatment for hyperbilirubinemia Ventricular shunt for newborn
1960s	Total parental nutrition
1970s	Regionalization of high-risk care Continuous positive air pressure (CPAP)
1980s	Pulse oximetry trials Open fetal surgery Neonatal surfactant therapy introduced Cryosurgery for retinopathy
1990s	Laser surgery for retinopathy
2000s	Nitric oxide

Source: Pinch, W. (2002). *When the bough breaks: Parental perceptions of ethical decision making in the NICU.* Lanham, MD: University Press of America, pp. 8–11.

when to initiate, and under what conditions to continue, ongoing treatment of ELBW infants in view of the potential but unpredictable complications resulting from their early birth.

Legislation

Understanding the history behind current laws pertaining to the care and treatment of critically ill and premature infants is an important aspect of an advance practice nurse's (APN's) knowledge base. This permits an appreciation of the complexity of the conflicts surrounding treatment decisions. The law honors the parents' rights to make medical decisions on behalf of their infant with two exceptions. The first exception is an emergency situation, where lifesaving treatment is required and parents are not available to give consent. This exception requires that healthcare providers determine and provide the most appropriate medical treatment. The second exception occurs when the court determines that parents are not acting in the best interest of their child. This

Table 7-2   Legislation Related to Newborn Infant Care

Law	Year	Implications
Rehabilitation Act Section 504	1983	Nontreatment equivalent to civil rights violation. Act not upheld in court
Child Abuse Amendments	1984	Nontreatment considered neglect
Emergency Medical Treatment and Labor Act Section 1867 of the Social Security Act	1997	Healthcare providers must offer emergency services, even when this is potentially futile
Born Alive Infant Protection Act	2002	Ensures that neonates are afforded legal status and protections under the law at birth

exception enables the court to override the parents' medical decisions for their child (Hurst, 2005) in the interests of protecting the child. Legislation related to medical treatment decisions for handicapped or prematurely born infants is provided in Table 7-2.

This legislative agenda evolved over three decades in response to increased public reporting of what were seen as troubling end-of-life decision-making practices by physicians and parental refusal of medical treatment for critically ill and handicapped infants (Anspach, 1993). Duff and Campbell (1973) first reported the end-of-life decision-making practices in their Yale, New Haven, NICU. They studied infant deaths over a 2-year period and identified two categories of infant deaths. Causes of death for infants in category 1 resulted from pathologic conditions. Category 2 infant deaths were associated with severe impairments usually resulting from congenital anomalies. The deaths of these infants resulted from withdrawal or discontinuance of treatment. This disclosure, along with others, prompted wide public and professional debate over treatment decisions for handicapped and extremely early born infants (Anspach, 1993; Singh, Lantos, & Meadow, 2004).

The "Baby Doe Rules" resulted from these widely publicized cases involving the death of handicapped newborns resulting from the withholding of medical treatment. The primary case, Baby Doe, occurred in 1982. This case involved the parents' refusal to allow physicians to treat medical conditions that were diagnosed at the baby's birth. Baby Doe was diagnosed with Down syndrome, tracheoesophageal atresia, and other problems. Conflict arose between the involved pediatricians regarding the most appropriate course of treatment, and legal action was eventually sought by the birth hospital. Baby Doe's pediatrician and parents elected not to repair the infant's atresia and to withhold fluids with the intention of not prolonging the infant's life. This decision was held up in court and Baby Doe died 6 days later (Munson, 2008). In 1983, a similar situation involving "Baby Jane Doe," an infant with spina bifida, an abnormally small head, and hydrocephaly, again brought public attention to the issue of withholding treatment for newborns with disabilities.

Responding to these and other cases, the Department of Health and Human (DHHS) Services amended regulations of the Rehabilitation Act Section 504 that included strict guidelines regarding the treatment of sick or handicapped newborns. The Baby Doe Amendments defined child abuse to include the withholding of fluids, food, and medically indicated treatment from disabled infants. This legislation stipulated that failure to provide medical treatment was a violation of the infant's civil rights (Kopelman, 2005). To enforce these regulations, hospitals were required to post notices with hotline numbers for any professional or lay person to report instances of suspected medical neglect. Investigations of reported neglect included medical record review, private investigations, and court orders to force medical treatment that had been refused by parents. The investigations revealed no instances of medical neglect, but the threat of federal investigations prompted many hospital administrators and healthcare providers to alter their practices regarding treatment decisions for these infants. Treatments were often given even where little hope of survival or quality of life existed.

The first set of Baby Doe Rules was challenged and invalidated in 1986 (Kopelman, 2005). A second set of Baby Doe Rules was enacted in 1984 as amendments to the Child Abuse and Protection and Treatment Act. This legislation forbade the withholding of indicated treatment. Healthcare providers were required to institute care to handicapped or preterm infants regardless of the infant's gestational age or the benefit or futility of treatment. These regulations distinguished between merely prolonging life with measures that are considered futile and care that was beneficial irrespective of the infant's probable handicap (Avery, 1998). The regulations along with definitions of the 1984 Child Abuse Amendments (CAA) are included in Table 7-3.

Controversy within the healthcare community regarding the Baby Doe Rules continues. Some professionals believe that the CAA regulations limit the parents' right to decide (Kopelman, 2005; Sayeed, 2005). Many physicians have altered their practices related to end-of-life decision making for the handicapped and critically ill newborn as a result of these rules, which in fact remain

Table 7-3   U.S.C.A. Title 42, Chapter 67, Sec. 5106a. Grants to States for Child Abuse and Neglect Prevention and Treatment Programs

(B) an assurance that the state has in place procedures for responding to the reporting of medical neglect (including instance of withholding of medically indicated treatment from disabled infants with life-threatening conditions), procedures, or programs, or both

(within the State child protective services system) to provide for

    (i)   coordination and consultation with individuals designated by and within appropriate health-care facilities;

   (ii)   prompt notification by individuals designated by and within appropriate health-care facilities of cases of suspected medical neglect (including instances of withholding of medically indicated treatment from disabled infants with life-threatening conditions); and

  (iii)   authority, under State law, for the State child protective services system to pursue any legal remedies including the authority to initiate legal proceedings in a court of competent jurisdiction, as may be necessary to prevent the withholding of medically indicated treatment from disabled infants with life threatening conditions;

untested. Others consider the regulations related to state funding for child abuse prevention grants (Hurst, 2005) stipulating that the language of the regulations contains no sanctions against medical providers for violating the law. The American Academy of Pediatrics (AAP) recommends individualized treatment decisions by clinicians and families using the best interest standard (AAP, 2007; Hurst, 2005). Application of the Baby Doe Rules is perceived as limiting clinician discretion and preventing individualized care (Kopelman, 2005; Sayeed, 2006). The guidelines recommended by the AAP are perceived by some as not consistent with the law (Sayeed, 2006), and this creates ambiguity for healthcare providers in the NICU.

The Emergency Medical Treatment and Labor Act (EMTLA), section 1867 of the Social Security Act enacted in 1997, imposed specific obligations on Medicare-participating hospitals to offer emergency services and medical screening for emergency medical conditions to all patients presenting themselves to their hospitals (Romesberg, 2003). This act was intended to prevent the dumping of poor and indigent patients by emergency departments. It allows for no exceptions, futile care or otherwise. The law stipulates that if a patient can be stabilized, then the healthcare providers must stabilize the patient (Hurst, 2005). Legal precedent has been established that enables parents to request the initiation of treatment even in cases where treatment may be incompatible with life (Romesberg, 2003).

The most current legislation affecting the neonate in our society is the Born Alive Infant Protection Act (BIPA) of 2001. This act defines being born alive as displaying signs of life including the following:

> breathing, beating heart, pulsation of the umbilical cord or definite movement of voluntary muscles, regardless of whether the umbilical cord has been cut, and regardless of whether the expulsion or extraction occurs as a result of natural or induced labor, cesarean section or induced abortion. (H.R. 2175 107th Congress 2nd session)

This regulation, initially understood as anti-abortion rhetoric (Sayeed, 2005), raised little concern among the healthcare community. Clinicians responding to the delivery of marginally viable newborns are instructed by the Neonatal Resuscitation Program (NRP) steering committee to retain their current approach to treatment for the care of the marginally viable newborn (AAP, 2007). However, it is evident from recent discussions in the literature that new concerns are being raised about the intent and potential effects of this legislation (Sayeed, 2005, 2006). One major concern is specifically related to the absence of language regarding standards of practice, best interest of the neonate, or the parents' decision-making authority. And although there is no mandate for medical treatment where none is currently indicated, the worry is that a "prudent" lay person attending a birth and seeing what he or she takes to be a viable infant in need of emergency medical care could call for care to be initiated. A further concern is that literal interpretations of the legislation could result in overtreatment of infants born at lower and lower gestations (Sayeed, 2006). Recent research regarding delivery room treatment decisions for marginally viable newborns and end-of-life decisions in the NICU is inconsistent with policy (Singh et al., 2004). Although the law continues to evolve, there are no clear legal answers (Hurst, 2005) especially related to the treatment of, or protection of, those at the margins of viability. The question also remains of what are the moral responsibilities of healthcare professionals related to the care and treatment for such infants. Treatment of very premature neonates continues to vary significantly across NICUs.

Role of Direct Care Neonatal Nurses

Direct care NICU nurses fulfill a unique role in caring for infants and their families. NICU nurses encounter ethical issues daily and are in a position to both understand the implications of a medical condition as well as be familiar with the family's customs, feelings, and attitudes (Catlin, 2007). The number and types of dilemmas that confront those involved with care of critically ill or premature babies are likely to increase as a result of advances in technology and pharmacology, parental involvement in decision making, and varying availability of resources (Spence, 2000).

The National Association of Neonatal Nurses (NANN) recognizes the NICU nurse as a contributor to the ethical decision-making process (Catlin, 2007) through direct care and family education. NICU nurses report they are more likely to be involved in clinical decision making than ethical decision making (Romesberg, 2003). In addition, the theoretical differences between physicians' and nurses' approaches to care (Catlin, 2007), along with the existence of a multicultural society where differing beliefs and values abound, are factors affecting the ability to reach consensus about the best course of action in ethical dilemma situations. APNs in all roles can mentor, counsel, and coach direct care nurses experiencing dilemmas in daily practice.

The parental role in the NICU has evolved over the past century to family-centered care (FCC) as best practice. The FCC framework is based on respect, information sharing, collaboration, and confidence building with collaborative partnerships as the foundation of encounters between nurses and parents (Fegran, Helseth, & Slettebo, 2006; Harrison, 1993). Although implementation of FCC is variable and NICU nurses have different experiences with the approach, both parents and nurses share a common concern—the vulnerable infant. NICU nurses provide a constant presence in the care of the infant, and the relationship developed with the family is crucial in determining how parents move from involvement to participation in the care of their infant. The parents are dependent on the nurse to help them integrate new knowledge, enabling them to act in their child's best interest. It is essential for NICU nurses to consider the vulnerability parents experience because they are dependent on nurses to care for their child. Parent participation can be achieved by encouraging nurses to create opportunities for participation. Nurses must also be alert and responsive when parents initiate caregiving activities. APN administrators, CNSs, and NPs can enable direct care NICU nurses to reflect on their competence and willingness to involve parents in their infant's care (Fegran et al., 2006).

In summary, the context in which the NICU nurse provides care to critically ill and premature infants is influenced by the geographical context, technologic capability, and the clinicians' interpretation of the laws regulating care. The direct care NICU nurse is in the crucial role of ensuring that parents receive appropriate information concerning the prognosis and treatment options for their infant. This can be achieved by facilitating discussions with all clinicians involved in care along with the family. Hurst (2005) encourages nurses to facilitate the transparent communication processes advocated by many national associations including the AAP and NANN.

One mechanism to enhance transparent communication among all clinicians in the NICU is regular multidisciplinary ethics rounds. In the context of ethics rounds, all members of the healthcare team can express their individual views and gain an understanding of the goals of other disciplines in the care of infants and their families.

BEST INTEREST STANDARD

Most, if not all, decisions made in the care of newborns utilize the best interest standard. It is derived from the ethical principles of beneficence and nonmaleficence (Steinberg, 1998). These principles, along with considerations of the value and quality of life, serve as the decision framework. This framework enables healthcare providers to determine which interventions will benefit the infant, produce the least amount of harm, and include the cultural traditions of the parents. Before describing the best interest standard decision-making model, I review the principles related to the standard so that you can develop a detailed understanding of the decision-making process affecting the care of both healthy and high-risk infants.

Beneficence

Beneficence refers to activities that assist others. Beauchamp and Childress (2001, p. 167) outline specific moral rules related to beneficence that include the following:

1. Protect and defend the rights of others.
2. Prevent harm from occurring to others.
3. Remove conditions that will cause harm to others.
4. Help persons with disabilities.

Beneficence requires positive actions, may include favoritism, and if not followed, seldom leads to legal challenges. Special relationships, such as the nurse–patient relationship, require specific beneficence related to role responsibilities. According to the ANA (2001), "The primary commitment of the nurse is to the health, welfare and safety of the client." See also the discussion of beneficence in Chapter 1.

Beneficence also includes the concept of utility. Utility in this context involves the use of analytic techniques applied in health policies that provide information regarding the benefits of a treatment compared to the detriment or costs of treatments (Beauchamp & Childress, 2001). Cost-effectiveness analysis (CEA) and cost-benefit analysis (CBA) are the two most commonly used analytic techniques to evaluate the impact on health and the safety of medical technologies. Both tools are utilized to identify the value of outcomes, one in monetary terms and one with both monetary and nonmonetary terms. QOL or cases describing cost of life years saved can be assessed utilizing CEA. Utilizing a monetary measurement, CBA provides outcomes of both benefit and cost. These analytic techniques are designed to provide information for health policy makers concerning the possible benefits and risks of medical treatments (Beauchamp & Childress, 2001).

Both risk and uncertainty are considered in the analytic techniques of CEA and CBA to determine which medical treatments or policies are beneficial. While both share the meaning that there is a lack of predictability or knowledge of future events, they are different concepts. Risk can be defined as the likelihood and extent of negative outcomes. A risk benefit analysis is the ratio of expected benefits to risks. It involves the probability of the individual experiencing harm and focuses on the acceptability of the harm related to the good that is anticipated (Beauchamp & Childress, 2001).

With insufficient evidence, there is an inability to predict or know an outcome resulting in uncertainty. There is always uncertainty in risk assessment. The challenge for the analysts in risk assessment is in knowing that their values and attitudes may determine a negative or positive prediction (Beauchamp & Childress, 2001). In the NICU, APNs must know that their values and attitudes contribute to their perception of potential benefits and harms of treatments. The APN must communicate the reasons for a specific plan based on this assessment with the direct care nurse and family.

Nonmaleficence

Nonmaleficence, described by Beauchamp and Childress (2001), refers to the obligation not to harm others by intentionally causing pain, disability, mental harm, and death. This principle focuses on a person's actions related to creating situations, participating in acts and/or not acting that result in tribulations or the risk of tribulations to others. Rules outlined by Beauchamp and Childress (2001), regarding nonmaleficence include; "do not kill, cause pain or suffering, incapacitate, cause offense or deprive others of the goods of life" (p. 117).

There are healthcare guidelines developed that specify requirements of nonmaleficence for treatment and nontreatment decisions. The guidelines include "distinctions related to withholding and withdrawing life-sustaining treatment, extraordinary (or heroic) and ordinary treatment, artificial feeding and life-sustaining medical technologies, and intended effects and merely foreseen effects" (Beauchamp & Childress, 2001, p. 119).

Beauchamp and Childress (2001) contend that the preceding guidelines may lead to over- and undertreatment. They advocate that healthcare providers consider a detailed assessment of the benefits and burdens of a treatment and determine individual medical treatment plans with the greatest benefits and least burdens to the infant, family, and society. Beauchamp and Childress (2001) provide the following descriptions of benefits and burdens related to treatment:

> If balance of benefits outweighs burdens, the obligation is to treat.
> If no reasonable hope of benefit exists, the obligation is not to treat.
> If a reasonable hope of benefit exists with significant burdensomeness,
> the treatment is optional. (p.133)

Other considerations regarding treatment decisions of the infant include the absolute value and QOL. Historically, societies and all major religions have considered the absolute value of life one of the most important values. The absolute value of life criterion is considered objective with a biologic and medical definition. However, this value is diminishing in importance. Ethicists currently are focusing their attention on the QOL criterion, which may not always benefit infants and small children (Steinberg, 1998). The QOL criterion can be considered biased, and not applicable to infants or young children who are incapable of verbally stating a personal QOL view. Dangers may exist in prioritizing the QOL definition over the "absolute value" leading to worries that a "slippery slope" might occur in the absence of precise boundaries regarding making life and death decisions (Steinberg, 1998). What is meant by "slippery slope" is that over time it might cause us to relax our view of the importance of human life and permit unjust deaths or inadequate treatment for some patients for whom benefit of treatment is possible. As Beauchamp and Childress (2001) note, "The best interest standard has sometimes been interpreted as highly malleable, thereby permitting values that are irrelevant to the patient's benefits and burdens" (p. 103). They give the example of parents giving permission for the donation of an organ from one child to a brother or sister in need where the rationale given is that it will benefit the donor to know that he or she has helped a sibling. The best interest standard is supposed to protect the interest of an individual who does not have decision-making capacity and for whom we do not know what their beliefs and values would or will be. A surrogate decisionmaker is appointed or approved to consider the benefits of various treatments and the alternatives to treatments for the infant or individual in question.

Thus, the Best Interest Standard protects another's interest by requiring a surrogate decisionmaker to consider the benefits of various treatments and the alternatives to treatments. "The surrogates consider pain, suffering and restoration, as well as loss of functioning when determining the highest benefit among available options" (Beauchamp & Childress, 2001, p.102). The Best Interest decision makers for the infant include the parents, the healthcare team, and if necessary the legal system. The decision-making framework requires the healthcare team to gather relevant medical data and to determine which treatment provides the most benefits with the least amount of pain and suffering.

Information must be shared with the family decision makers or others who have been granted the decision-making responsibility in a way that takes into account the knowledge and educational level of the ultimate decision maker. Long-term benefits and burdens are important aspects of the consideration. In addition, the healthcare team must establish and maintain therapeutic relationships with parents and include the sociocultural and religious preferences of the family in the decision-making process (Steinberg, 1998).

In summary, the best interest standard of decision making for handicapped and critically ill infants is derived from the ethical principles of beneficence and nonmaleficence. The principle of beneficence describes the obligations to protect from harm, prevent harm, and remove conditions that will cause harm to others, although this last obligation applies more to those who have the physical capacity to harm others. The principle of nonmaleficence describes the obligation to refrain from actions that intentionally cause harm and to take into consideration possible harm when making treatment decisions. The decision makers must consider all possible treatments and select the treatments that provide the highest benefit and the least harm. The QOL and the absolute value of life are to be integrated into the treatment decisions as well. Thus, the APN in the NICU is required to act positively by protecting infants and their families from harm, removing the conditions that cause harm, and helping persons with disabilities. This is facilitated by enabling positive acts by other health team members in the care of infants in the NICU.

CASE STUDY: BEST INTEREST

The transport team of Robynhood Hospital was contacted to transport a term infant with possible seizure activity for a workup from a community newborn nursery. While the transport physician obtained necessary and relevant medical data, other members of the team including the nurse and respiratory therapist prepared the transport equipment for departure. The time of the transport call was 6:30 p.m., and the staff for the night shift was arriving on the unit.

The region was experiencing a severe snowstorm with blizzard conditions reported in several areas. The oncoming nurses reported treacherous weather conditions and extreme difficulty driving. The nurse assigned to transport that night witnessed several cars and small trucks that skidded off the roads. Other nurses arriving reported many car accidents. The arriving transport nurse questioned the safety of the transport and strongly suggested that the team delay or refuse the transport completely because she believed that traveling would endanger the team. The attending physician disagreed with the transport nurse's suggestion and directed the team to proceed with the transport.

The transport physician obtained a current medical history of the infant at the community hospital. The male infant, now 12 hours old, presented at delivery with clear amniotic fluid, a nuchal cord times one (one loop of the umbilical cord wrapped around the neck during delivery), Apgar scores of 6 at 1 minute and 8 at 5 minutes of life. He was taken to the newborn nursery of the delivery hospital, where he was noted as having nonsignificant physical and clinical course. The baby was described by nurses as vigorous and after the initial evaluation spent the majority of time in the mother's room. The parents reported, and this was subsequently observed by community hospital medical and nursing staff, time-limited jerky movements consistent with seizure activity. Oxygen saturations were noted to be greater than 98% in room air, and the infant remained vigorous after the episode. After the initial episode, no further jerky movements were noted; however, the referring pediatrician requested the infant be transferred to further evaluate the possible seizure activity. No information regarding the parents' concerns was available for discussion with the physician.

The options for the transport team of Robynhood Hospital were to risk the transport in treacherous conditions or refuse the transport. The ethical dilemma the team faced was deciding what on balance was in the best interest of this newborn infant and the transport team. The NICU nursing director was contacted by the transport nurse to discuss her concerns and resolve the situation.

Using the Best Interest Standard to Explore the Case

According to the best interest standard, this situation requires the NICU nursing director to facilitate the discussion regarding the transport of this otherwise healthy infant with neurological symptoms during a severe snowstorm. The discussion needs to include the benefits of transport to a NICU with the diagnosis of suspected seizures as well as the burdens of remaining in a hospital that may not be equipped with technology and personnel to care for him. In addition, the discussion requires the consideration of the risks of transport during a severe snowstorm. Possible risks to the infant include potential weather-related accidents and harm related to the slow traveling time if he should become compromised during the journey. Additionally, an accident could damage the transport vehicle and the special equipment in which the infant is housed during transport. This type of damage could cause physiologic instability and possible harm to the infant. The speed with which the infant is returned to the NICU may create a situation where the transport team is unable to optimally provide needed interventions such as intubations for mechanical ventilation.

The NICU nursing director also must consider the benefits and burdens for the transport team. The reported travel conditions indicated that travel was dangerous, and the oncoming shift witnessed many travel accidents. This transport would require the team to travel in severe storm conditions twice, increasing the chances of harm to the team. Whereas harm to the team members is and of itself an ethical consideration, the loss of services to other infants that might accrue is an additional burden to be factored into the decision-making process. To make a decision that considers the best interests of the team and the infant, the NICU nursing director requires more information before determining how the transport team will respond to this request.

Relevant Facts

The male infant is 12 hours old. He was delivered by spontaneous vaginal delivery with Apgar scores of 6 at 1 minute and 8 at 5 minutes. He had a nuchal cord times one and weighs 8 pounds and 6 ounces. He is noted to be a vigorous infant with good tone and has voided and passed stool. His neurological exam revealed no negative findings, and no further episodes of jerky movements have been observed. His oxygen saturations remain at 98–100%. The nursing director at Robynhood Hospital contacted the NICU physician to further discuss this transport. Specifically, the nursing director was interested in what data regarding the infant were so concerning to the physician that a transport was considered urgent enough to risk traveling in the severe weather.

The nursing director also requested to speak with the ambulance company that provides the transport and obtained an updated weather forecast. By collecting all of the relevant data regarding the ability of the transport team to respond, the healthcare team can make the best decision for the infant and transport team. The nursing director requests a conference call with the NICU physician and transport nurse.

Who Are the Decision Makers?

The healthcare providers in both NICUs along with the parents are the decision makers for this infant. All are in agreement that it is in the infant's best interest, all things being equal, to be transported to the NICU for further evaluation of his neurological symptoms, but not all agree on the urgency of the transport. However, the severe snowstorm in progress alters the situation and must be factored into the decision making. The NICU transport nurse has rightly questioned the decision regarding the safety of the transport. The NICU physician informs the NICU nursing director that there is no other information concerning the medical history of this infant. The infant continues to room-in with the mother and is breastfeeding uneventfully. The lack of specialty physicians at the community hospital is the reason the NICU physician is adamant that the transport occur. The nursing director informs the physician that the storm is expected to decrease in severity in about 2 hours. The NICU physician and community hospital physician discuss the coverage that will be needed for at least 2 more hours and reach agreement regarding physician availability in the community hospital and the possibility of a consult from the specialists at Robynhood Hospital should there be changes in the infant's status. The transport team is in agreement that the infant will remain at the community hospital until the storm lessens in intensity, and then he will be transported to the NICU at the larger hospital.

After the problem is resolved, the nursing director decides that it is important to put into place a policy that will guide future similar decisions. She will convene a meeting for the purpose of policy making related to transport safety. She involves the NICU physicians, members of the transport team, the NICU CNSs and NPs, the shift charge nurses, and a member of the hospital ethics committee who serves as the NICU resource for difficult cases. Although policy making cannot anticipate all problems that can occur, guidelines are helpful in pointing to possible resources and avenues of action. Additionally, discussion of such issues after the fact is educational and permits insights about important considerations in such situations.

COLLABORATIVE DECISION MAKING

Collaborative decision-making in the NICU means that all pertinent voices are encouraged and heard as an important part of the data necessary for good (beneficent) or least harmful (nonmaleficent) care of the infant that takes into account the long- as well as the short-term implications. Important perspectives are those of the involved physicians, APNs, direct care nurses, and family members or guardians. The importance of collaboration has not always been, and is not always, understood. A collaborative environment is difficult to institute and maintain under the best of circumstances when all are willing to participate (Grace, Willis, & Jurchak, 2007). It involves trust and respect for a variety of viewpoints and the treatment of each perspective as equally relevant.

As with other aspects of neonatal care, decision making is in the process of evolving from a process of closed communication that tends to leave out family members and paternalism, where healthcare professionals determine appropriate actions, to one of transparency and collaboration. Although the importance of family involvement is in general more valued than previously, it is still not always honored currently. The following discussion provides an argument for the importance of family involvement and the role that APNs can play in encouraging this.

In earlier years, parents assumed a more passive role in the care of their critically ill and/or premature infant. They tended not to be involved in clinical decision-making processes because of barriers in communication and the hierarchical structure of the NICU (Pinch, 2002). The barriers parents faced included a lack of pertinent medical knowledge and an inadequate understanding of information provided to them by professionals, including the short- and long-term implications of treatment. In addition, in some studies aimed at gaining clarity about this problem, parents reported being overwhelmed by the technology, the terminology, a lack of continuity of relationships, and reluctance to voice concerns (King, 1992; Penticuff, 2005; Pinch & Spielman, 1990). The reluctance to participate in the process or to voice concerns stems, in part, from a fear of being labeled a difficult parent and the consequences that may have for their baby (Hurst, 2001). In addition, the decision-making process for most aspects of an infant's care became part of the medical decision-making agenda as technologic advances were made and the ability to save very premature and critically ill infants became possible. The parents' point of view was ignored or neglected. Harrison's (1993) publication of the FCC principles and the AAP endorsement of these principles created momentum for parents and professionals to achieve a more active partnership regarding the care of high-risk infants. The FCC principles are listed in Table 7-4.

Several studies conducted both in the United States and elsewhere have pointed to the desire and need of parents to participate in decision making related to their infant (Brinchmann, Førde, & Nortvedt, 2002; McHaffie, Laing, Parker, & McMillan, 2001; Orfali & Gordon, 2004; Wocial, 2000). These studies reported that parents actively sought out the opportunity to participate in all aspects of their newborn's care including ethical discussions related to withholding or withdrawing life support. All parents desired to be involved with the discussions regarding their infant but varied in their desire to participate in

Table 7-4   Family-Centered Care Principles

1. Family-centered neonatal care should be based on open and honest communication between parents and professionals on medical and ethical issues.
2. To work with professionals in making informed treatment choices, parents must have available to them the same facts and interpretation of those facts as the professionals, including medical information presented in meaningful formats, information about uncertainties surrounding treatments, information from parents whose children have been in similar medical situations, and access to the chart and rounds discussions.
3. In medical situations involving very high mortality and morbidity, great suffering, and/or significant medical controversy, fully informed parents should have the right to make decisions regarding aggressive treatment for their infants.
4. Expectant parents should be offered information about adverse pregnancy outcomes and be given the opportunity to state in advance their treatment preferences if their baby is born extremely prematurely and/or critically ill.
5. Parents and professionals must work together to acknowledge and alleviate the pain of infants in intensive care.
6. Parents and professionals should work together to ensure the safety and efficacy of neonatal treatments.
7. Parents and professionals should work together to develop nursery policies and programs that promote parenting skills and encourage maximum involvement of families with their hospitalized infant.
8. Parents and professionals must work together to promote meaningful long-term follow-up for all high-risk NICU survivors.

Source: Harrison, H. (1993). The principles for family-centered neonatal care. *Pediatrics, 92,* 643–650.

the final decision to withdraw or withhold medical support. As one parent in Brinchmann and colleagues' (2002) Norwegian study stated:

> One has to distinguish between information and discussion. Discussing is something different from making a decision. One can listen to arguments for and against. In making a decision one does not necessarily include all the things one has discussed. But anyway, I think it is important to be part of the discussion. (p. 396)

Although many complex decisions are made in the NICU regarding the care of high-risk infants, parents report their involvement tends to be considered superfluous until the question of redirection of care arises (King, 1992; Pinch, 2002). The ANA *Code of Ethics for Nurses with Interpretive Statements* (2001) describes the nurse's opportunity and responsibility to preserve, protect, and support the rights and interests of families. Informed parental consent is essential in the delivery of good care for infants and their families.

Direct care NICU nurses, through their close contact with parents, are in pivotal positions to ensure that parents receive information about what is known and is not known regarding outcomes. They are in a position to understand the family's needs for information and what is required for their comprehension of the information. Through the process of transparency, NICU APNs can model for other healthcare professionals and new nurses the delivery of appropriate information to parents. Transparent communication requires APNs to disclose to the parents the healthcare team's reasoning process along with the meaning and implications of the technical information. Through the process of transparency, parents are prepared for their decision-making role and enabled to provide informed consent when necessary for their infant.

Neonatal APNs can help parents be adequate decision makers for their infants in the NICU by discussing the burdens and benefits of treatments with parents. Penticuff (2005) reports improved parental understanding with use of an educational process aimed at explaining the types of treatment as well as the burdens associated with treatments. Parents reported increased understanding of the goals of treatment as well as the implications of those situations in which infants were not meeting the goals of treatment. These shared understandings of goals of treatment empower parents to participate more fully in the treatment decisions for their infants. Challenges to the view that parents are the ideal decision makers for their infants come from worries that they may not always make decisions that consider all of the following: their infant's QOL, their own QOL, and the value of their child's life within society. However, whenever possible, parents' wishes should be honored when medically reasonable and legally appropriate (King, 1992).

Hurst (2001) describes "empowering information" (p. 46) as a determining factor that contributes to collaborative decision making in the NICU. Empowering information is easily accessible, pertinent, and understandable. In addition, empowering information includes the descriptions of the unit's philosophy of care and practice along with how care is organized and delivered to foster supported parental independence. This is achieved through the establishment of trust that has evolved from the development of caring relationships. The APN is in the unique position to model transparency with both the medical team and the direct care nurses. In this influential position, the APN can reduce the barriers parents face in participating in the decision-making process for their infants. APNs play an important role in fostering collaborative decision making in the NICU by ensuring regular meetings, especially when goals of treatment between disciplines conflict.

Case Study: Collaborative Decision Making

Natalie Smith is a former 29-week gestation infant, now corrected to 38 weeks gestation. Natalie is preparing for discharge home after a complicated course including intubation for 2 weeks resulting from prematurity and sepsis along with a cardiac lesion that will be repaired when she is 6 months old. Natalie is now in an open crib maintaining her temperature and has not recently had any apneic or bradycardiac episodes. The main challenge for Natalie is to obtain adequate nutrition from her oral feedings. Her cardiac condition causes her to fatigue easily, and occasionally she requires supplemental gavage feedings to ensure that she receives adequate nutrition and hydration.

Natalie's parents have been very involved in her care and have participated in many meetings with the healthcare team to discuss her medical course and health needs. Natalie's healthcare team and parents are concerned that she is still not able to consistently feed by bottle. A meeting is called with the purpose of discussing the options available to ensure that Natalie will receive the necessary nutrients and hydration for her development and eventual discharge home. It is hoped that she can be discharged to her home soon. Present at the meeting are Natalie's mother and father, her primary nurse, as well as the neonatal nurse practitioner (NNP) assigned to her case. In the course of discussion, the NNP reviews Natalie's progress to date and identifies the single barrier to discharge as Natalie's inability to obtain all necessary fluids via a bottle. Natalie's parents are in agreement that Natalie is not able to complete her bottle feedings. The NNP describes possible options to consider including keeping Natalie in the hospital until she is able to bottle feed or placing a gastrostomy tube in her stomach. Natalie's parents can be taught how to care for the feeding tube and administer the amount of feeding that Natalie is not able to take orally. Natalie's parents listen to the options and both agree that neither is acceptable to them. They do not want their daughter to have a surgical procedure because of the risks of reintubations and the possibility of a prolonged ventilator requirement because of a previous experience of this. Their perception of the current problem is that Natalie will be able to achieve full feedings soon after she gets home. They inform the team that they believe that Natalie is not consuming the necessary amounts of her bottle feedings because of inconsistencies in approach used by the variety of nurses who care for her. The NNP considers the information the parents are sharing and suggests that they review her entire medical course to put into context their concerns. At the conclusion, the parents again share that they are not interested and will not consent to a gastrostomy tube.

What Are the Relevant Facts?

Natalie is unable to obtain adequate feedings via the bottle to meet her needs. This is a problem involving the principles of beneficence and nonmaleficence for the healthcare team. Professional obligations include promoting the well-being of the infant and avoiding harm. However, there are also responsibilities to the parents to help them find a solution that will meet their needs and concerns. Viewing this as a family problem rather than just a problem of avoiding harm to Natalie permits the envisioning of alternatives that could work to the benefit of all. The parents have concerns about the course of action proposed and do want Natalie home with them as soon as possible, which is understandable after the long hospitalization that she has had and the future hospitalization that she will face. We do need more information about the parents and what they are or are not willing to accept, why they seem so adamant, and whether compromise is possible. It is implied from their concerns about the different feeding styles of the nurses that there may be some trust issues. More information is needed about this. Additionally, it would be important to know how often Natalie requires extra feedings and how capable the parents are of monitoring her hydration and nutritional needs should she go home. Would they be capable of learning the gavage techniques used by the nurses? Could a homecare agency provide this service?

Who Are the Decision Makers?

Once Natalie is discharged, her parents will be the ones who make decisions for her. Currently, however, decision making is presumably a team effort. The healthcare team members are the ones who evaluate Natalie's nutritional status, who place the tube, and supply the tube feedings when necessary. Indeed if Natalie's parents objected to a necessary tube feeding, their decision would be overridden if this posed a significant risk to Natalie and there were no other options. However, the ideal is a collaborative endeavor where all parties are willing to listen to each other and try to work out a compromise. Knowing who the parents are, what their fears are, and what their needs for support are both short and long term would be helpful. Their fears about the gastrostomy tube placement and possible side effects, including needs for long-term endotracheal intubation, may not be warranted. But if they are making this connection, it is not surprising that they object. Their interest is in protecting their daughter from harm.

Collaborative Resolution

Several possibilities suggest themselves. First, if a long-term gastrostomy tube placement has not been considered while she was hospitalized, the implication is that her nutrition needs were able to be met by other means. The parents may be wrong that the different bottle feeding styles of the nurses contribute to the problem, but this could be addressed. Understanding the pattern of her fatigue, when it occurs, and what precursors exist may be helpful. This would also be useful information for the parents to have as they take her home. Another option is to have the parents consistently do the feedings themselves and be involved in monitoring her nutritional and hydration status. This way they could see for themselves what is entailed. Nurses have a responsibility to prepare the parents to care adequately for her at home anyway, and this would include the parents learning how to monitor her nutrition and hydration status. Although such problems might initially be viewed as dilemmas, they are usually not. Other options may well be available, and thus the challenge is to try to envision what these might be.

APNs with their advanced education and expanded knowledge base know how to access resources. The NNP in this case has a responsibility to work with the family on discovering options. Possible options are Natalie remains in the unit long enough to train the parents how to monitor her hydration status and safely give gavage feedings as indicated; Natalie goes home and is monitored by the parents with the adjunct assistance of visiting nurses to help monitor her nutrition and hydration and provide supplemental feedings. Natalie is brought back for insertion of a gastrostomy tube if her nutritional and hydration status is not maintained.

Questions to Consider

1. Under what conditions might we seek to override the parents' decision:
   As the NNP?
   As the visiting nurse once Natalie goes home?
2. Identify other aspects of collaboration not discussed in the case.
3. In your view what are the limits of collaboration? Give rationale.

MEDICAL FUTILITY

Futility may be defined as the inability to achieve a stated purpose. Beauchamp and Childress (2001) note that *medical futility* has several meanings that can be derived from the literature. Two pertinent meanings in the NICU setting are "the procedure cannot produce the intended physiological effect" and "the procedure cannot reasonably be expected to produce the benefit that is sought" (Beauchamp & Childress, 2001, p. 192). Additionally, the term *futility* has been divided into "quantitative futility," that is, the likelihood of benefit is extremely small, and "qualitative futility" where the quality of benefit is likely very meager (Jecker, 1998). The idea of futility has been used over the last several decades as a clinical criterion in unilateral decisions about prolonging life (Romesberg, 2003). Penticuff (1998) describes futility in the NICU as a synthesis of medical and humanistic elements. The medical element is the inability to achieve specific physiologic responses. The humanistic element is the inability to achieve elemental quality of life goals. As Truog, Frader, and Brett (1992/1998) note in their cautions about an overreliance upon futility as a reason to limit care, "A clear understanding of futility has proved to be elusive" (p. 323). Determinations of futility can be especially difficult in the NICU because it is not always possible to predict the likely long-term sequelae of a brain injury.

Although Truog and colleagues (1992/1998) argue that only certain "narrowly defined physiologic" criteria can point to a determination of futility, the concept of futility can be helpful in decision making as long as we understand that there are often no clear delineations that can be made. For example, one QOL goal for ELBW infants would be to eventually establish a reciprocal relationship with parents or guardians. If the infant is neurologically devastated from a severe intracranial hemorrhage and is blind and deaf, the infant may not have the capacity to establish meaningful relationships with parents. The philosophical arguments for this are complex and intricate and are beyond the scope of this chapter to discuss in detail. They hinge on the idea that children should be able to experience a meaningful life and not be exposed to a life where the burdens of living outweigh the benefits. Munson (2008) gives an illustrative example of when the burdens of maintaining a life might outweigh the quality of that life. He describes the short life of a child born with Hallopeau-Siemens syndrome. This terrible collagen deficit disease, which is genetic in origin, causes intractable pain and discomfort from continual blistering of the skin and mucous membranes. There is no treatment for the disease and life is usually short and very painful.

The three interacting factors involved in the analysis of futility in the NICU include (1) the impact of treatment on the probability of mortality, morbidity, and QOL, (2) the extent that treatment produces less pain and discomfort and increased comfort and benefit, and (3) the involvement and decision-making prerogative of the infant's parents (Penticuff, 1998). The use of futility as a clinical criterion in the NICU must be determined individually by each infant's response to treatment and other supportive data. In the case of the ELBW infant, decisions to redirect the goals of care, from that of prolonging life with pharmacologic and technologic interventions to providing comfort measures only, should be based on the infant's response to treatment and the parents' QOL goals for their infant, not solely the infant's gestational age or birth weight.

Case Study: Medical Futility

Mrs. M. experienced an uneventful early pregnancy but ruptured her membranes at what was estimated to be 24 weeks gestation and began to labor. She was admitted to the labor and delivery unit by her obstetrician. A NICU consult was requested. The consulting neonatologist met with Mr. and Mrs. M. while Mrs. M. was in early labor. The neonatologist informed them of the medical course their infant would likely experience and some of the possible complications of such an early delivery. In addition, they were informed that the NICU team would respond to her delivery and provide the necessary treatment for her baby.

Mr. and Mrs. M. requested that no medical treatment be administered because they did not believe their prematurely born infant would survive. Mrs. M. had no previous experience with prematurely born infants and did not want her child to suffer because she could not carry her infant to term. The information Mr. and Mrs. M. received from the neonatologist only confirmed that their wishes of no intervention at delivery were reasonable. However, the neonatologist informed Mr. and Mrs. M. that the technology to sustain the infant's life was available and that some infants born this early do survive in the NICU with the highly advanced technologic and nursing care provided there. Moreover, Baby Doe and related laws have caused many providers and institutions to be nervous about the legal ramifications of delivery practices when the delivery is very premature. Thus, a neonatologist may be moved by personal or institutional policy to attend those births suspected to be problematic for whatever reason, including prematurity. The neonatologist in this case saw herself as being legally required to attend the birth and to provide care if the baby seemed "like it could live," and she conveyed this message to the family. She went on to note that many babies survive with minimal handicaps if the necessary interventions are initiated. However, she assured the couple that she would communicate the consult findings and request of no intervention to the NICU delivery team.

Mrs. M. delivered a 560-gram female infant. The infant emerged pink, crying, and a heart rate was noted to be greater than 100 beats per minute. Based on the current legislation and the infant's condition at birth, the NICU team provided warmth and cardiopulmonary support in the form of ventilation, oxygen, and fluid though intravenous catheter for this ELBW infant.

Nurse S. admitted Baby M. to the NICU and assumed the role as the baby's primary nurse. She was aware of the neonatology consult and parents' request, as well as the reasons given for instituting treatment. Initially, Baby M. responded to treatment and required minimal interventions—Mr. and Mrs. M. started to become more optimistic. Nurse S. proceeded to establish a therapeutic relationship with Baby M.'s parents. She communicated with them daily and included them in aspects of care they were interested in such as obtaining their daughter's temperature and changing her diaper and discussed the baby's status. She talked with them about their lives and expectations, and they told her about their cultural backgrounds and beliefs. Nurse S. was concerned that the family receive the external supports they needed because they had no support structure in the area. Unfortunately, on day 7 of life, the baby suffered a severe intracranial hemorrhage that extended well into the brain as identified on ultrasound. Nurse S. requested a family meeting to inform the parents of this finding. During this meeting, the parents requested that the treatment to their daughter be stopped and that comfort measures only be offered.

Case Analysis—Discussion Questions

Using Table 2-5 as pertinent and the preceding discussion, explore this case in class or with colleagues.

1. What data would support a determination of futility and a redirection of care toward comfort measures?

2. As the NNP on duty, if a determination of futility is made, what are your responsibilities:

   To the baby?
   To the parents?
   To Nurse S.?

3. Suppose the team concludes that it is too early to determine whether the continuation of treatment is futile. How would you approach the family?

   What would your role be related to Nurse S.?

4. Given the ambiguous status of the laws governing the treatment of babies who are born at the borderline of viability (500 g or 22 weeks approximately) and the arguments that these laws can limit our ability to serve the babies' best interests, what if any are APNs' responsibilities to be politically active in challenging these laws?

5. What strategies can be used by APNs to inform the public?

SUMMARY

Advanced nursing practice in neonatal settings can be both very rewarding and very difficult. It is rewarding when an infant begins to thrive and is eventually discharged with minimal injury. It is difficult when one is faced with ambiguity and uncertainty about the infant's short- and long-term prognoses or when the infant is suspected to be experiencing ongoing suffering. Not only are these infants extremely vulnerable physically, their parents are faced with emotional turmoil and crisis during what for many others is a time of anticipation and joy. For this reason, ethical NICU practice is concerned with the needs of the family unit. Paradoxically, in the United States at least, although we are beginning to take seriously the parental interests in the child's well-being and understand the importance of involving the parents in the decision-making process, concerns about the law may trump ethical concerns about the good of the baby and the good of the family unit.

Much more could be said about ethical issues associated with NICUs. Questions have been raised about the antecedents of the current increase in premature births and whether more money should be diverted to this area of concern than is currently. There is concern about the issue of nurses being able to maintain their sense of personal integrity and about issues of moral distress and burnout. These problems were not discussed in great detail in this chapter but were discussed earlier in the book and later related to other specialties. When nurses experience prolonged distress in their workplace, they may leave their jobs or become more resistant to noticing ethical issues. Either case is liable to contribute to the problem of providing good care for these infants and appropriate support for their families.

DISCUSSION QUESTIONS

In the collaboration case presented earlier in this chapter, the parents would not consent to a gastrostomy tube for their baby. Although there were options available to redress the issue in that case, alternative scenarios might be more difficult to resolve. Suppose the mother does not speak English. She and her husband are here for a year related to his lecturing appointment. The baby has been in the NICU for several weeks. Usually, the husband serves as the translator. He has to go back to Turkey (they are of Kurdish origin). The baby is almost ready for discharge, but in this case a gastrostomy tube is necessary if the baby is to go home. The mother is unable to understand the request for consent to the procedure, which the nurse thought the husband had explained to her. The only available interpreter who speaks her language is Turkish. When the interpreter arrives and the mother discovers his origin, she is horrified (this is reported by the interpreter) and will not talk to him.

1. What are the important issues here?
2. How would you take into account cultural beliefs and values in discharge planning?
3. What avenues of action are available?
4. For a culture for which you are not aware of the beliefs and values, how would you go about gathering information about these?
5. What is the role of empathy or self-reflection in such cases?

REFERENCES

American Academy of Pediatrics. (2007). Non-initiation or withdrawal of intensive care for high-risk newborns. *Committee on Fetus and Newborn Pediatrics 2007, 119*, 401–403.

American Nurses Association. (2001). *Code of ethics for nurses with interpretive statements.* Washington, DC: Author.

Anspach, R. (1993). *Deciding who lives: Fateful choices in the intensive care nursery.* Berkeley: University of California Press.

Avery, G. B. (1998). Futility considerations in the neonatal intensive care unit. *Seminars in Perinatology, 22*(3), 216–222.

Beauchamp, T., & Childress, J. (2001). *Principles of biomedical ethics* (5th ed.). New York: Oxford University Press.

Born Alive Infant Protection Act. (2001). Retrieved January 23, 2008, from http://www.nrlc.org/Federal/Born_Alive_Infants/Baipatext.pdf.

Brinchmann, B. S., Førde, R., & Nortvedt, P. (2002). What matters to the parents? A qualitative study of parents' experiences with life-and-death decisions concerning their premature infants. *Nursing Ethics, 9*(4), 386–404.

Brinchmann, B. S., & Nortvedt, P. (2001). Ethical decision making in neonatal units—the normative significance of vitality. *Medicine, Healthcare & Philosophy, 4*, 193–200.

Catlin, A. (2005). Thinking outside the box: Prenatal care and the call for a prenatal advance directive. *Journal of Perinatal & Neonatal Nursing, 19*(2), 169–176.

Catlin, A. (2007). Commentary on NANN position statement 3015: NICU nurse involvement in ethical decisions (treatment of critically ill newborns). Ethical issues in newborn care. *Advances in Neonatal Care, 7*(5), 269.

Duff, R., & Campbell, A. (1973, November 12). Shall this child die? *Newsweek*, 70.

Fegran, L., Helseth, S., & Slettebo, A. (2006). Nurses as moral practitioners encountering parents in neonatal intensive care units. *Nursing Ethics, 13*(1), 52–64.

Grace, P. J., Willis, G. G., & Jurchak, M. (2007). Good patient care: Egalitarian inter-professional collaboration as a moral imperative. *American Society of Bioethics and Humanities Exchange, 10*(1), 8–9.

Grundstein-Amado, R. (1992). Differences in ethical decision-making processes among nurses and doctors. *Journal of Advanced Nursing, 17*, 129–137.

Hack, M., Flannery, D., Schluter, M., Cartar, L., Borowski, E., & Klein, N. (2002). Outcomes in young adulthood for very-low-birth-weight infants. *New England Journal of Medicine, 346*(3), 149–157.

Harrison, H. (1993). The principles for family-centered neonatal care. *Pediatrics, 92*, 643–650.

Hurst, I. (2001). Vigilant watching over: Mothers' actions to safeguard their premature babies in the newborn intensive care nursery. *Journal of Perinatal & Neonatal Nursing, 15*(3), 39–57.

Hurst, I. (2005). First rule: Choose your battles wisely. *Pediatrics, 116*, 288.

Jecker, N. (1998). *Futility.* University of Washington, School of Medicine Ethics Website. Retrieved February 9, 2008, from http://depts.washington.edu/bioethx/topics/futil.html.

King, N. (1992). Transparency in neonatal intensive care. *Hastings Center Report, 22*(3), 18–25.

Kopelman, L. (2005). Are the 21-year-old Baby Doe Rules misunderstood or mistaken? *Pediatrics, 115*, 797–802.

Lantos, J. D., Mokalla, M., & Meadow, W. (1997). Resource allocation in neonatal and medical ICUs . Epidemiology and rationing at the extremes of life. *American Journal of Respiratory and Critical Care Medicine, 156*, 185–189.

McHaffie, H. E., Laing, I. A., Parker, M., & McMillan, J. (2001). Deciding for imperiled newborns: Medical authority or parental autonomy. *Journal of Medical Ethics, 27*, 104–109.

Meadow, W., Lee, G., Lin, K., & Lantos, J. (2004). Changes in mortality for extremely low birth weight infants in the 1990s: Implications for treatment decisions and resource use. *Pediatrics, 113*(5), 1223–1229.

Munson, R. (2008). *Intervention and reflection: Basic issues in medical ethics* (8th ed.). Belmont, CA: Wadsworth/Thomson Learning.

Orfali, K. (2004). Parental role in medical decision-making: Fact or fiction? A comparative study of ethical dilemmas in French and American neonatal intensive care units. *Social Science & Medicine, 58*, 2009–2022.

Orfali, K., & Gordon, E. J. (2004). Autonomy gone awry; a cross-cultural study of parents' experiences in neonatal intensive care units. *Theoretical Medicine, 25*, 329–365.

Penticuff, J. H. (1998). Defining futility in neonatal intensive care. *Nursing Clinics of North America, 33*(2), 339–352.

Penticuff, J. (2005). Effectiveness of an intervention to improve parent-professional collaboration in neonatal intensive care. *Journal of Perinatal & Neonatal Nursing, 19*(2), 169–176.

Pinch, W. (2002). *When the bough breaks: Parental perceptions of ethical decision making in the NICU.* Lanham, MD: University Press of America.

Pinch, W., & Spielman M. L. (1990). The parent's perspective: Ethical decision-making in neonatal intensive care. *Journal of Advanced Nursing, 15*, 712–719.

Pinch, W., & Spielman, M. L. (1993). Parental perceptions of ethical issues post NICU discharge. *Western Journal of Nursing Research, 15*(4), 422–440.

Rebagliato, M., Cuttini, M., Broggin, L., Berbik, I., de Vonderweid, U., Hansen, G., et al. (2000). Neonatal end-of-life decision-making. Physicians' attitudes and relationship with self-reported practices in 10 European countries. *Journal of the American Medical Association, 284*, 2451–2459.

Romesberg, T. L. (2003). Futile care and the neonate. *Advances in Neonatal Care, 3*(5), 213–219.

Sayeed, S. A. (2005). Baby Doe redux? The Department of Health and Human Services and the Born-Alive Infants Protection Act of 2002: A cautionary not on normative neonatal practice. *Pediatrics, 116*(4), 577–585.

Sayeed, S. A. (2006). The marginally viable newborn: Legal challenges, conceptual inadequacies, and reasonableness. *Journal of Law and Medical Ethics, 34*(3), 600–610.

Singh, J., Lantos, J., & Meadow, W. (2004). End-of-life after birth: Death and dying in a neonatal intensive care unit. *Pediatrics, 114*, 1620–1626.

Spence, K. (2000). The best interest principle as a standard for decision making in the care of neonates. *Journal of Advanced Nursing, 31*(6), 1286–1292.

Steinberg, A. (1998). Decision-making and the role of surrogacy in withdrawal or withholding of therapy in neonates. *Clinics in Perinatology, 25*(3), 779–790.

Truog, R., Frader, J., & Brett, A. (1998). The problem with futility. In J. Monagle & D. Thomasma (Eds.), *Health care ethics: Critical issues for the 21st Century* (pp. 323–329). Gaithersburg, MD: Aspen. (Reprinted from *New England Journal of Medicine, 326*(23), 1560–1565, 1992.)

Vohr, B., Wright, L., Dusick, A., Perritt, R., Poole, W., Delaney-Black, V., et al. (2004). Site differences and outcomes of extremely-low-birth-weight infants. *Pediatrics, 113*, 781–789.

Wilson-Costello, D., Freidman, H., Minich, N., Fanaroff, A., & Hack, M. (2005). Improved survival rates with increased neurodevelopmental disability for extremely low birth weight infants in the 1990s. *Pediatrics, 115*, 997–1003.

Wocial, L. D. (2000). Life support decisions involving imperiled infants. *Journal of Perinatal & Neonatal Nursing, 14*(2), 73–86.

CHAPTER 8

Nursing Ethics and Advanced Practice: Children and Adolescents

Nan Gaylord

So many people feel so overwhelmed and disempowered by the stresses of modern life that they convince themselves they can't make a difference. So they don't even try. They bury their talents in the ground and let their spirits wither on the vine of life. I hope they will bestir themselves at least to say every day as an anonymous old man did, "I don't have the answers, life is not easy, but my heart is in the right place."
—*Marian Wright Edelman*

. I've learned that people will forget what you said, people will forget what you did, but people will never forget how you made them feel.
—*Maya Angelou*

INTRODUCTION

The health care of the child requires the child's parents' involvement for success. Children are integrally dependent upon their parents for their physical care, emotional support, transportation, and nutrition; parents are ultimately responsible for their children and their children's well-being. Therefore, ethical concerns of children involve their parents. Caretakers for children are most often their parents; however, it is acknowledged that there are other persons who care for children besides parents. This chapter uses the term *parents* to encompass all of those persons who may assume the primary responsibility for children, whether those are grandparents, aunts, foster parents, or appointed guardians. Assurance of who does have legal custody, and thus is legally permitted to give consent for interventions or other actions on behalf of the child in the absence of a parent, should be ascertained where healthcare-related interventions are needed.

Parents have a vested interest in, and generally the legal capacity to consent for, the care provided to their children. Parents generally care about their children and are ultimately responsible for addressing the health needs of their children. For the most part, this means parents make healthcare decisions that are in the child's best interest. Therefore, overriding the parents' request for, or denial of, care for their child should not be undertaken lightly because the consequences of those decisions are ones with which parents must live.

The rights-based autonomous person ethical stance in health care for adults (as discussed in earlier chapters) is not appropriate in the care of children because the one-to-one relationship with the healthcare provider is not possible when caring for children. Additionally, inclusion of as many support persons as necessary into the child's care, upon request of the child or parent, is advantageous for children who require significant adaptation in the home or community. It has been noted that to nurture a healthy, happy child in today's world may take a village. "And we have learned that to raise a happy, healthy and hopeful child, it takes a family, it takes teachers, it takes clergy, it takes business people, it takes community leaders, it takes those who protect our health and safety, it takes all of us" (Clinton, 1996). Therefore, inclusion of family members and family supporters is a component of the health care of children, and those invited persons are not excluded from information or care as they may be in the autonomous patient model of care.

Related to the care of children, the principle of autonomy centers around informed consent, and the question to be answered is, "Is the healthcare decision made knowing all the risks and benefits?" Therefore, the major ethical concerns evidenced in the care of children are parental consent or refusal, adolescent consent or refusal, and child assent or refusal. The outcomes of healthcare decisions in the ethical care of children should be to promote the parents' ability to care for the child, the child's ability to care for him or herself, and collaboration between the healthcare provider/system and the family.

Although Gilligan's (1982) ethical feminist perspective has received criticism in the rights-based healthcare arena (as discussed in Chapters 1 and 3), an ethic of care is applicable to the care of children. This perspective emphasizes responsibilities and relationships. Cockburn (2005) promotes this perspective because it allows children to be active social players with a voice rather than passive recipients of care and rights. Additionally, communication in this ethical stance is valued because it is the foundation of stable, caring relationships. This relationship focus gives rise to the moral orientation of care. The pediatric provider, including the advanced practice nurse (APN), with this ethical focus strives to be the kind of person who fosters relationships by presenting a caring attitude when others such as pediatric patients and their families are encountered. This interest and concern are manifested through "attentiveness to the other's particular needs and unique life circumstances and through the expression of compassion when faced with great need or vulnerability on the part of the other" (Keller, 1996). Communication about health information within the context of relationships and responsibilities is important, and adversarial encounters diminish the capacities of such relationships (child to provider, parent to provider, child to parent) to promote healing and growth. It is essential that the pediatric healthcare provider values, maintains, and promotes those relationships that the child is physically and emotionally dependent upon as well as other relationships by which the child's sense of self and security is nurtured.

FREQUENTLY ENCOUNTERED CONCERNS

Two case studies follow. They demonstrate frequently encountered ethical concerns in the care of children.

Case 1: Immunizations

John is brought to the health center by his mother for a pre-kindergarten physical examination and health assessment. The nurse practitioner ensures that the child's hearing and vision are normal, the physical examination reveals no concerns, and the child is free from contagious diseases at this visit. Immunizations that are due between the ages of 4 and 6 years are generally administered during this health screening visit. However, when the nurse practitioner begins to discuss the recommended immunizations, the mother responds, "We are not giving John any immunizations." Upon further questioning as to her rationale for not immunizing John against the covered childhood diseases and tetanus, his mother states that she does not want to expose John to the multiple serious risks posed by the vaccines (Fictional case provided by J. Gladson, MSN).

Questions

1. When can parents refuse immunizations?
2. How can the ethics of care model assist in the resolution of these issues?
3. When does the greater good for the population outweigh parental (individual) rights?
4. In what cases do interventions for the child override parental rights/consent?

Discussion

The risks of the diseases that are prevented by the recommended immunizations are higher than the risk of receiving the vaccines. For instance, if the measles, mumps, and rubella (MMR) vaccine is refused and the child acquires measles, the possible sequelae of the disease include the following:

> Ear infection, pneumonia, seizures (jerking and staring), brain damage, and death. A vaccine, like any medicine, is capable of causing serious problems, such as severe allergic reactions. The risk of MMR vaccine causing serious harm, or death, is extremely small. Getting MMR vaccine is much safer than getting any of these three diseases. Most people who get MMR vaccine do not have any problems with it. (Centers for Disease Control and Prevention, 2003)

All healthcare providers who administer immunizations through the Vaccine for Children program are required to provide parents with the vaccine information sheet (VIS) relative to the vaccine received. The information provided by the Centers for Disease Control and Prevention (CDC) in the MMR VIS goes on to state that some persons may experience the following:

Mild Problems

- Fever (up to 1 person out of 6)
- Mild rash (about 1 person out of 20)
- Swelling of glands in the cheeks or neck (rare)

  If these problems occur, it is usually within 7–12 days after the shot. They occur less often after the second dose.

Moderate Problems

- Seizure (jerking or staring) caused by fever (about 1 out of 3,000 doses)
- Temporary pain and stiffness in the joints, mostly in teenage or adult women (up to 1 out of 4)
- Temporary low platelet count, which can cause a bleeding disorder (about 1 out of 30,000 doses)

Severe Problems (Very Rare)

- Serious allergic reaction (less than 1 out of a million doses)
- Several other severe problems have been known to occur after a child gets MMR vaccine. But this happens so rarely, experts cannot be sure whether they are caused by the vaccine or not. These include:
  - Deafness
  - Long-term seizures, coma, or lowered consciousness
  - Permanent brain damage (CDC, 2003)

When a parent reads the VIS with all the preceding potential problems listed, concern is frequently generated, yet parents still for the most part provide consent for administration of the vaccines. Consent, however, has been found in one research study to rely heavily on the trust built with the child's primary caregiver (Benin, Wisler-Scher, Colson, Shapiro, & Holmboe, 2006) rather than an understanding of information. The study found that mothers who wish to vaccinate their infants and those who wished not to vaccinate both lacked sufficient information regarding immunizations for them to qualify as being informed. Smith, Kennedy, Wooten, Gust, and Pickering (2006) found that healthcare providers were able to influence parents positively in regards to vaccination safety. Healthcare providers who spend more time and effort discussing vaccine safety concerns as well as vaccine benefits with parents are likely to improve immunization rates. Parents refuse immunizations for multiple reasons including religious beliefs, cultural, and safety concerns. There have been clinical monographs and studies (Diekema & Committee of Bioethics, 2005; Fair, Murphy, Golaz, & Wharton, 2002) describing parents' rationale for vaccine refusal, and most propose that additional health information and education is needed for parents to make fully informed choices regarding vaccines. Most parents and grandparents of today are not familiar with vaccine-preventable diseases and the morbidity and mortality associated with those diseases, so their focus is on the possible side effects of the vaccines for their own child.

Refusing Immunizations

Once fully informed of the pros and cons of vaccines, the parents still have the right to refuse immunizations for their child. Indeed there are certain high-risk children who should not receive vaccines, but, for those who are eligible, the vaccine is highly recommended. So, what is the concern if parents refuse the vaccinations that are recommended for their child? Yes, the unimmunized child will probably not acquire the vaccine-preventable disease in a community where the immunization rates are high. In fact, it may be in the individual child's best interest not to receive the vaccine and expose the child to vaccine-associated risks. Yet that child is benefiting from the actions of other children's parents who consent for their children to receive the vaccine and expose them to vaccine-associated risks. When the incidence of the disease is low because of a high community immunization rate, an occasional parental refusal is not problematic. Because more parents, however, are beginning to refuse vaccines, the vaccine-preventable diseases will increase in incidence and even some of those children who are vaccinated will contract the disease because no vaccine is 100% effective.

Although immunizations are required upon school entry, immunization refusal is acceptable if parents sign a waiver stating they are refusing immunizations for their child based on personal or religious reasons. In 2003, about

38,000 children received exemptions from state vaccination requirements. A study by Omer and associates (2006) revealed that the mean exemption rate has increased an average of 5–6% per year for those states with nonmedical/personal or religious exemptions during the years of 2001–2004. State policies granting personal belief exemptions and states that easily grant exemptions are associated with increased pertussis incidence. Another study (Feiken et al., 2000) concluded that schools with outbreaks of a certain infectious disease had more children in attendance that had exempted immunizations than other schools. It was found that children who were exempted from immunizations were 22.2 times more likely to acquire measles and 5.9% more likely to contract pertussis when compared to those who were vaccinated. A similar study (Salmon et al., 1999) found that the risk of measles was 35 times greater in unvaccinated than in vaccinated children. Another study (Parker et al., 2006) examined the 2005 measles outbreak in Indiana and found that 94% of the people who contracted measles were unvaccinated and 88% of those were under the age of 20 years. All parents should be aware of the increased risk of contracting measles and pertussis when requesting immunization exemptions for school entry. Additionally, between the years 1992 and 2000, 12 out of the 15 cases of tetanus in children were in children who had not been vaccinated against tetanus (Fair et al., 2002). Parents should also be advised of the risk of not vaccinating their children against tetanus. Tetanus, although relatively rare, is a very dangerous disease with a risk of mortality.

The Supreme Court has ruled on several occasions that requiring vaccination by the state is permissible, and that "the very concept of ordered liberty precludes allowing every person to make his own standards on matters of conduct in which the society as a whole has important interests" (Malone & Hinman, 2003). That is, restrictions on personal liberty are sometimes permissible when the possibility of serious or widespread harm exists within a society. There is no state that has mandated, nor has the nation been willing to mandate, immunizations for children as yet. A community dialogue has been proposed to resolve, or at least discuss, the ethics of a national immunization policy. To increase immunization rates several issues need to be considered (Feudtner & Marcus, 2001) including equal access to immunizations for all children, fair share of the benefits and risks of immunizations, and due respect for those families who refuse to have their children vaccinated. At this point in the United States, we have made vaccines available for all children via the National Vaccine for Children program. Access to the vaccines is facilitated via local health departments and private healthcare offices. The United States has attempted to protect children from vaccine-associated risks by reporting reactions to the Vaccine Adverse Event Reporting System (VAERS). This national program is a postmarketing safety surveillance program.

That is, it keeps track of vaccines that have received Food and Drug Administration (FDA) approval to be widely distributed. If a vaccine seems to be causing unanticipated or serious problems, the FDA and the CDC will investigate further. Compensation to persons injured by vaccines is available through the National Vaccine Injury Compensation Program (VICP). For adverse reactions to vaccines, there is reimbursement for healthcare expenses, payment for projected healthcare expenses, and compensation for pain and suffering. Therefore, it is the case that vaccines are not without side effects and some do have serious adverse effects. Therefore, we cannot reassure families that there is no risk, but we can discuss the risk versus benefits of immunizations. We can try to determine what the needs and capacities of the child's decision maker are related to comprehending information and exchange information with them accordingly.

Ethics of Care Model

At this point, the decision whether or not to vaccinate one's child is a decision to be made by parents, hopefully after being adequately informed. The transfer of this information by healthcare providers, specifically APNs, requires knowledge and time (Hansson, Kihibom, Tuvemo, Olsen, & Rodriguez, 2007). It has been demonstrated that the time to explain the targeted diseases, the rationale for the development of the vaccine, the potential sequelae of the disease process, the vaccine-associated risks, and the anticipated side effects of the vaccine affects the decision of parents. It may be, too, that the parent does not consent to vaccines at that visit, but the relationship of the APN or other provider with the child and parent is ongoing and the discussion can continue at the next visit.

As the child develops understanding of health issues, pressure is frequently put on the parent by the child, and the child requests the vaccine in the presence of the parent. However, if it is the case that the parent consents and the child refuses, then it becomes important to explain to the child in age and developmentally appropriate language why the vaccine is important. The use of an ethic of care means that the provider enlists the child's cooperation and involvement through open honest communication about possible discomforts and how these will be relieved. However, if the child fails to assent, this does not trump the parents' consent and their request for vaccine administration, although patience and explanation by the provider are essential to maintenance of the relationships involved.

The American Academy of Pediatrics Committee on Bioethics (1995) stresses the importance of trying to gain a child's assent and encourages involving children in discussions about their health care to "foster trust and a better physician [provider]-patient relationship, and perhaps improve long-term health outcomes." Although, they do also recognize that there may be occasions when one does not try to elicit a child's assent if the treatment is necessary and will be provided. In such cases, it is the healthcare provider's responsibility to lessen the child's fear and apprehension and minimize the child's distress. The process of gaining a child's assent should include at minimum all of the following elements:

1. Helping the patient achieve a developmentally appropriate awareness of the nature of his or her condition.
2. Telling the patient what he or she can expect with tests and treatment(s).
3. Making a clinical assessment of the patient's understanding of the situation and the factors influencing how he or she is responding (including whether there is inappropriate pressure to accept testing or therapy).
4. Soliciting an expression of the patient's willingness to accept the proposed care. Regarding this final point, we note that no one should solicit a patient's views without intending to weigh them seriously. In situations in which the patient will have to receive medical care despite his or her objection, the patient should be told that fact and should not be deceived. (American Academy of Pediatrics Committee on Bioethics, 1995, p. 316)

Although assent is important, it is also important not to view consent simply as a one-time event involving a test of the child's understanding or ignorance. The consent *process* can nurture and enlarge children's understanding, trust, and confidence in caring for themselves, and this is especially true in children with chronic illnesses. Over time as children learn about their diseases and in the process of maturing, they begin to acquire more and more responsibility for their care. Through the child's personal growth and in the process of parental–child, healthcare provider–child interactions, the responsibility for managing the illness may be transferred from parent to child over time. In a study by Alderson, Sutcliffe, and Curtis (2006), children and parents repeatedly showed "an awareness of their own responsibilities and capabilities that suggests they would regard parents' overruling of children's responsible health care decisions as a violation of parental responsibility and loving family intimacy" (p. 33).

In the case of vaccination refusal for a minor child by his or her parent, when the unimmunized person reaches the age of consent (18 years of age in most states), he or she will of course be free to seek immunizations independently. In some states and some health departments, immunizations may be provided to adolescents as young as 14 without parental consent. The American Academy of Pediatrics Bioethics Committee (1995) introduces another concept, parental permission, into the consent discussion, stating that children of these ages may actually provide consent for their own treatment and parents by law are informed of their child's decision; however, parental consent is not required. Discussion around the age of consent for immunizations is now complicated by the human papillomavirus (HPV) vaccine because an adolescent may seek care for sexual health at the age of 14 without parental consent and this vaccine was developed to prevent cervical cancer. The question of whether this vaccine falls into sexual health care or the traditional immunization schedule that requires parental consent is presently being debated (Farrell & Rome, 2007).

Overriding Parental Consent for the Greater Good of the Community

With the passage of time and because vaccine-preventable diseases are no longer common, thus familiar to the public, it is anticipated that the numbers of persons refusing vaccines will continue to increase. When outbreaks of these diseases do occur as they almost inevitably will, persons who are not vaccinated will seek the vaccine but not before many more will acquire the disease. At some point, we may need to reevaluate our more lenient school exemption policies or introduce mandatory immunizations for school entrance as was the intent of mandatory immunization laws when originally instituted. Parents today have a choice, and providers should continue to ensure that this decision is well informed and that the long-term as well as short-term risks and benefits are understood. This is important both to protect the children from future problems and also others for whom acquiring these infectious diseases could be deadly, such as those with compromised immune systems.

A child is required to attend school (or receive home schooling) until he or she is 16 years of age, whether parents agree that education is important or not. This requirement is for the community's good as well as the individual's, but permission or consent is not required by the individual or his or her parents. Thus, a precedent exists for ensuring a good by limiting the liberty to dissent. In health care, one example of when parental consent for treatment is not required is when the child has tuberculosis. Treatment for tuberculosis is mandated for the common good whether the parents agree or not because treatment is required to prevent the disease's spread to others. Thus, the risk of likely and serious harm to others, as discussed in earlier chapters, is a valid limit on the freedom to act according to one's own will. Generally, superseding the parental right to consent or refuse health care is reserved for cases when the best interests of the child are at risk. For the most part, parents are left alone to nurture their children in accordance with their own values and beliefs.

Overriding Parental Rights/Consent in the Best Interest of the Child

In cases where the child's life is threatened by the parents, parental neglect exists, the parent is making an obviously poor choice that will affect the child's well-being, or the parent's beliefs are endangering a child's physical health, healthcare providers, child protection professionals, and ultimately the courts will step in and override the parents' rights to make decisions for or sometimes even to care for the child. Most frequently, this occurs in the community setting and as a consequence of child abuse or neglect. However, in the healthcare setting, if parents are refusing lifesaving interventions, healthcare providers can request that the courts give them permission to intervene with those measures necessary for the safety, well-being, or benefit of the child. The reason for this is that the child is considered to have the right to live long enough to be able to decide for him- or herself what beliefs are acceptable. The following is a case that exemplifies this particular problem—a parental belief system that may put the child at risk of death or serious impairment.

Case 2: Parental Refusal of Blood for a Child

A 7-year-old male presented with his parents to the outpatient surgery unit for a tonsillectomy. After preoperative arrangements were complete, the patient was taken to surgery. A tonsillectomy was performed without difficulty, but a substantial amount of blood was lost during the procedure. After the patient was taken to the postanesthesia recovery room, a complete blood count (CBC) was drawn from a blood sample and revealed normal results, with the exception of a hemoglobin (8.2 gm/dL) and hematocrit (30.4%), which had decreased in comparison to the baseline results of a hemoglobin (12.0 gm/dL) and hematocrit (40.0%). After the results were evaluated, the surgeon ordered 1 unit of packed red blood cells (PRBC) to be given. However, when the surgeon, Dr. J., went to discuss the blood transfusion with the parents, they became very upset and told Dr. J. that a blood transfusion would not be possible because of their religious beliefs. The surgeon explained the risks for the patient not receiving the blood transfusion, including the possibility of hypovolemic shock resulting from inadequate circulating blood volume. Inadequate circulation decreases tissue perfusion and can result in organ failure and death. The parents continued to be adamant that their son not receive the blood transfusion despite the surgeon's medical advice (see Chapter 12 for further discussion of the beliefs of Jehovah's Witnesses and the anesthesia provider). The parents were informed that, unfortunately, a court hearing would be necessary to overrule their authority and permit this intervention, which was seen as necessary for their son's safety. However, they continued to be adamant that their son not receive a blood transfusion.

During the emergency court hearing, the presiding judge ruled in favor of giving the patient a blood transfusion. The judge stated that although he respected the religious beliefs of the parents, the life of a child had to be considered more important. Thus, the child received the blood transfusion. However, at a difficult time the family was exposed to further distress. This may have been unavoidable, but often such problems can be anticipated.

Discussion

In primary care settings, healthcare providers would usually know what a family's beliefs and values are. These are good places to have discussions with families about what their beliefs and values mean in the context of highly technologic healthcare settings and how they can best communicate these to providers should they ever need to be hospitalized. In this case, surgery was elective and scheduled ahead of time. Thus, problems could have been anticipated and alternatives or options explored. Cases such as these can, however, be prevented or at least anticipated if parents express their beliefs prior to the intervention, especially if the intervention is nonemergent. Communication between the surgeon, the preoperative nurse, the parents, and the child could elucidate the religious beliefs of the family. Autologous or family-member-directed blood donation may be permissible, depending on the belief system. In such cases, blood could be garnered ahead of time and stored for use if needed (storage is time-sensitive). Anticipation of problems can lessen the possibility of conflict between the family and the healthcare professionals. Additionally, a decision to override the parents' wishes should be made only after careful consideration and with a reasonable certainty that the child really is at risk. Other surgeons may have been willing to observe for evidence of circulatory compromise rather than treat immediately, although a court order may still need to be obtained for precautionary purposes (in the event of an emergency or deterioration). The child may be admitted for observation and monitoring of the hematocrit/hemoglobin levels for the next 24 hours because these levels are reported as borderline indications for transfusion after acute blood loss (Carson, Noveck, Berlin, & Gould, 2002; Guay, de Moerloose, & Lasne, 2006; Lacroix & Corwin, 2007), although not enough information is provided in the clinical scenario to determine if that is the case. There are, however, probably no surgeons willing to chance losing a child from excessive bleeding from a tonsillectomy, and they would err on the side of providing the lifesaving measure by overriding the parents' refusal to consent.

Other examples of court intervention for lifesaving healthcare interventions include effective treatments for cancer that the parents are refusing, minor interventions in the intensive care nursery for infants who will live with minimal impact from their prematurity (see Chapter 7), and parents who are incompetent to make decisions for themselves or their children for whatever reason. APNs who suspect child abuse are obligated to report the abuse to the appropriate authorities, and parents lose their rights as parents if the children are judged to be in danger and/or neglected. These children are removed from the home and placed in foster care or with another family member until appropriate intervention is decided.

For parents to lose their ability to consent for healthcare decisions or to have the court mandate care of a particular child requires that the intervention is life-saving and the child will die without the intervention. Until that point, parents can decide what care is and is not appropriate for their own child. Again, for the most part parents are left to nurture their children in accordance with their own values and beliefs.

ADOLESCENTS

Case 3: The Request for Birth Control

Julie, a 15-year-old high school freshman, comes into the healthcare setting and requests a pregnancy test and birth control. She is also complaining of a sore throat and cough. You have not seen Julie before and know nothing about her, her family, and current situation. No one has accompanied her to the visit. What should your response be to Julie's request?

Questions

1. Based on Julie's age, what services is the APN able to provide?
2. What services may not be provided?
3. What other consent/assent issues are confronted when caring for adolescents?
4. How can the ethics of care model assist in the resolution of these issues?

Discussion

Confidential assessment, pregnancy testing, and provision of a birth control method for adolescents seeking contraception as in the preceding situation are permitted in every state. For all women, including adolescents, reproductive health services are accessible and confidential based on the Title X of the Public Health Service Act, which was signed into effect in 1970 by President Nixon. In 1977, family planning services, including the availability of contraception, were extended to minors under the age of 16 as a result of the Supreme Court's decision in *Carey v. Population Services International* (Planned Parenthood, 2005). As a result, clinics supported by Title X funds have been able to serve adolescents requesting these services since 1977 without parental consent or permission.

Services the APNs Can Provide

However, only 36 states have laws that allow the provision of contraceptive services to adolescents without parental consent, even though it has been approved at the national level. Fourteen states require parental permission or notification for adolescents seeking contraceptive services (Guttmacher Institute, 2008). All 50 states legally permit the treatment of sexually transmitted diseases (STDs) in adolescents without parental consent or notification.

New parental notification laws (PNL) have recently been initiated by lawmakers at the urging of conservative parents and interest groups. These parents were concerned about not knowing when their children sought these services and believed it to be a parent's right to know. Additionally, the proposed PNL were intended to help adolescents by increasing adolescents' social and emotional support in sexual decision making. However, in a recent study (Eisenberg, Swain, Bearinger, Sieving, & Resnick, 2005), researchers asked parents their views on (1) PNL when minor children seek to obtain prescription contraceptives, (2) the exceptions to PNL parents would endorse, and (3) the consequences they would expect if PNL were instituted. Only 42.3% of the parents originally asked completed the telephone questionnaire. Fifty-one percent of those parents thought PNL were a good idea when teens sought reproductive care. However, 96.1% expected at least 1 negative consequence to result with the enactment of PNL and 47.6% expected 5 or more negative consequences. The more negative consequences that were expected, the more reticent the parents were about enacting such laws. The study concluded that parents could be educated about the need for confidentiality in the delivery of these services if consequences could be delineated. One such consequence is reported by Reddy and colleagues (2002) who found that 59% of the girls who received reproductive health care would stop using the care if their parents were informed when they sought prescription birth control. Jones and colleagues (2005) found that 60% of the 1,526 adolescent females surveyed by a research team had parents who knew about their accessing of contraceptive services. If parental involvement was mandated, however, adolescents responded with several actions they would consider. Forty-six percent would use an over-the-counter method, and 18% would go to a private physician. Seven percent said that they would stop having sex as one response, but only 1% indicated this would be their only reaction. One in 5 adolescents would use no contraception or rely on withdrawal as one response to mandated notification.

PNL have not been supported by professional organizations for these reasons and the Association of Women's Health, Obstetric and Neonatal Nurses (AWHONN, 2000) states that "the health risks to the adolescents are so impelling that legal barriers and deference to parental involvement should not stand in the way of needed health care." The American College of Obstetrics (2003) reinforces this by stating, "The potential health risks to adolescents if they are unable to obtain reproductive health services are so compelling that legal barriers and deference to parental involvement should not stand in the way of needed health care for patients who request confidentiality (p. 2)."

Services Not Able to Be Provided

If Julie is pregnant and is considering an elective termination of the pregnancy, 35 states require parental involvement (Planned Parenthood, 2007), 21 states require parental consent, and 11 states require parental notification when an adolescent seeks abortion services. In addition, Julie cannot consent to the evaluation and treatment of her complaints of sore throat and cough. Full legal consent for healthcare interventions, other medical procedures, and pharmacologic therapeutics is given to all persons at 18 years of age, so evaluation and treatment, if indicated, would require parental consent.

According to the American Academy of Pediatrics (1995):

> Laws designate two settings in which minors have sole authority to make health care decisions. First, certain minors are deemed "emancipated" and treated as adults for all purposes.
>
> Definitions of the emancipated minor include those who are:
>
> 1. self-supporting and/or not living at home;
> 2. married;
> 3. pregnant or a parent;
> 4. in the military; or
> 5. declared to be emancipated by a court.

Second, many states give decision-making authority (without the need for parental involvement) to some minors who are otherwise unemancipated but who have decision-making capacity ("mature minors") or who are seeking treatment for certain medical conditions, such as sexually transmitted diseases, pregnancy, and drug or alcohol abuse (p. 2).

In those health centers where a majority of the patients are adolescents, parental consent may be acquired in the form of a blanket consent, meaning that the available services are listed and the parent acknowledges with a signature that the child may receive the listed services. This arrangement acknowledges the adolescent's ability to make healthcare decisions and to be responsible for so doing. It also permits the adolescents' confidentiality to be maintained over a wide range of services that are normally available only with parental consent as required by law.

Other Consent/Assent Issues

Another consent issue to be explored in Julie's case is that of sexual activity: is her sexual activity voluntary? Most of the time, adolescent sexual activity is voluntary; not planned, but voluntary. It is important, however, to ask how old the boy/man is that she is having sexual relations with to assess voluntariness. Significant age differences change the power differential, and voluntariness can be questioned even when the adolescent says the sex is consensual. When the male is 5 years older than the minor, statutory rape should be considered and reported to the police and the sexual assault crisis center if concerns are raised (or as the law of the state requires). When the minor female is reporting sexual activity as voluntary but the activity involves another family member and is an incestual relationship, a report should be made to the child protection agency. Any nonconsenting sexual activity is reported to the police and sexual assault crisis team as rape and appropriate support given to the adolescent.

OVERRIDING PARENTAL RIGHTS

Parental rights to make healthcare decisions for adolescents can be overridden as they can for younger children. For example, anorexia nervosa is a condition that sometimes involves family complicity or influence. As such, it may require family therapy to address the complex issues inevitably involved. This requires clinical judgment on the part of the APN to evaluate and communicate concerns appropriately and allow early interventions. The child may need to be admitted to the hospital for treatment and observation whether the parent agrees with the APN or not. Or the family may need to be referred for counseling to a professional who has expertise in the evaluation and treatment of eating disorders.

Case 4: The Adolescent at Risk

For example, an adolescent girl 13 years of age presented to a private primary care health center in an affluent neighborhood for a well-child check. At the initial well-child visit, however, the APN, a pediatric nurse practitioner (PNP), became concerned because the health history and physical exam, as well as her interactions with the girl, and answers given to questions about her diet and activities all indicated the possibility of anorexia nervosa. Additionally, the girl's father and mother had recently divorced and her father moved overseas with his job. The PNP discussed her worries with her physician colleague who, while acknowledging that the family was under stress, discounted her concerns about an eating disorder, saying, "It's 'genetic' in that family; all the women in the family are thin—look at her mother."

The physician had for several years served as the primary provider for the father (before he moved overseas), the mother, and the daughter but had wanted the nurse, an experienced PNP, to assume the ongoing care of the adolescent because "she is difficult." The PNP, however, was puzzled by the explanation of the girl's weight as genetic and was worried that her colleague was missing the boat. The issue of conflicts among professionals is discussed in more detail in Chapter 5 along with strategies to resolve collaboration problems, and the PNP will have to address this problem with her colleague eventually. However, for current purposes the conflict is about doing the right thing for the girl and this means raising a sensitive issue with her and her mother.

Despite the sensitive nature of issues such as weight and mental health, a responsibility exists to address them with patients and, in the case of adolescents, with the adolescent and the family. A tactful, empathetic, and nonjudgmental approach is required. The approach should be tailored to knowledge of the persons in question and introduced in ways that are most likely to permit a therapeutic course of action. When the problem involves an adolescent, the situation is complicated by having to address entrenched parental attitudes and possibly the parent's facilitation of the adolescent's behavior. In this case, the APN discussed some of her concerns with the mother and daughter, although she did not label her concerns as anorexia nervosa. She did, however, discuss the stresses of adolescence, introduced some information about ways adolescents try to cope with the anxieties related to their development, and suggested that the daughter might benefit from both nutritional and psychological counseling.

Despite the PNP's carefully considered discussion, the mother became very indignant. "We don't want her getting too fat, she'll become unpopular. I know, I have seen what happens when you can't control your weight. You're just fine, aren't you?" At this point, the daughter nodded but didn't say anything. The PNP was worried but did not think she had enough evidence to pursue the issue further at that point, and the adolescent did not seem to be in any imminent danger. She was able to get the two to agree to a follow-up visit in one month.

Two weeks later the mother and daughter returned. The adolescent was now suffering from respiratory symptoms, fatigue, and was diagnosed with mononucleosis. At 5 foot 4 inches and 98 pounds, her weight at the first visit had been a little worrying, but though thin, she had not seemed emaciated. Now her weight had dropped to 93 pounds and she looked pale and listless. The PNP's concerns about anorexia were strengthened by this second visit and her current evaluation. She discussed with them the nature of and possible contributors to mononucleosis, effective treatment options, exercise limits, and a nutrition plan before raising the issue of the daughter's weight again and her seeming unhappiness. This time the daughter did not disagree about being unhappy and the mother seemed worried. The PNP's approach based on a developing understanding of both the mother and daughter and their relationship was empathetic, and when the PNP was alone with the mother she acknowledged the fact that it must be very difficult for her to be raising her daughter alone. They reached agreement that the daughter needed help, which permitted further options to be explored.

This is the best-case scenario where an understanding of professional responsibility to address difficult issues, along with clinical judgment and compassion, facilitates a parent to act in the best interests of her child. It will not always be the case that the parent or the child will agree to accept the help that is needed. At the end of the chapter, a discussion question related to the problem of reluctance to receive appropriate help is raised for further exploration. When APNs encounter difficult problems that seem beyond their capacity to address, it is important that they seek the counsel of an expert colleague rather than avoid dealing with the problem. In this case, consultation with and possible referral to a colleague who has expertise in the diagnosis and treatment of eating disorders would be helpful.

Discussion

The mortality (6%) and morbidity of anorexia nervosa (U.S. Department of Health and Human Services, 2006) is significant and the cure rate estimated as low as 50% (National Alliance on Mental Health, 2003). Early intervention is thought to improve cure rates, so the time to intervene with families assertively, despite their reticence to discuss the situation, is at the diagnosis, or possible diagnosis, because the psychological aspects and family component of this disease process also require intervention. In addition to healthcare services, outpatient management of anorexia nervosa should include individual counseling, family counseling, and nutrition counseling. The ethical ramifications of anorexia revolve around many patients' refusal to acknowledge the diagnosis and needed treatment.

Although wishing to promote autonomous decisions among adolescents and parents, APNs must also seek to protect the patient's best interests. Compulsory treatment, however, has proved ineffective in long-term management of anorexia because many patients view anorexia as a part of their personal identity, making treatment a difficult choice for them (Tan, Hope, & Stewart, 2003). Nevertheless, the APN cannot avoid discussing sensitive topics, whether that be weight or sex or smoking, but the discussion should proceed from an attitude of concern and interest for intervention to be helpful.

Enacting an Ethic of Care

A 16-year-old female patient accompanied by her grandmother presented with the chief complaint of nausea and vomiting. A urine sample was collected to rule out a urinary tract infection based on the vagueness of some of her complaints. After leaving the room, the APN decided to run a pregnancy test on the collected urine. The grandmother and patient were told that the purpose of the urine was to ensure no infection, but there was no mention of a pregnancy test, nor were questions about sexual activity asked of the patient. It was determined the patient had acute gastroenteritis and was treated appropriately.

Several weeks later, the grandmother called very upset because a pregnancy test was done on her granddaughter without either of them knowing about it. She complained that no one discussed this test with her at the time of the visit and her granddaughter was not asked about having sex. She also pointed out that she was sure she wasn't sexually active and she wasn't paying for the test. It was explained to her the purpose of the test and reasons for needing to perform it and how this is part of the workup for menstruating females presenting with nausea and vomiting. The grandmother was still upset.

This could be handled differently by being honest with patients about the tests ordered and the rationale for the order. Asking for a sexual history in front of parents/grandparents opens the door for them to talk with their adolescent about it when they arrive home. Yes, parents/grandparents/legal guardians have the right to refuse the test, but the concern about pregnancy being a cause of the presenting symptoms has been mentioned, and if the female patient is pregnant, the chart should reflect the discussion and refusal of the test. Adolescents may not always tell the truth in front of their parents, and therefore, if possible, evaluation of adolescents without parents at some point during the visit is preferable. If that opportunity is not possible or refused by one or the other, then the provider cannot avoid sensitive topics. In the ethic of care model, the trust relationship between provider and patient/parent was damaged in the clinical case given, but it could have been avoided with an open, frank discussion of possible concerns.

Another similar concern is when the adolescent is seen alone and the parents receive the healthcare bill outlining exactly what services were provided. Payment for services may need to be addressed with the adolescent prior to being seen. In states where it is legal for the adolescent to seek sexual health care without parental consent, sending the bill or insurance statement to the house may be problematic. Adolescents may need counsel on the financing of healthcare services, and referral to health department/free clinics may be appropriate for the adolescent population if it is requested that parents not know about services received.

When confronting healthcare concerns with adolescents, the adolescents' web of relationships must be considered. Requirements for parental notification do not encourage supportive family relationships but demand information about an adolescent when the adolescent might not be ready to share it. There are adolescents who would never enlist parental participation in their care, and some parents are more helpful than others in difficult situations. If the adolescent is encouraged to talk about who will help with the presenting problem, most will name a supportive adult, but it is not always a parent. Frequently, the APN is enlisted to talk with the designated adult in the presence of the adolescent about the problem at issue. Whether that adult is the parent or not, it is helpful that assistance has been enlisted willingly by the child, and the other adult can facilitate parental involvement if it is deemed appropriate or important. The APN's understanding of the issue can actually be distorted if the only perspective available is that of the adolescent in question. The adolescent may have misinterpreted parental concerns or attitudes as interfering, judgmental, or punitive. In the ethic of care model, the maintenance and encouragement of significant supportive relationships available to the adolescent are important. Such relationships permit uncovering the nuances of the situation and allow the concerned provider to work in concert with the adolescent and his or her support system toward a satisfactory outcome for difficult problems.

The adolescent, however, needs to know under what circumstances parental consent is required and what information will be given to the parent regarding the treatment needed. Consent for treatment may be required, but confidentiality regarding the adolescent's healthcare visit can be maintained with the adolescent as long as the adolescent is not in danger of harming self or others. The AWHONN states in its policy position statement (2000) on Confidentiality in Adolescent Health Care that "health professionals have an ethical obligation to provide the best possible care and counseling to respond to the needs of their adolescent patients (p. 1)." When providing health care to adolescents with or without parental consent, there is a higher level of accountability to ascertain their consent for treatment is fully informed.

As patients progress through their teen years, the responsibility for consenting to health care gradually becomes more the adolescent's than the parents', even when parents are present and the official consenters. The adolescent, in the absence of cognitive problems, will be legally responsible for personal healthcare decision making at 18 years of age if not earlier, but being responsible and informed does not happen when the birthday candles are blown out. Development of the necessary maturity for making sound decisions is gradual. It is facilitated by the existence of supportive others and with opportunities to practice decision making in safe environments. Unfortunately, not all adolescents will have the benefit of ideal circumstances. APNs are ideally situated to understand this and to provide the needed resources and assistance.

CONCLUSION

APNs and all healthcare providers who are caring for children serve as advocates for children. Children vary in their developmental stages and levels of maturity, and they cannot legally represent themselves, except in specific circumstances, so often their voice is heard only when others express their needs on their behalf. The provision of health care for children in any setting requires attention to (1) the web of relationships in the child's life, (2) the parents' interests, and (3) the child's needs. Consideration of the parents' and child's understanding of healthcare decisions is important in both parental informed consent and the child's consent at times/assent at others.

Inherent in the communication style between APNs, other healthcare providers, the child, and the family is the ethical term *respect for persons*. Communication with both parents and children is important, and it may guide interaction patterns in healthcare encounters throughout life. Analysis of one's communication style is important, and there are styles that demonstrate more caring attitudes than others. One study (Hansson et al., 2007) looked at nonverbal communication of physicians. The more positive styles (general politeness, actively showing efforts to set the stage for a respectful encounter, and showing sensitivity by responding to parents' needs in a respectful manner) were associated with a respect for integrity when parents were interviewed after healthcare encounters with their children. The study had only 21 subjects, but it is significant in that it acknowledges that nonverbal communication is important in the healthcare encounter. Additionally, the study also recognizes that time and communication skills are required of the healthcare provider for informed decision making by parents.

Excellent communication skills with children and families are important because in ethical concerns, problems, and dilemmas with children there is frequently no good answer and the best answer is often not good. The answer may not be decided immediately and it may require days, months, or years of conversation for everyone to reach consensus. The plan of care is agreed upon by all involved parties—it is not that one side wins or loses. APNs and other health providers cannot make children or parents act/behave/perform as prescribed or as we would ourselves; therefore, achieving consensus on the plan of action may take effort by all involved.

Other clinical cases with ethical components could have been discussed in this chapter. Examples include children as organ donors, parental/family presence during procedures and resuscitation, complementary therapies, withdrawal of support in the pediatric intensive care unit (PICU)/neonatal intensive care unit (NICU), end-of-life care for children, substance abuse screening in schools, growth hormone administration, increasing use of psychostimulants in children, and technology-dependent children in the home and community and the moral obligation of parents to care for them. This latter issue is increasingly important in relationship to the resources available or unavailable to these children and their families. The case studies chosen and discussed, however, set an ethical framework for discourse and evaluation of other moral concerns in the care of children.

The final ethical principle guiding the care of children is that of justice. It is our moral responsibility as APNs to ensure that our most vulnerable population, our nation's most treasured resource, has access to care. Access ensures the health of our nation's children so that they may develop their full potential as our nation's future leaders and workforce. The Code of Ethics for Nursing Plank 3 (American Nurses Association, 2001) states that "the nurse promotes, advocates for and strives to protect the health, safety and rights of patients." Health care for children includes access to (1) well-child care to detect and intervene in healthcare concerns early and receive vaccines to prevent disease, (2) timely intervention into acute illnesses to prevent long-term sequelae of illnesses, and (3) coordinated care and interventions for children with special healthcare needs.

> Better the occasional faults of a government that lives in a spirit of charity than the constant omissions of a government frozen in the ice of its own indifference.
> —*Franklin D. Roosevelt*

DISCUSSION QUESTIONS

1. Case number 4—*The Adolescent at Risk*—had the possibility of a good resolution because of the considered actions of the PNP and the receptiveness of the family. However, the mother may well have continued to deny the need for assistance based on her own problems and issues. With colleagues or classmates, discuss what would be required if the mother and/or daughter continued to deny that a problem existed.
2. How have your own attitudes toward stigmatized issues such as psychiatric illness and eating disorders changed over time? Or have they? What rationale can you give for your beliefs?
3. What does it mean to say parents are responsible for their child's health behaviors? What does it mean to say adolescents are responsible for their health behaviors?
4. There is an ongoing debate about the relationship of autism to vaccines. The debate persists despite the fact that there is little to no supporting evidence of a relationship. What is the APN's responsibility related to understanding the status of knowledge related to such controversial issues? How do you address healthcare-related questions that patients raise and that have not yet been satisfactorily answered in the literature?

ACKNOWLEDGMENTS

The author would like to acknowledge Juliet Gladson, MSN, for her assistance with the review of the literature and research for this chapter. Her contributions and persistence were invaluable in the writing. The case studies in this chapter were provided by graduate students at the University of Tennessee in the PNP program: Juliet Gladson, Lori Heston, Andrea Heaton, and Miriam Allman.

REFERENCES

Alderson, P., Sutcliffe, K., & Curtis, K. (2006). Children's competence to consent to medical treatment. *Hastings Center Report, 36*, 25–34.

Angelou, M. (2000). Interview with Maya Angelou by Oprah Winfrey reprinted in the *The Oprah Magazine*, December 2000.

American Academy of Pediatrics Committee on Bioethics. (1995). Informed consent, parental permission, and assent in pediatric practice. *Pediatrics, 95*(2), 314–317. Retrieved January 19, 2008, from http://www.cirp.org/library/ethics/AAP/.

American College of Obstetrics. (2003). Access to reproductive health care for adolescents. *Health care for adolescents: Policies and Materials on Adolescent Health of the American College of Obstetricians and Gynecologists*. American College of Obstetrics, Washington, DC. Retrieved April 20, 2008 from http://www.acog.org/departments/dept_web.cfm?recno=7.

American Nurses Association. (2001). *Code of ethics for nurses with interpretative statements*. Retrieved January 20, 2008, from http://nursingworld.org/mods/mod580/cecdevers.htm.

Association of Women's Health, Obstetric and Neonatal Nurses. (2000). *Confidentiality in adolescent health care: Policy position statement*. Retrieved April 20, 2008 from http://www.awhonn.org/awhonn/content.do?name=05_HealthPolicyLegislation/5H_PositionStatements.htm.

Benin, A. L., Wisler-Scher, D. J., Colson, E., Shapiro, E. D., & Holmboe, E. S. (2006). Qualitative analysis of mothers' decision-making about vaccines for infants: The importance of trust. *Pediatrics, 117*, 1532–1541.

Carson, J. L., Noveck, H., Berlin, J. A., & Gould, S. A. (2002). Mortality and morbidity in patients with very low postoperative hemoglobin levels who decline blood transfusion. *Transfusion, 42*, 812–819.

Centers for Disease Control and Prevention. (2003, January 15). *Vaccine information statement for MMR*. Retrieved January 20, 2008, from http://www.cdc.gov/vaccines/pubs/vis/downloads/vis-mmr.pdf.

Clinton, H. R. (1996). Speech made on Tuesday, August 27, 1996, at the Democratic National Convention in Chicago, IL. Retrieved January 20, 2008, from http://www.pbs.org/newshour/convention96/floor_speeches/hillary_clinton.html.

Cockburn, T. (2005). Children and the feminist ethic of care. *Childhood: A Global Journal of Child Research, 12*, 71–89.

Diekema, D. S., & Committee of Bioethics. (2005). Responding to parental refusals of immunization of children. *Pediatrics, 115*, 1428–1431.

Edelman, M. W. (2000). *Guide my feet: Prayers and meditations for our children*. New York, NY: Harper Collins Perennial.

Eisenberg, M. E., Swain, C., Bearinger, L. H., Sieving, R. E., & Resnick, M. D. (2005). Parental notification laws for minors' access to contraception: what do parents say? *Archives of Pediatrics & Adolescent Medicine, 159*, 120–125.

Fair, E., Murphy, T. V., Golaz, A., & Wharton, M. (2002). Philosophical objection to vaccination as a risk for tetanus among children younger than 15 years. *Pediatrics, 109*, 1–3.

Farrell, R. M., & Rome, E. S. (2007). Adolescents' access and consent to the human papillomavirus vaccine: A critical aspect for immunization success. *Pediatrics, 120*, 434–437.

Feikin, D. R., Lezotte, D. C., Hamman, R. F., Salmon, D. A., Chen, R. T., & Hoffman, R. E. (2000). Individual and community risks of measles and pertussis associated with personal exemptions to immunizations. *Journal of American Medical Association, 284,* 3145–3150.

Feudtner, C., & Marcus, E. K. (2001). Ethics and immunization policy: Promoting dialogue to sustain consensus. *Pediatrics, 107,* 1158–1164.

Gilligan, C. (1982). *In a different voice.* Cambridge, MA: Harvard University Press.

Guay, J., de Moerloose, P., & Lasne, D. (2006). Minimizing perioperative blood loss and transfusions in children. *Canadian Journal of Anesthesia, 53,* S59–S67.

Guttmacher Institute. (2008). Minors' access to contraceptive services: State policies in brief. Retrieved January 19, 2008, from http://www.guttmacher.org/statecenter/spibs/spib_MACS.pdf.

Hansson, M. G., Kihlbom, U., Tuvemo, T., Olsen, L. A., & Rodriguez, A. (2007). Ethics takes time, but not that long. *BMC Medical Ethics, 8,* 1472.

Jones, R. K., Purcell, A., Singh, S., & Finer, L. B. (2005). Adolescents' reports of parental knowledge of adolescents; use of sexual health services and their reactions to mandated parental notification for prescription contraception. *Journal of the American Medical Association, 293,* 340–348.

Keller, J. (1996). Care ethics as a health care ethic. *Contexts: A Forum for Medical Humanities, 4.* Retrieved January 19, 2008, from http://www.uhmc.sunysb.edu/prevmed/mns/imcs/contexts/care/carejean.html.

Lacroix, J. R., & Corwin, H. L. (2007). Transfusion strategies for patients in pediatric intensive care units. *New England Journal of Medicine, 356,* 1609–1619.

Malone, K. M., & Hinman, A. R. (2003). Vaccination mandates: The public health imperative and individual rights. In R. A. Goodman, M. A. Rothstein, R. E. Hoffman, et al. (Eds.), *Law in public health practice* (pp. 262–284). New York: Oxford University Press.

National Alliance on Mental Health. (2003). Anorexia nervosa. Retrieved January 19, 2008, from http://www.nami.org/.

Omer, S. B., Pan, W. Y., Halsey, N. A., Stokley, S., Moulton, L. H., Navar, A. M., et al. (2006). Non-medical exemptions to school immunization requirements: Secular trends and association of state policies with pertussis incidence. *Journal of the American Medical Association, 296,* 1757–1763.

Parker, A. A., Staggs, W., Dayan, G. H., Ortega-Sanchez, I. R., Rota, P. A., Lowe, L., & et al. (2006). Implications of a 2005 measles outbreak on Indiana for sustained elimination of measles in the United States. *New England Journal of Medicine, 355,* 447–455.

Planned Parenthood. (2005). *Fact sheet: America's family planning program: Title X.* Retrieved January 20, 2008, from http://www.plannedparenthood.org.

Planned Parenthood. (2007). *Fact sheet: Laws requiring mandatory parental involvement for minors' abortion.* Retrieved January 20, 2008, from http://www.plannedparenthood.org.

Reddy, D. M., Fleming, R., & Swain, C. (2002). Effect of mandatory parental notification on adolescent girls sexual health care services. *Journal of the American Medical Association, 288,* 710–714.

Salmon, D. A., Haber, M., Gangarosa, E. J., Phillips, L., Smith, N. J., & Chen, R. T. (1999). Health consequences of religious and philosophical exemptions from immunization laws: Individual and societal risk of measles. *Journal of the American Medical Association, 282,* 47.

Smith, P. J., Kennedy, A. M., Wooten, K., Gust, D. A., & Pickering, L. K. (2006). Association between health care providers' influence on parents who have concerns about vaccine safety and vaccination coverage. *Pediatrics, 118,* 1287–1292.

Tan, J. O. A., Hope, T., & Stewart, A. (2003). Anorexia nervosa and personal identity: The accounts of patients and their parents. *International Journal of Law Psychiatry, 26,* 533–548.

U.S. Department of Health and Human Services. (2006). *Anorexia nervosa.* National Women's Health Information Center. Retrieved January 19, 2008, from http://www.womenshealth.gov/faq/easyread/anorexia-etr.htm#a.

CHAPTER 9

Nursing Ethics and Advanced Practice: Women's Health

Katharine T. Smith

INTRODUCTION

The advanced nursing practice specialty of women's health concentrates its focus on addressing health issues of particular concern to women. However, many of the issues that arise in women's health clinical settings are also encountered in other areas of advanced practice nurse (APN) practice; thus, this chapter provides insights, approaches to care, and strategies facilitative of health that have broad applications. Adult health and family nurse practitioners (NPs) are educated to be knowledgeable about women's health and have many of the same professional skill sets as women's health nurse practitioners (WHNPs), and our scope of practice often overlaps with theirs. What, then, differentiates women's health advanced practice nursing from other specialty practice? It is the concentrated focus permitted by our scope of practice on the experiences associated with being female and the ways in which this cultural identity affects a patient's health and well-being.

Through studies in nursing, women's health nursing, ethics, and clinical practice, I have encountered problems stemming from two societal influences on women as a group. Because of their ties to the cultural identity of women and their implications in many of the ethically difficult cases encountered by WHNPs, understanding the bases of these influences is important, not only for women's health practitioners, but also for practitioners of all advanced practice settings who care for women. The first influence is that of historically and culturally established gender-based power imbalances that are pervasive throughout our society. When people feel powerless, they may not be able to discern what their own needs and wishes are and consequently are not able to articulate these to others. There are degrees of powerlessness; however, many issues encountered both in women's health and primary care settings prove especially difficult to resolve because their roots are deeply embedded in the culture of many societies. Issues faced by APNs include patients experiencing interpartner violence (IPV), those who have been sexually assaulted, those who have reproductive control issues, or those who live in poverty yet have children for whom they are the sole support. The second influence often affecting ethical issues in women's health, regardless of setting, is rooted in the societal expectations of women to fulfill certain roles and identities. Women's health issues are inherently tied to women's expected roles as mothers, professionals, caregivers, wives, and friends. Many ethical issues in women's health arise from the complicated factors involved in women negotiating their identity through a balance among these roles.

As discussed in Chapter 1, feminist ethics approaches are aimed at exposing the power imbalances and underlying assumptions present in a case, based on gender, race, class, or other factors. Additionally, philosophical understandings of nursing and its purposes in concert with a feminist ethic of care direct us to engage with our patients in a process that permits a holistic understanding of the person as a unique individual inseparable from his or her context. Thus, adopting these perspectives to explore women's health concerns yields a fuller account of the issues. For, if our practice is interested in caring not just for female patients, but for patients who are affected by their cultural identity as women, then we must work to understand the complex ways in which this identity has influenced each patient's life, experiences, and healthcare needs. Traditional principles of healthcare ethics are helpful for further clarifying specific issues and in moral decision making within this feminist care perspective but will not be the primary approach. Therefore, this chapter analyzes ethical issues in women's health in a way that is based on the value of an ethic of care; first attempting to understand the complexities of a woman's unique experience, and then applying both feminist and traditional ethical principles to develop possible courses of ethical action.

It would be impossible to address every ethically difficult issue or clinical situation that WHNPs may encounter. Instead, I have chosen two case studies from my clinical practice because of their distinct focus on the issues of patient empowerment and women's societal roles. Each case study represents a composite patient situation. They are presented and analyzed using the ethical decision-making guidelines proposed in Chapter 2. Major issues central to the case and relevant to other areas of women's health advanced practice nursing are identified and discussed further. An ethic of care, which guides the nurse to engage in a process of knowing the patient to understand her as an individual within her context, underpins case explorations, and ideas of traditional ethics and feminist ethics, will be used to further explore the issues and develop courses of action. Finally, practical strategies that can be used by APNs in addressing ethically difficult situations are presented. An additional case for in-class or solo exploration is provided along with some questions for further discussion.

SARA'S CASE

Nineteen-year-old Sara presents to an adolescent obstetrical clinic for a routine visit. She is at 30 weeks gestation. This is her first pregnancy and she has been consistent in her prenatal care since she discovered that she was pregnant. The pregnancy was unplanned but is now welcomed by Sara, who lives with her father and her two younger siblings. The father of the baby is her boyfriend of several months who lives nearby in her neighborhood. On a previous visit, it was noted that Sara had bruises on her arms, back, and shoulders. When asked about them, Sara admitted that her boyfriend became angry and hit her. This has become a recurring pattern. At this particular visit, Sara tells her NP about a recent incident in which her boyfriend grabbed her violently and pushed her to the floor. She explains that her family is concerned about the abuse and is urging her to move in with her mother, who lives many states away. When Sara was 6 years old, the department of social services removed her from her mother's custody and placed her with her father. Since then, she and her mother have had a strained relationship, talking with each other only a few times each year. Sara explains to the NP that she is fearful of moving somewhere unfamiliar, but thinks that maybe she should move because her family insists it would be best for her and the baby. However, her boyfriend does not want her to leave and if she does has said that he will not be present for the birth of the child and he will refuse to take part in the child's upbringing. She states she wants to do what is best for the baby, but that her boyfriend is "all I've got" and she does not want to lose him. It is clear that Sara has less than ideal support systems and coping mechanisms, but what she does have, her family, friends, and the adolescent clinic staff, are located here. Sara asks her NP, "What should I do?" The NP responds by asking Sara what it is she "wants" to do. Sara is unable to answer decisively, responding only by shrugging her shoulders, as if to suggest that she does not know. The NP knows that the violence is likely to increase but is also aware that for Sara to move to a faraway state at this crucial time in her pregnancy would mean losing what few support systems she has.

Background on IPV and Pregnancy

Current statistics regarding IPV tell us that such violence is, unfortunately, all too common during pregnancy. According to the U.S. Department of Health and Human Services, homicide is the leading cause of maternal death in the United States and maternal abuse is more common than either gestational diabetes or preeclampsia, both conditions being ones that are routinely screened for throughout prenatal care.

IPV during pregnancy has been shown to contribute to chronic health problems and complications during pregnancy such as low weight gain, anemia, infections, first- and second-trimester bleeding, and maternal depression, as well as tobacco, alcohol, and illicit drug use (Family Violence Prevention Fund, 2004).

Evidently, there is a critical need for healthcare providers to screen for and address domestic violence as a routine component of prenatal care. Many organizations and researchers have recognized this need for increased assessment for IPV during pregnancy. The American College of Obstetricians and Gynecologists (2007) has developed a screening tool for domestic violence and recommends that providers screen pregnant women for domestic violence at the initial prenatal visit, once per trimester, and at the postpartum visit. In addition, the Family Violence Prevention Fund (Warshaw & Ganley, 1996) has published a resource manual for healthcare providers aimed at helping providers identify, assess, and intervene on behalf of victims of domestic violence. The authors suggest that an appropriate intervention would include (1) validating the patient's experience; (2) providing the patient with pertinent information regarding domestic violence; (3) aiding the patient in creating a safety plan; and (4) questioning whether the involvement of law enforcement is appropriate (Warshaw & Ganley, 1996).

A wealth of research has investigated the gap between these recommendations and current practice, suggesting that addressing domestic violence within the clinical setting is made difficult by many complicated factors. Hertzig and colleagues (2006) conducted focus groups with obstetricians, NPs, and certified nurse midwives to investigate their methods of addressing the behavioral risk factors of alcohol, tobacco, and illicit drug use and IPV in pregnant patients. Their results suggest that IPV was the only risk not routinely screened for by the providers. In addition, participants expressed that their screening for IPV may have been hindered by their own pessimism, as well as feelings that they were ill equipped to intervene and that they would have difficulty identifying relevant cases.

Although IPV in pregnancy is a well documented threat to maternal and fetal well-being, evidence shows that addressing individual cases on the part of a healthcare provider may be much more complicated than expected. The research suggests that the NP in Sara's case is not alone in being uncertain of how to proceed. She is aware that no single approach will work for all victims of domestic violence and must instead try to establish a relationship with Sara to understand her values, beliefs, and experiences to develop with Sara an ethical plan of action.

Using Decision-Making Guidelines

Chapter 2 offered a set of guidelines to be used by APNs when evaluating ethically difficult situations. The steps that ask us to determine who is involved, determine the prevalent values, and identify gaps in information are particularly useful for ensuring that we are considering all aspects, influences, and possibilities involved in the case. In addition, these steps aid us in extracting the major issues central to the case. When evaluating a hypothetical case such as Sara's, we may find that we do not have access to as much information as would be ideal. In a real-life situation, it would be important to return to the patient to gather as many details as possible. Although there may be many questions in this case for which we do not have answers, working through the framework permits a detailed exploration that brings out otherwise hidden facets, highlights nuances, and thus clarifies ethical implications for the WHNP. This process allows us to form a more complete understanding of the issues involved so that a truer range of possible actions can be considered. The following exploration identifies possible contributing factors, discusses major issues using supporting literature, and formulates possible courses of action. Some questions useful for the purposes of self-reflection and further discussion are suggested.

Major Ethical Principles Involved

The major issue at first consideration is the conflict between the NP's responsibility to beneficence, that is, the nurse must work to produce a good for his or her patient, and nonmaleficence, the nurse must not cause harm to his or her patient. In Sara's case, the good that the NP is required to promote is that of a physically and psychologically healthy pregnancy and transition into motherhood. This appears to require Sara to stay near her social and psychological supports. Yet, simultaneously, the NP must also maintain her responsibility to protect Sara from the violence that she may be subjected to if she remains in the current abusive environment. At first glance, this conflict appears to pose an ethical dilemma. It seems that the NP cannot both protect Sara from the abusive environment and maintain her psychosocial supports. However, by using the decision-making considerations and guidelines provided earlier, it becomes obvious that the conflict may not be a true dilemma after all, and the possibility of other options is revealed. In reality, instead of the problem appearing as requiring one or the other of two seemingly conflicting courses of action, we can see that taking a different perspective reveals the problem as both more complex and open to different avenues of action. These potential actions may allow for both promotion of a healthy pregnancy and Sara's protection from further violence.

Who Is Involved?

The most obvious stakeholder is Sara. Unfortunately, it is difficult to determine Sara's needs because she is unable to assert her own autonomy by expressing her priorities in regards to the current situation. Thus, the WHNP will need to establish a relationship with Sara that will permit discovering acceptable options. We do know that Sara has evidenced a hesitancy to let the relationship with her boyfriend dissolve. However, up to this point she has been unable to express what motivates this hesitancy. From a professional standpoint, we can identify that Sara has many other needs at this point in her pregnancy, even though she has been unable to express them herself. Among these are the need for a physically and emotionally safe environment for her and her fetus, psycho-social supports to help contribute to healthy transitions into motherhood, and economic supports to allow for more independence within her environment.

Although we can assume that Sara needs certain social and physical supports, it is problematic that she is unable to articulate her desires and priorities. The NP does have a responsibility to provide an intervention that promotes Sara's safety, but she also has a responsibility to provide care in a way that promotes Sara's autonomy. Unless Sara can be assisted to verbalize what her needs are, it will be very difficult for the NP to act in a way that promotes Sara's autonomy. This problem is probably reflective of Sara's deep disempowerment. Understanding the nature and effects of powerlessness upon people is important for the goal of meeting Sara's health needs. The concept of patient empowerment is discussed shortly.

The fetus constitutes another stakeholder. As a fetus, it is at risk of trauma within the womb, and as a potential human being, it is at risk of emotional and physical violence if it is born into an abusive environment. For optimal development, the fetus is in need of a physically safe and developmentally supportive home throughout the gestation period and after birth. This adds another level of complication to the case. The WHNP is responsible for the health of Sara as well as the health of the fetus. This could be perceived as an ethical conflict for the NP if Sara's choice is to stay within the abusive environment. This issue of perceived conflict between the interests of mother and fetus will also be explored shortly.

Sara's boyfriend also has a stake in the outcome of this situation. He has expressed that he would be angry if Sara moved away, as well as his desire to be active in the child's life, conditional on Sara's decision not to move. Other than that, we do not know much about his situation and therefore cannot make assumptions about what underlies his behavior. He may genuinely care for Sara, be both excited and fearful about having a child, and be hurt that Sara has threatened to move away. He may regret his violence toward Sara but not know how to gain control of his emotions. Thus, he may need support in exploring and resolving these issues. It is possible that he would be receptive to, or interested in, seeking counseling to attempt to change his behavior. Although, some authors suggest that it is inappropriate for couples to seek joint counseling to resolve issues of IPV (Warshaw & Ganley, 1996), he may be willing to seek counseling independently. Although we do not have a lot of information about Sara's boyfriend, he is an important character in this case and knowing more about his situation could prove helpful in resolving the issue.

Sara's family and friends have shown that they care for her and do not want to see her or her fetus physically injured. Sara's father has encouraged her to move to her mother's home ostensibly to protect her safety and remove her from her boyfriend's influence. Yet it is possible that he has other motives for suggesting that it would be best if Sara moved. He could be fearful of assuming responsibility for yet another child in addition to his own three children and a new grandchild. He may be feeling overwhelmed and not know how he could secure the resources to care for them all. He may see Sara's move to her mother's as a way of solving many problems. Still there may be other influences and factors that are contributing to his current situation. A more contextual view of Sara's life and situation highlights the fact that there may be alternate avenues of action to facilitate her in getting her health needs met.

Prevalent Values

The presence of certain personal as well as institutional values are important considerations in resolving this case. Sara seems to value her relationship with her boyfriend more than do others in her life, including the NP. It appears to be difficult for others to understand her desire to keep her relationship intact. It is important for the NP and other providers involved to explore their personal experiences, beliefs, and values regarding IPV. A provider may have previous experience with IPV or may know a close friend or relative who has. One may have preconceived ideas regarding perpetrators and victims of IPV. Such factors work to shape the ways in which one can frame and think about situations involving IPV. Ethical care requires the WHNP to understand his or her own experiences and examine his or her beliefs and values so that he or she can set them aside in exploring the current situation. Additionally, familiarizing oneself with available literature on a subject that one encounters frequently in practice helps to widen one's perspective and reveal different possibilities.

Major Issues Involved

Two major issues central to Sara's case can be identified. The first is Sara's seeming lack of empowerment. The second is the possible conflict between maternal and fetal interests. A third issue, related to what the provider's legal responsibilities are, was not identified directly in the preceding discussion but requires further evaluation as well.

Patient Empowerment

As previously discussed, a major issue involved in the case is the NP's inability to support Sara's choices because Sara is either unwilling or unable to articulate these. One reason for this may be maturational—at 19 years of age she can still be considered an adolescent. Another reason may be that Sara feels powerless. For the purpose of this case, we'll suppose that Sara is so disempowered within her own situation that she is unable to verbalize, or possibly even determine, what her individual needs and priorities are. This situation is very problematic for the NP because her practice goals are to provide patients with the information, resources, and support to meet their health needs. This requires understanding what their health needs are, at least partly from their perspective; that is, respect for patient autonomy is an important practice value. It is questionable to what extent a disempowered person can exercise his or her right to self-determination. Therefore, the NP must first discover ways whereby Sara can be empowered to make informed decisions that are most likely to be in line with her desires and aspirations for the future. A first step toward this is to understand what is known about IPV and powerlessness.

In a review of the literature regarding IPV in the 1990s, Johnson and Ferraro (2000) identified control as one of the two main themes present within IPV research. They report that the majority of both feminist and nonfeminist analyses of IPV identify the dynamics of power and control as being central to the abusive relationship. Although individual complexities and types of violence among relationships differ, their review suggests that, in general, IPV serves to give the perpetrator some measure of control over the victim and the relationship. Based on the theme of control, many researchers and theorists argue that disempowerment is a key player within abusive relationships and that victim empowerment ought to be at the crux of interventions for victims of IPV.

In her article aimed at guiding nursing practice in identification and treatment of victims of IPV, Nancy Chez (1994) suggests that patient empowerment should be the primary goal of interventions. She offers practical strategies for promoting patient empowerment, which emphasize validation of the patient's experiences and support for her priorities, such as listening in a supportive and understanding way and forming a safe environment in which the patient can express her feelings and tell her stories of abuse (Chez, 1994). These interventions, aimed at validation and support, are common in many practice guidelines developed for practitioners working with victims of IPV and are an important and necessary component of an optimal course of action. However, for Sara, as for many other patients who are seen in women's health practice settings, these strategies represent only a beginning; they do not unearth one of the core questions. How does the NP promote patient empowerment if Sara is unable to express her needs? The NP is charged with the difficult task of trying to make a connection with Sara that permits her to start to identify what Sara's preferences are.

WHNPs are often faced with women that are in similar situations of disempowerment. For instance, it is not uncommon for an NP to encounter a patient presenting to the clinic with questions regarding contraceptive methods. When the options are explored, it becomes clear that the patient is unable to express her own desires or priorities for a method; often she will defer either to her partner's opinion or that of the provider. This lack of voice may lead to the sacrificing of a woman's own reproductive health and safety. For example, she may not be able to insist on the use of condoms when she knows that her partner has multiple partners.

Women's health as a specialty also has an interest in understanding the influence of women's disempowerment caused by oppressive societal values and customs, including questions of who should control women's reproductive choices and why a disproportionate number of women and children are currently living in poverty. Regardless of the specifics of each case involving a need for patient empowerment, a deeper understanding of the concept of empowerment may allow us to develop practical strategies to address these issues within the constraints of the clinic setting.

Theories about gender-based power imbalances and power dynamics within relationships offer further insight into Sara's case. There have been several nursing and other research studies investigating the influence of relationship power. These include the recent development of the Sexual Relationship Power Scale (Pulerwitz, Amaro, De Jong, Gortmaker, & Rudd, 2002), the theory of gender and power (Connell, 1987), and aspects of social exchange theory (Emerson, 1981) and were designed to add to the knowledge base related to interpersonal dynamics involved within heterosexual relationships. In his discussion of social exchange theory, Emerson (1981) defines the concept of power as a dynamic within a dyad relationship that is exercised through the ability of one partner to control decision-making processes whether or not the outcomes of the decision benefit the other partner. Connell's (1987) theory of gender and power is a social theory of gender relations, which suggests that the social structure of gender-based power inequalities leads to male-favored power over decision-making processes at the societal level as well as within individual heterosexual relationships.

These theoretical approaches suggest that increasing a patient's sense of personal power would lead to more autonomous and independent behavior on the part of women and within their relationships. These forms of autonomous behavior would be exercised through control over decision-making processes, many of which deeply affect reproductive health and well-being. Likewise, if power within a relationship is essentially control of decision-making processes, then interventions aimed at supporting and facilitating patients' decision-making capabilities would empower patients. This suggestion has important implications for Sara's case as well as for other cases involving a need for patients to exercise more personal power over their choices.

In Sara's case her inability to verbalize her own desires for action permits her family members, boyfriend, and now the NP to take over her decision-making processes. If decision-making processes are a method through which to exercise power, then it is crucial that Sara be encouraged and supported to make this decision on her own, to exercise her individual autonomy and gain some, albeit small, degree of power over her own situation. Although she may not currently have all the social resources necessary to fully exercise her autonomy in decision making within her environment, in the clinic environment she can safely explore her needs and desires, deliberate regarding a desired outcome, and verbalize an autonomous decision in favor of that particular outcome. The NP can then respond in a manner that validates Sara's decision-making process and allows the power to remain in Sara's control. By providing Sara with support to learn and develop skills to gain control over decision-making processes, the NP is not simply promoting Sara's empowerment, but providing Sara with the tools necessary to empower herself in the future.

In a qualitative study investigating nursing interventions aimed at supporting female patients who are victims of domestic violence, Curry, Durham, Bullock, Bloom, and Davis (2006) come to a similar conclusion regarding promoting empowerment within the clinic setting. They identify victim empowerment as a key component involved in IPV. They suggest that patient empowerment can be promoted within the clinic setting if the provider attempts to allow the patient to feel in control at the clinic, respect the patient's autonomy within the clinic, encourage the patient to verbalize her own feelings and desires, and then support her in a manner that respects these.

An exploration of the current theory and research regarding patient empowerment in its relation to IPV suggests that interventions aimed at promoting patient empowerment may be a key component aimed at addressing the underlying issues of several ethical dilemmas in women's health advanced practice nursing. Appropriate interventions would be ones that work to validate the patient's experience, use the clinic environment as a safe space in which the patient can practice exercising decision-making processes, support and encourage her to explore her needs and priorities until she is able to independently choose a favored course of action, and support her choices and priorities.

Maternal-Fetal Conflict

What if Sara's choice is to stay with her abusive partner? The NP would then be faced with the dilemma of supporting Sara's autonomy while simultaneously bearing responsibility for the well-being of the fetus, which may now be exposed to harm resulting from the abusive environment in which Sara has chosen to remain. Traditionally, this type of ethical dilemma is titled a "maternal-fetal conflict." However, this language can be constrictive because it depicts a situation in which the unique aspects of dependence and interconnectedness inherent in the pregnant state are ignored and a view of the fetus and mother as two distinct individuals in direct conflict with each other is adopted. It creates an adversarial dichotomy in which the autonomy of one individual cannot be honored without risking the welfare of the other; it proposes mother versus fetus. Approaching such a dilemma from this perspective can be a disservice because it diverts our attention from the details and context of the case, precludes us from deciding upon a course of action that honors the needs of both stakeholders, and makes it seem as if one must choose between patients. If this situation were viewed through a feminist ethic of care lens, it would lead to an evaluation of the details of the experiences within the case so that the practitioner could develop a course of action that may benefit both mother and fetus (Marcellus, 2004).

Shanner (1998) offers an alternative conceptualization of the relationship between mother and fetus: the pregnant embodiment model. This perspective allows us to evaluate discourses between the welfare of women and their pregnancies in a way that is more consistent with the approach offered by an ethic of care. Pregnant embodiment removes the "mother or fetus dichotomy" suggested by "maternal-fetal conflicts" and replaces it with a "both and" view of pregnancy. The pregnant embodiment model suggests that a better way of understanding the maternal-fetal relationship is to avoid viewing the mother as providing housing for an individual entity within her, but rather to view a pregnant woman as transcending the boundaries of her original, nonpregnant identity to become something greater than her previous self. She is becoming mother and fetus. Inherent in this model is a view of pregnancy as a process. Events from quickening to birth allow the fetus to be slowly viewed more and more as an individual "other." "Both babies and mothers come into being gradually, over time and through tiny, imperceptible changes" (Shanner, 1998, p. 762). Pregnant embodiment asks us to view pregnancy as an ongoing progression of the maternal-fetal unit, discouraging us from identifying a distinct moment during gestation when a woman and her fetus can be viewed as separate entities with conflicting agendas. It requires us to seek ethical decisions that address the needs of the pregnancy as a whole; to assess the details of the case to develop an optimal course of action that would benefit the maternal-fetal unit.

The model of pregnant embodiment is especially apt for evaluating ethical issues in advanced practice nursing because of its consistencies with maternal nursing theory. Rubin (1967) proposes the theory of maternal role attainment, which describes progressive stages through which women move throughout pregnancy and enter into the postpartum period to achieve new identities as mothers. Maternal role attainment is achieved through the psychosocial work that pregnant women undertake throughout pregnancy. Many researchers and theorists have further developed and added to Rubin's concept of maternal role attainment in attempts to describe the transformative processes that women undergo during the experience of pregnancy. Theories of "becoming a mother" and "transitions to motherhood" (Mercer, 2004; Nelson, 2003) among others have been added to the maternal role attainment theory and serve to guide current practice in prenatal, intrapartum, and postpartum nursing. Although these theories speak mostly to a woman's experience of coming into a new identity and not directly to the conceptualization of the maternal-fetal relationship, they are similar to the pregnant embodiment model in the ways in which they describe pregnancy as a dynamic and transformative experience that is based on the concepts of process, transcendence, and commitment. This consistency with the pregnant embodiment model suggests that the conceptualization of pregnant embodiment may be appropriate for APNs to adopt when evaluating this type of ethical dilemma instead of the traditional perspective offered by "maternal-fetal conflict." Viewing the maternal-fetal relationship through the pregnant embodiment model provides new opportunity for solving problems of discourse in pregnancy. The pregnancy embodiment model removes the emphasis from the fetus alone, thereby allowing us to focus on the comprehensive, long-term well-being of the mother (Marcellus, 2004).

At this point let's return to the details of the individual case in order to determine what resources and support Sara needs to put herself and her fetus into a healthier situation. IPV, perhaps not surprisingly, has been found to be highly associated with depression, anxiety, lack of social supports, housing problems, inadequate prenatal care, and feelings of little or no control over the current situation (Campbell, Harris, & Lee, 1995). The incidence of these factors suggests that it is as important for interventions to address these complex issues as it is for them to address the violence. If there is no attempt to change the conditions that have caused Sara to find herself and remain within a situation of IPV, then, even if she and her fetus are removed from the current situation, nothing has been done to prevent her and her future children from entering into similar relationships in the future. Curry and colleagues (2006) conducted investigations to evaluate nursing interventions aimed at supporting victims of domestic violence. Their results support this hypothesis and suggest that optimal interventions focus on identifying an individual patient's priorities, and then supporting these choices. The majority of participants identified the pregnancy, housing needs, and relationship issues with family members as their priorities.

Adopting an alternative perspective to the maternal-fetal conflict that reflects the implications of Curry et al.'s (2006) research when evaluating Sara's case directs us to develop a course of action that provides Sara with the psychosocial support and outside resources that she needs. Only when the NP encourages Sara to gain independence in her environment does he or she enable Sara to access an environment that does not expose her fetus to the violence present in the current relationship.

Liability and Mandated Reporting

The consideration of the involvement of law enforcement has been identified as a necessary part of an intervention aimed at aiding a victim of IPV (Warshaw & Ganley, 1996). If the NP deems that the patient or patient's family is in immediate danger because of the threat of violence, it may be appropriate to involve law enforcement agencies to ensure protection. Making this decision is always a complicated one, and it should be discussed and decided upon in collaboration with the patient to maintain the NP's obligations to confidentiality, loyalty, and patient–provider trust. However, for many practitioners this process is further complicated by the presence of laws mandating that healthcare providers report incidences of domestic abuse to law enforcement agencies with or without the permission of the patient.

At this time, six states have laws that specifically mandate practitioners to report cases of domestic violence or adult abuse. The particular laws vary among these states, from requiring anonymous reporting for data collection purposes to requiring the practitioner to report to law enforcement agencies and include identification of the victim, the victim's whereabouts, and place of residence. In addition, the majority of states have mandates requiring that healthcare providers report cases of an injury that appear to have been inflicted by a gun, knife, firearm, or other deadly weapon (Family Violence Prevention Fund, 2004). It is important to contact your state for up-to-date information on mandated reporting of IPV. Proponents of such mandated reporting laws—especially those laws that deal specifically with IPV—argue that such laws hold perpetrators accountable for their actions and provide a means of tracking IPV, thereby decreasing the incidence. Opponents of such laws cite ethical complications and increased risks of violence associated with mandated reporting as evidence against the efficacy of such laws (Sullivan & Hagen, 2005).

Exploring the topic of mandated reporting in cases of domestic violence, Lewis-O'Connor (2004) discusses issues involved in legally requiring healthcare providers to report cases of domestic violence. Currently, the effectiveness of state-mandated reporting has not been evaluated, and it is therefore impossible to use quantitative data to assess the effects. However, she elucidates the most common arguments against such laws. First, it is feared that mandated reporting by healthcare professionals may lead to retaliation by the abusive partner. This effect not only increases the risk of harm to the victim, but also may inhibit him or her from seeking medical care for fear of being reported. Mandated reporting also puts practitioners in an ethically compromised situation. Reporting a case of domestic violence without the consent of the patient may be perceived as a breach of confidentiality and may lead to the patient feeling betrayed and losing trust in the provider and/or healthcare system (Lewis-O'Connor, 2004). In addition, reporting by an NP without the consent of the patient, although legally required, may violate the ethics of nursing practice. As stated by the American Nurses Association in its *Code of Ethics for Nurses with Interpretive Statements* (2001), "The nurse's primary commitment is to the recipient of nursing care and health care services—the patient. When conflict persists, the nurse's commitment remains to the patient" (ANA, 2001, provision 2). If nurses are required to report cases of IPV to law enforcement agencies with or without the consent of the patient, a conflict of interests arises. In a case where a patient refuses to consent to reporting, a nurse cannot be loyal both to her patient and to the law. If a conflict arises, then as stated in the provisions for ethical practice, the nurse must remain committed to the patient. However, the nurse then makes himself or herself vulnerable to the legal ramifications of forgoing reporting. She must evaluate the risks to the patient and weigh these against the risk to herself and to future patients.

In a state that legally mandates healthcare professionals to report IPV, focus groups with survivors of such violence were conducted to explore their opinions on mandated reporting laws (Sullivan & Hagen, 2005). An overwhelming majority of participants expressed disagreement with such laws, citing the resultant increased risk of retaliation by the perpetrator and eventual harm to the victim as reasons. Participants also reported that they desired an end to the violence and wanted healthcare providers to take part in that process, but believed that including law enforcement agencies was too great of a risk. Still, most participants did agree with the goal of mandated reporting: that the perpetrator be held accountable for the abuses. However, they suggested improvements to the system that would allow victims to be more comfortable with mandated reporting. These suggestions included adding provisions to protect the victim's safety and provide the victim and perpetrator with resources that would be facilitative of longer-term solutions. One participant elaborated, "Before I would tell, I would have to know for sure that (a) he would not just be jailed overnight, (b) he'd be sent to some kind of treatment, (c) he'd be told by a judge that there would be serious consequences if he did it again, and (d) he'd receive at least six months of treatment" (Sullivan & Hagen, 2005, p. 358). These insights suggest that interventions aimed at protecting and supporting victims of domestic violence need to incorporate more than punishing perpetrators and encouraging separation of victims from their abusive partners. As articulated previously by a survivor, it is necessary to provide comprehensive interventions such as treatment and therapy that are aimed at treating several issues involved in the abuse.

This discussion is helpful when considering Sara's case because it provides insight into the difficult conflict between an NP's responsibility to his or her patient and the NP's legal responsibilities. Although the nurse may feel responsible to protect himself or herself legally by encouraging Sara to leave her boyfriend, the NP is supported and required by her professional code of ethics to be first and foremost committed to promoting a good for the patient. Therefore, if the NP deems that Sara's option of moving to leave her boyfriend will cause more harm than good, then she is ethical in not encouraging Sara to move. Finally, the insight provided by survivors of IPV reminds us that optimal interventions for victims focus on several aspects of the victim's and perpetrator's conditions. More than the threatened punishment of perpetrators or encouraged separation of partners, interventions must offer aid in healing the factors that contribute to the abusive environment on the part of both the victim and perpetrator.

Implications for Sara's Case

Interventions aimed at supporting victims of domestic violence should incorporate the current recommendations for healthcare providers. As previously discussed, these include (1) validating the patient's experience, (2) providing the patient with pertinent information surrounding IPV, (3) aiding the patient in developing a safety plan, and (4) questioning whether the involvement of law enforcement is appropriate (Warshaw & Ganley, 1996). In addition, through the use of the ethical decision-making guidelines and the discussions of major issues in Sara's case, we can develop additional courses of action that ought to be incorporated into interventions to support Sara.

The discussion of the concept of empowerment suggests that an appropriate intervention would be aimed at facilitating and supporting Sara's decision-making capabilities. The NP could use the clinic setting as a safe environment in which Sara can practice autonomous decision-making processes—she may have to be creative in arranging the time for Sara to do this and for building a trust relationship with her. Because of Sara's inability to express her needs and priorities, this will not be simple. But the NP should encourage Sara in an exploration of her needs and desires. Once she has established a relationship with Sara, ways of eliciting her input will become clearer. Guided by her knowledge of Sara, one possibility might be to prompt Sara to an informative response by asking nonthreatening questions first such as ones regarding her general likes and dislikes. Then, the NP can ask her to envision what life would be like if she had already made one decision or the other. Then, perhaps asking questions such as: "What do you think you would miss if you moved to your mother's?" "What do you think it would be like if you stayed near your boyfriend?" "Who do you want to help you take care of the baby after it is born?" "What are you most afraid of or nervous about?" Using questions such as these to spark conversation, the NP could then guide Sara through a decision-making process to choose a course of action that Sara deems helpful for her current situation. The NP should then support this decision and the priorities that Sara has identified to promote her empowerment. During future visits, similar strategies could be used so that the clinic would continue to serve as a safe environment in which Sara is able to practice her decision-making capabilities and develop a greater sense of empowerment over her situation and life condition.

Through the discussion of the possible maternal-fetal conflict present within Sara's case, we have learned the importance of considering alternative perspectives of the maternal-fetal relationship and investigating the details of the case to provide interventions that treat the complex social factors that contribute to the current situation. This means that in Sara's case it is necessary for the NP to provide interventions that focus on increasing social supports, aid Sara's financial and housing needs, and provide support for others involved in the case so that Sara will have the resources necessary to put both herself and her fetus in the healthiest environment possible. This is an important point at which to collaborate with other professionals. The NP could collaborate with or refer Sara to a social worker, who would be able to aid Sara in accessing social and financial supports such as new employment and housing opportunities, a temporary shelter for victims of IPV, and other community supports for victims of IPV. In addition, a social worker or psychiatric APN will be able to provide Sara with counseling and support to address the emotional and psychological factors associated with abuse. It is also important for the NP to explore with Sara the possibility of her partner seeking counseling or treatment. If this appears to be a possible intervention, it is necessary for the NP to fulfill her responsibility to provide an appropriate referral for Sara's partner to seek counseling or treatment.

Finally, it is necessary for the NP to reflect on whether it is appropriate to incorporate law enforcement into her plan. If the patient or her family appears to be in immediate danger, the NP has a responsibility to discuss with the patient whether she deems that notifying law enforcement agencies would provide her with the protection needed or if it would expose her and her family to an increased risk of violence. A decision must be made in collaboration between the nurse and the patient. The nurse must act in collaboration with his or her professional responsibilities of loyalty, confidentiality, and nonmaleficence and an ethic of care. However, if the NP is practicing in a state that mandates reporting of IPV, it may be more complicated to initiate an ethical course of action. The NP again has a responsibility to be honest with Sara and inform her that he or she is required to report the situation to law enforcement agencies. Then, as suggested by Sullivan and Hagen's (2005) research, it is important for the NP to address other factors involved to promote Sara's long-term safety such as providing access to safe housing, new employment opportunities, and referral to treatment for her boyfriend.

In summary, an optimal course of action in Sara's case would be one that tries to understand who Sara is as a person, helps her to articulate her desires and values, validates her experience, educates her about IPV, aids her in developing a safety plan, encourages her to use the clinic as an environment to practice her decision-making abilities, addresses the complex social influences, and questions the appropriate way to include the use of law enforcement agencies.

ROBYN'S CASE

The following composite case explores ethically difficult situations, which often arise when providing infertility or other technologically advanced treatment for women. After discussing the details of the specific case using the decision-making guidelines, ideas around stereotyping, women's societal expectations, the effects of stigma, and patient autonomy are explored further. Finally, specific practice implications and suggestions are offered.

A 37-year-old woman presents for an intra-uterine insemination. She is married, has never been pregnant before, and has no children. At her initial intake visit into the fertility clinic, she met with a physician for a complete physical and to discuss her treatment options and the usual protocols. Although morbidly obese, weighing 400 pounds, her initial physical exam and laboratory tests indicate that she is generally healthy. She does not suffer from diabetes, hypertension, hypercholesterolemia, or abnormal thyroid levels. Her hormone levels do suggest polycystic ovarian syndrome (PCOS) a relatively common problem, for which she is prescribed metformin to aid in the insulin resistance that is associated with PCOS. She was told that at 400 pounds, her body mass index (BMI), a measure of weight compared to height, was too high to be eligible for in-vitro fertilization because of the increased risks of anesthesia use in obese patients. The physician discussed with her the increased risks associated with obesity in pregnancy as well as the part obesity may be playing in her infertility. The recommendation was that to undergo infertility treatment, she must first lower her BMI. She refuses the option of bariatric surgery prior to fertility treatment, stating that she is increasing in age and could not wait the year it would take to undergo and recover from such a procedure. The physician and patient agree that she will attempt to lose weight through lifestyle modification and will return for her first trial of intrauterine insemination in 3 months.

Today, she presents for her insemination procedure. She has lost 10 pounds since her intake visit. This is the first time the NP has met this patient, and when the NP reviews the patient's health history, she feels uncomfortable continuing with the insemination because of the risks associated with obesity in pregnancy. However, there is no precedent set at this fertility center for denying treatment to women based on an increased BMI, nor is there a standard protocol for addressing such issues. The NP identifies that there is clearly much wrong in this case, including inadequate patient education and information.

Concepts of informed consent are discussed in depth in Chapter 3. The following discussion focuses on other aspects of the case and addresses informed consent through questions of ensuring patient autonomy.

Background on Obesity and Pregnancy

Catalano and Ehrenberg (2006) summarize the short- and long-term implications of obesity on maternal and fetal well-being. Risks to the pregnancy include a higher risk of miscarriage both for pregnancies conceived naturally and those conceived with the aid of fertility therapies. Maternal obesity is also associated with increased risks for gestational hypertension, preeclampsia, and gestational diabetes, which were determined to be 2.5 to 3.3 times more likely to develop in women who were obese prior to conception. The prevalence of these complications contributes to a significantly increased risk of preterm delivery before 37 weeks gestation for pregnancies affected by maternal obesity. In addition, maternal obesity, studied independently from the influence of maternal diabetes or folic acid intake, has been linked with increased incidence of fetuses affected by neural tube defects.

In addition to the risks posed to the pregnancy, maternal obesity increases one's likelihood for having to undergo a cesarean section and the associated complications. These complications include increased difficulty of spinal or epidural placement, possibly requiring multiple attempts, and those associated with the use of general anesthesia such as difficult intubation and an increased incidence of postpartum sleep apnea. Furthermore, obese women undergoing cesarean sections are exposed to a significantly greater risk of suffering from postoperative complications, including wound infection, excessive blood loss, and postpartum endometritis (Catalano & Ehrenberg, 2006).

Obesity has also been identified as a factor predisposing women to problems with infertility (Kelly-Weeder & O'Connor, 2006). "Obesity predisposes women to fertility impairment, particularly menstrual disorders, infertility, miscarriage, poor pregnancy outcomes, impaired fetal well-being and diabetes mellitus," (p. 271). It is suggested that the link between obesity and impaired fertility is compelling, recommending a need for obesity prevention and weight-loss support as a mechanism to promote fertility status and healthy pregnancies.

The research surrounding maternal obesity, pregnancy, and fertility supports the NP's concerns about providing aided conception in an extremely obese patient. The conflict between the good that would be provided for the patient and the real and possible harm that may be created through aided conception must be closely evaluated to arrive at an optimal course of action for Robyn. This will mean doing more than questioning whether the procedure is safe for her; it will also require the NP to gain an understanding of Robyn within the context of her life, learning her story and how her life and environmental influences have led to obesity and to her urgently wanting a pregnancy. Using the ethical decision-making guidelines proposed in Chapter 2 as well as the principles suggested through an ethic of care approach, we may be better able to understand Robyn's experience and the nuances of the issues involved to develop a course of action that is well suited for Robyn and her family.

Using Decision-Making Guidelines

Major Problems Involved

Similar to the previous case, the fundamental problem is the conflict between nonmaleficence and beneficence. The NP must negotiate between providing a good for Robyn, aiding her in conceiving a biological child, and preventing the harm that may be caused by facilitating a pregnancy in a woman with an extremely high BMI. If we look further, we can tease out other issues that may be contributing to the difficulties in this case. First, the NP has not met Robyn before this visit. It is therefore impossible for her to know the details of Robyn's experience without further opportunities to discover these. Yet a holistic nursing approach based in a feminist care perspective requires her to know more about Robyn's situation so that alternative courses of action can be developed. Additionally, although the NP recognizes the limits of her own knowledge related to this particular issue, there are no policies or other available resources within her practice setting that she can draw upon. Finally, the NP may be discouraged from developing new ways to intervene with Robyn by the presence of common stereotypes and stigma surrounding both infertility and obesity.

Who Is Involved?

What we do know about Robyn's situation is that she has expressed a strong desire to conceive a pregnancy. However, it is not known what motivates such a desire or her feeling that she does not have time to delay treatment. Additionally, we do not know what information Robyn has been given and how she has processed this. Countless factors could be at play other than desire for a family. Giving birth to a genetic offspring may be very important to her, she may feel that giving birth will make her socially more acceptable, she may be pressured by her husband, or she may have experienced social and cultural pressures to bear children before a certain age. Additionally, she may have already experienced difficulties attempting to create a family through alternative methods such as adoption.

If Robyn has an involved partner or family, it is important to assess their stakes and influences in the case as well. It is possible that they may not have been adequately informed regarding the risks to Robyn or her pregnancy if she were to become pregnant at her current weight. They may also have their own motivations or feelings regarding the desires for a family created through assisted reproductive technologies. Finally, their influences on Robyn's decision-making processes must also be considered.

A case involving new technologic therapies such as those that assisted reproductive technologies offer is influenced by the ethos of the particular medical institution. As a center focused on fertility treatments, the clinic has an interest in providing safe and comprehensive care to patients to develop a reputation for offering quality patient care. They often have financial incentives to provide services, which can cause a conflict of interest for their medical and nursing staff (see Chapter 3). The motives of such institutions may include advancing scientific knowledge and ensuring its application; thus, they have to strike a balance between scientific goals and the goals of ethical patient care.

The NP's responsibilities are to ensure that Robyn's health needs receive primary consideration. This means discovering what pregnancy means to Robyn and providing the resources and support she needs to make good choices for herself. This result may still be a desire for pregnancy, in which case the goals are for Robyn to experience a physically and psychologically healthy pregnancy, gestation, and birth. Alternatively, other courses of action that will facilitate Robyn's health will be envisioned. For these reasons, the clinician has a particular interest in understanding both the underlying factors that have contributed to Robyn's morbid obesity and those that have resulted in this strong desire for pregnancy.

Prevalent Values

What information we do have about Robyn's situation tells us that she seems to value the ability to carry and birth her own biological child. NP values include ensuring a psychosocially and physically healthy transition to motherhood, if this is determined to be what is best. The medical and scientific disciplines value the possibility of scientific progress as demonstrated by the ability to "cure" infertility with assisted reproductive technologies. As discussed in Sara's case, the presence of these varying but strong values emphasizes the necessity for providers to understand what their own values are—this requires reflecting upon those values. Unexamined values can lead to biased approaches to patient care. They obstruct the ability of healthcare providers to discover and address the fundamental issues that underlie patients' presenting problems.

As previously discussed, any ethical decision-making framework cannot be used as a recipe applied to all ethically problematic situations. Instead, there is often a nonlinear process of exploration where emerging details of a particular case give rise to, or suggest, further questions. Decision-making guidelines are tools that are helpful to begin an exploration of the nuances of a particular case and provide assurance that no perspective has been overlooked. As quickly became apparent during this exploration, the decision-making guidelines do not directly lead us to a possible course of action in Robyn's case. Instead, we have identified many areas lacking in information. However, this helps us to identify a major issue central to the case: very little information is known about Robyn or the details of her situation. Unfortunately, this is not an uncommon situation for many WHNPs who are challenged with trying to provide support, treatment, and care that addresses the real needs of the women who present for infertility treatments. In evaluating the issues central to Robyn's case, it may be helpful to think, "In an ideal situation, what knowledge and strategies would need to be available to the NP to prevent such an ethically difficult situation from arising?" The following section addresses some issues associated both with women's health and implied by Robyn's situation, including societal stereotyping of infertility, the effects of stigma, and issues of informed consent and autonomy.

Major Issues

A Stereotype of Infertility

It is difficult for the NP to form any type of conclusion or judgment regarding an optimal course of action for Robyn because fairly little is known concerning the details of Robyn's story, priorities, experiences, or the reasons she has for pursing a course of treatment that appears to pose many risks to her health. An ethic of care guides us to seek an understanding of the details of a woman's unique experience to better develop a course of action that serves to promote a good that is consistent with her priorities (Marcellus, 2004). Unfortunately, Robyn, has progressed through several phases of the process without having her unique experience understood.

In Susan Sherwin's seminal book, *No Longer Patient: Feminist Ethics and Healthcare* (1992), she offers an explanation that can be used to understand why cases such as Robyn's are all too common in the field of reproductive technologies. Practitioners, critics, and arguably society at large assume that involuntary childlessness leads to desperation. We accept the notion that it is "natural" for a woman to feel incomplete without conceiving and giving birth to her biological offspring. We are thereby simultaneously creating and reinforcing a stereotype of infertile women as naturally desperate to become pregnant. By accepting this stereotype, we as providers are disregarding the complex feelings and varied responses that are actually involved in the experiences of women and their partners (Pfeffer, 1987). Without participating in a process to better understand the complicated factors unique to each patient, we cannot attend to the real health needs of an individual patient. Instead, we help perpetuate culturally based assumptions.

Feminist critiques of assisted reproductive technologies result from analyses of the cultural values, social assumptions, and the historical context in which women are asked to make decisions regarding motherhood, childbearing, and ultimately reproductive technologies. This context has been described as overwhelmingly pronatalist because it encourages women to bear children "beyond all else" (Meyers, 2001). Evidence for this is found in widespread religious support for procreative heterosexuality. A variety of religions use strong imagery coupling womanhood with motherhood.

Additionally, historical political discourse in the United States supports the notion of childbearing as a woman's destiny, and current popular media outlets depict motherhood as the road to fulfillment for women (Meyers, 2001). Through her research of women's decisions to become mothers, Meyers (2001) discovered a common theme—that childbearing had always been accepted as an inevitable part of participants' lives. She notes, "(M)ost people presume that children are necessary to personal fulfillment and never consider not having children" (Meyers, 2001, p. 746).

Sherwin (1992) suggests three conditions prevalent in the current cultural structure that aggravate the grief of childlessness and that may contribute to the intense drive to seek infertility treatments that is depicted in the stereotype of infertile women. The first is a social structure that inhibits adults from forming family relationships or intimate interactions with children that are not their own. Involved in this structure is the complicated, emotionally trying, and expensive nature of most adoption processes in the United States. The second condition is the cultural persuasion that a woman's most important purpose in life is to bear children, and thus the work of motherhood is persistently judged as valuable. Finally, a cultural condition in which many individuals are searching for true intimacy and attachment to others and the only method through which to achieve this appears to be childbirth is described (Sherwin, 1992). These analyses of a pronatalist and socially restricting culture draw attention to some of the complexities that inevitably affect a woman's feelings and decisions surrounding reproductive technologies. They provide insights for clinicians and assist in the development of a more profound understanding of the culturally based experiences of women.

This is not to suggest that infertility is not a devastating experience for women and their partners or that a woman's intense desire to bear her biological offspring is intrinsically invalid. Furthermore, many women may experience other underlying factors that contribute to their decision to undergo infertility treatments such as a desire to experience pregnancy and childbirth for itself. In addition, it should not be assumed that these cultural influences may be implicated in all women's experiences or that such influences devalue the profound experience and loss that is associated with infertility. They are simply examples of the complicated social context in which women must make decisions about reproductive technologies and provide evidence that the stereotype of the desperate, infertile woman is one-dimensional and overly simplified. By developing a better understanding of the cultural subtleties involved in women's choices to undergo reproductive technologies, NPs will be better enabled to explore with each patient her unique experiences and ultimate goals. This process is the most likely to result in a plan of care that addresses the patient's distinctive situation.

The Effects of Stigma

An important question to ask when evaluating Robyn's case is, "Why has she not yet received care that appropriately addresses her obesity? How has it gotten to this point?" It is important to consider what barriers may have interfered with her getting appropriate treatment in the past. Part of an ethical exploration requires us to ask, What could have been done differently so as to prevent this situation in the first place?

Research has been unable to identify any one specific cause of obesity. Some researchers suggest obesity is a result of genetic and metabolic factors and is only somewhat related to dietary factors. Others identify complicated interactions between physical and environmental influences (Crandall, 1994). Some research has looked into emotional and psychological effects on obesity, suggesting a correlation between some obese individuals and a history of childhood sexual abuse. Similarly, overeating as a reaction to symptoms of post-traumatic stress disorder in some patients has also been proposed (Bell, 2005). What is clear from the research on obesity is that it is a condition affected by varying complex influences and is much more complicated than simply overeating and lack of self-control on the part of the obese individual.

Unfortunately, healthcare professionals overwhelmingly attribute controllable factors to the cause of obesity in their patients, such as lack of self-control and lifestyle choices (Drury & Louis, 2002). Crandall explains the negative impact of such stereotypes and assumptions. "If ideology leads a person to chronically attribute controllable causality to others, he or she will tend to blame fat people for their weight and stigmatize them for it" (Crandall, 1994, p. 884). Research on obesity stigma and healthcare professionals suggests that obesity is a characteristic that evokes negative responses among a large percentage of physicians and that many healthcare providers falsely attribute negative characteristics to obese patients such as "weak-willed," citing overeating and lack of self-control as the main cause of obesity (Drury & Louis, 2002). It has been argued that nurses in particular have contributed to the unhelpful responses offered to obese patients by accepting a behaviorist focus on obesity that identifies assumed bad eating habits and lack of willpower as the causative agents (Carryer, 2001). Nurses thereby have traditionally offered interventions that are falsely aimed at ideas of insufficient knowledge, poor motivation, and lack of intelligence.

It is important to consider the impact of such common assumptions and stereotypes on Robyn's case. It is possible that Robyn has not received the full range of resources that she has needed in the past because her obesity has been viewed by her healthcare providers as resulting from a lack of self-control. She may have been offered little more than diet plans as help. It is the NP's responsibility to self-reflect on her own biases and assumptions regarding obesity before meeting with Robyn so that she can approach Robyn with an open mind and desire to understand Robyn's unique experience. Only by doing this will the NP be able to achieve a holistic understanding of Robyn's experience and offer intervention options that are aimed at the complicated factors contributing to Robyn's obesity. She may find it suitable to not only offer Robyn support and guidance in making lifestyle and diet changes, but also to make appropriate referrals to therapists, nutritionists, and specialists.

It is also important to consider, on a larger scale, how the stereotypes and assumptions present within our practice affect vulnerable populations, such as obese persons, and can lead to population-based health disparities. Obese individuals report different responses to the stigma they face from health-care providers. Obesity stigma and its effects on healthcare utilization have been investigated (Drury & Louis, 2002). Results suggest that as body weight increases, the rate of healthcare avoidance or delay also increases. Participants report delaying treatment or preventative care for specific reasons such as having gained weight since their last visit, not wanting to be weighed, being embarrassed about weight, and planning on losing weight before their next visit. Such research illuminates the ways in which our practice may be further marginalizing obese patients.

Three-step strategies for healthcare providers to decrease the healthcare barriers faced by clients who are members of marginalized populations have been suggested (Spinks, Andrews, & Boyle, 2000). First, healthcare providers need to examine their own beliefs and values regarding the specific population of patients and compare these with current understandings available from research and philosophical inquiry and documented in professional literature to identify false assumptions that they may hold. Second, professional education should be used as a necessary tool to increase awareness and sensitivity to issues of stigmatization and marginalization. Finally, healthcare providers should work to communicate a validating and nonjudgmental attitude to all patients (Spinks et al., 2000).

It is possible that even if the NP identifies and sets aside her own biases, provides an affirming and nonjudgmental environment, works to understand Robyn's unique story, and offers strategies and resources that speak to the complex nature of Robyn's obesity, Robyn may still insist on continuing with the insemination in an urgent manner. The NP would then be left to question whether Robyn's obesity is a valid reason for denying treatment. In considering such an action, it is important to be cognizant of the history of and arguments concerning the regulation of access to fertility procedures. Considering the impact of stigma, stereotyping, and biases on limiting access will allow the practitioner to be more aware of the cultural context in which such a decision would be made, and the ways in which stigma has traditionally led to injustices.

Controversies about who should have access to reproductive technologies have existed since the invention and inception of such technologies. Crossley (2005) describes several studies surveying infertility clinics and their beliefs regarding screening for and regulating of reproductive technologies. A majority of providers expressed a belief that they had a responsibility to screen patients and turn away individuals who demonstrated personal attributes that, in the provider's opinion, would cause them to be unfit parents. Between 20% and 50% of clinics polled reported that they would refuse treatment to patients who planned on parenting the child in a single-parent home. Similar percentages reported that they would turn away patients who were members of same-sex partnerships. Other reasons for turning away patients were the mother's health or disability status. More than 50% specifically cited a positive human immunodeficiency virus (HIV) status of either parent as a reason to deny treatment (Crossley, 2005). In addition, much attention has been paid to the questions of whether older women or postmenopausal women ought to be allowed access to assisted reproductive technologies (Parks, 1999). The most common reasons suggested for such restrictions on access to reproductive technologies are the welfare of the potential child, prevention of harm to stakeholders involved, acceptable levels of risk, and the ethical obligations of providers (Spriggs & Charles, 2007).

However, the ethical standing of such claims is questionable when we consider the roles of discrimination, stigma, individual values, and the paternalistic nature of determining what patients make "suitable parents." There exists no quantifiable measure or standard with which to adequately predict whether a person will become a suitable or unsuitable parent (Spriggs & Charles, 2007). Such a measure would be extremely contentious to develop because it is impossible to determine what ideas and philosophies of parenting should be supported and which should be discouraged. Ideas about what types of individuals make suitable parents are inevitably contaminated by preexisting cultural assumptions and biases regarding optimal parenting and families. Another question could be raised about the appropriateness of screening of infertile couples for their suitability for parenthood because fertile couples are not subjected to such scrutiny. People who can conceive naturally are not required to justify their reasoning for becoming parents, their suitability to be parents, or demonstrate the absence of illness or disability (Spriggs & Charles, 2007). Crossley (2005) explains the discriminatory nature of such restrictions on access to reproductive technologies and the danger that they pose.

> Those individuals who are able to conceive a child in the "usual and customary manner" are not subject to scrutiny regarding their fitness to parent, while those who are infertile may be blocked in their efforts to achieve parenthood by the fitness judgments of medical providers or policy makers. While some fitness judgments may be widely accepted, others may tend to reflect suspect biases and any imposition of such judgments may create a slippery slope. (p. 106)

These arguments pertain to Robyn's case because they emphasize the need for any provider to reflect on and identify his or her own biases regarding obesity to decrease the likelihood that Robyn's care will be negatively affected by cultural assumptions about her suitability for pregnancy. In addition, understanding such arguments helps us be aware of the implications and possible injustices that could result from denying Robyn infertility treatment based on the risks associated with her obesity.

Autonomy and Informed Consent

As discussed in Chapter 2, the principle of autonomy is complex and easily affected by influencing factors. Decisions that may appear to have been made autonomously may actually have been highly influenced by contextual factors. Unfortunately, in the field of women's health, autonomy is all too frequently looked upon simply as a quest for personal choice, which facilitates ignoring the subtle and sometimes coercive influences of the context in which decisions are made. Within this view, a woman is deemed autonomous in her reproductive life if she is granted the ultimate power to give the final consent to treatment. Based on this concept, requiring informed consent is a process through which most healthcare professionals ensure that patients are making autonomous decisions. However, feminist critiques of the principle of autonomy demonstrate that this understanding may not be comprehensive enough for all instances

(Meyers, 2001; Sherwin, 1992). "Most nonfeminist bioethics treat reproductive freedom as if it were the consumer freedom to purchase technology" (Sherwin, 1992, p. 134). Sherwin suggests that autonomy is not something that can be determined on an isolated case basis but must be considered in light of the individual's entire life situation. Other scholars argue that there are forces present within the promise of new technologic advances that bear great influence on a patient's choice to pursue treatment, creating constraints on individual autonomy. The effect of such influences must be considered if we are to work to ensure patient autonomy.

The area of technologic advances in medicine has spawned much discussion regarding the assurance of patient autonomy and the many influences that affect a patient's right to self-determination when consenting to or choosing to undergo certain medical procedures. Because of the high growth rate of new medical procedures offered to women, such as reproductive technologies and prenatal screening technologies, the issues that this discussion raises are particularly salient to consider within the realm of women's health advanced practice nursing as well as Robyn's case. Scientific healthcare advances do not necessarily imply quality health care for individuals. Good patient care means considering whether, and which, technologic advances might be important adjuncts in light of our holistic understanding of a patient's needs. Therefore, as our practice of science progresses, we must consider whether our practice of care has progressed comparably to ensure that we are practicing ethically when we offer new treatment protocols.

Arguments regarding the ambiguity of choice (Davies, 2001) and the subtle coercive nature of offering technologically advanced treatment options (Sandelowski, 1991) have been made in regards to reproductive technologies as well as prenatal genetic screening. These instances and arguments are similar in nature and provide us with a point of view that asks us to consider whether a particular decision to pursue treatment has been based on a patient's autonomous decision-making capabilities or on the coercive nature of specific treatment options that make them inherently difficult to refuse.

Sandelowski (1991) goes beyond critiques of the cultural issues that influence a woman's decision to have infertility treatments and suggests that reproductive technologies are particularly compelling because of the nature of technology itself. Sandelowski (1991) studied the transcripts of interviews with women and couples facing infertility, whether or not they chose to undergo assisted reproductive technologies as well as the literature regarding infertility and conceptive technologies to investigate persistence in pursuit of infertility treatments. Major themes were identified that described women's experiences of choosing reproductive technologies. Examples included a feeling of an obligation "to try," a strong attraction to reproductive technologies because of their seemingly magical promise to cure, and an impetus to repeat and pursue treatments. Sandelowski (1991) concludes, "My own research with infertile couples and my reading of the literature on conceptive technology suggest that conceptive technology, by its valence toward repeated applications and comparison of its outcomes to natural conception, reinforces and mobilizes a cultural faith among couples and their doctors that persistence in the pursuit of a goal ultimately pays off" (Sandelowski, 1991, p. 41).

Similar arguments are cited in debates surrounding prenatal genetic testing, informed consent, and ensuring patient autonomy. Although it is often suggested that new technologies work to increase patient autonomy by offering more choices to women and their partners, many scholars argue that the act of offering an increased number of treatment options may present coercive influences itself. Davies (2001) refers to what she terms the "ambiguity of choice" in regard to decision-making processes over prenatal genetic testing. She contends that although these screening opportunities are offered to increase choice for women, the choice may be more of an illusion than originally understood. She explains that the more choices that are offered to a patient, the more necessary it is for the patient to explain and defend her decision, thereby making it difficult to say no to an offered procedure. In addition, other scholars suggest that women will accept prenatal screening options and other technologically advanced treatment options because they perceive an imperative to "do whatever they can" (Lippman, 2001). These subtle coercive influences that may be present in the offering of treatment options, whether they are prenatal or assisted reproductive, make it difficult for an NP to determine whether a patient has accepted to undergo treatment out of her own autonomy, out of a pressure to conform to the values of the medical institution, or as a result of coercion (Lippman, 2001).

To address issues of patient autonomy in decision-making processes, NPs have typically attempted to provide treatment options in a "nondirective" way so as not to persuade patients toward one decision or another. However, the previous discussion highlights the ways in which simply providing treatment options in a nondirective manner may not preclude the presence of all coercive influences when offering treatment options. Instead, it is imperative for an NP to know the patient, to engage in an exploration with the patient of her ultimate goals for her treatment, and then to use that knowledge to aid her in developing a plan of action that will support the patient's identified priorities.

When a practitioner has gained this knowledge about a unique patient, the practitioner is able to see how a plan of action may be discussed in a way that is suited to that individual patient's needs. For instance, some patients may clearly express a desire to utilize every possible treatment option. For these patients, it is appropriate to offer education about all possible options, the ways the treatment protocol may look down the line, and what they can expect in the future. For other patients, an NP may sense their hesitancy to refuse treatment options. In these cases, it may be necessary for the NP not to simply provide education regarding the possible options, but also to discuss common feelings about deciding to accept or refuse treatment. In some situations, practitioners may need to give permission to patients to discontinue or refuse treatment to reassure them that it is okay to make such a decision. This process will be different for each patient, clinical situation, and practitioner and will depend heavily on the relationship formed between provider and patient.

In addition to knowing the patient, it is necessary for NPs to understand the subtleties that are involved in offering technologically advanced treatment options and to reflect on their own values and beliefs regarding such treatments. Only after all of these have been explored can a practitioner offer treatment options in a way that encourages a patient to exercise her own autonomy to choose a plan of action that best suits her unique situation.

Implications for Robyn's Case

The previous discussion allows us to arrive at a course of action that provides more than simply denying or providing treatment to Robyn. In Robyn's case especially, we see the need for enacting an ethic of care and working to know Robyn as a unique individual. First, the NP must abandon any stereotypes of infertility and set forth to engage with Robyn to better understand the factors contributing to her desire to undergo intrauterine insemination. An NP is an aptly suited healthcare provider for this intervention because nursing theory that guides our practice directs us to seek a holistic understanding of a patient within the patient's context. The NP in this case could begin a conversation with Robyn to explore these issues prior to proceeding with the insemination. Exploration of Robyn's experiences and priorities could be promoted through questions such as: "What is your story of trying to conceive up to this point?" "How did you decide to pursue infertility treatments?" "What are your goals and priorities for treatment?" "What is your biggest fear in regards to this procedure?" This information could then be used by the NP to better understand Robyn as an individual patient complete with the complexities and environmental influences that bear on her desire to conceive. After a better understanding is developed, the NP would then be equipped to guide a discussion surrounding the possible options for delaying treatment, seeking weight loss or lifestyle modifications, or continuing with treatment in a way that would support Robyn's priorities. She may need to refer Robyn to other providers as indicated. As noted, this type of discussion would promote Robyn's autonomy and minimize the presence of coercive influences that may play a role in offering treatment options alone.

In addition to working to know Robyn and the details of her experience, the NP is also obligated to act in a way that reduces the effect of stigma and works to decrease the likelihood that this situation would occur again. As suggested in the discussion surrounding the effects of stigma, the NP can work to reduce these effects by examining her own beliefs and values regarding obese patients on a personal and professional level as well as communicate a validating and nonjudgmental environment when interacting with Robyn. After doing so, it is necessary for the NP to enact an ethic of care and to hear Robyn's story in attempts to understand the complicated influences that have led to her obesity. After forming a better understanding of Robyn's situation, the NP can offer resources and strategies that address the many factors contributing to Robyn's obesity, including appropriate referrals when necessary. Finally, it is necessary for the NP to work with colleagues to change the current structure of the clinic to develop an institutional forum in which providers can discuss their feelings and concerns, and educate themselves regarding ethically difficult cases such as Robyn's. Institutional change will provide support for providers so that situations such as this do not occur in the future.

SUMMARY

This chapter explores issues that are unique to women's health advanced practice nursing, focusing on a feminist ethic of care and utilizing traditional and feminist ethics approaches to explore two clinically-based cases. Issues that are prevalent in many discussions of women's health ethics and that are critical to each case are comprehensively discussed. These issues include patient empowerment, maternal-fetal conflicts, legal responsibilities, a stereotype of infertility, the effects of stigma and patient autonomy, and informed consent. Possible courses of action for each case were offered. Strategies emphasize the need for the NP to engage in a process with each patient to form a holistic understanding of the patient as a unique individual. Only by partaking in this process can the NP in each case provide interventions that support the patient's individual priorities instead of priorities based on cultural influences and assumptions.

DISCUSSION QUESTIONS

1. After engaging in this process, if Robyn still asserts that she wishes to pursue treatment, what should the NP do?
2. What additional issues are implicated in the cases of Sara or Robyn that were not discussed in this chapter?
3. Using an example from your practice setting or personal experience, explore the impact of bias or stigma.
4. Use the decision-making guidelines proposed in Chapter 2 and the principles of a feminist ethic of care to explore the following case. Reflect on the discussions of major issues in women's health in this chapter to guide your development of an appropriate course of action.

You are working as a WHNP in an ob/gyn private practice in a rural area. There is an ultrasound machine and trained technician at the office. However, many of the other luxuries that are easily available in more urban areas such as genetic counselors, level-two ultrasounds, amniocentesis, and termination procedures are not readily available to patients. You are caring for a pregnant patient who reports for her initial obstetrical visit. She is 10 weeks pregnant. She tells you that her sister, who lives in an affluent urban area, recently had a prenatal genetic screening test that told her she had a very low risk of carrying a fetus affected with Down syndrome or a neural tube defect. The patient wants to know if this is an appropriate test for her. Knowing that the appropriate follow-up resources may not be available and understanding the complex subtleties involved in offering technologically advanced treatment options to women, how would you address her question?

REFERENCES

American College of Obstetricians and Gynecologists. (2007). *Screening tools: Domestic violence.* Retrieved June 11, 2007, from http://www.acog.org:80/departments/dept_notice.cfm?recno=17& bulletin=585.

American Nurses Association. (2001). *Code of ethics with interpretive statements.* Retrieved April 1, 2007, from http://nursingworld.org/ethics/code/protected_nwco e303.htm.

Bell, S. (2005). Current issues and challenges in the management of bariatric patients. *Journal of Wound, Ostomy and Continence Nursing, 32*(6), 386–392.

Campbell, J., Harris, M., & Lee, R. (1995). Violence research: An overview. *Scholarly Inquiry for Nursing Practice, 9*(2), 105–126.

Carryer, J. (2001). Embodied largeness: A significant women's health issue. *Nursing Inquiry, 8*(2), 90–97.

Catalano, P., & Ehrenberg, H. (2006). The short- and long-term implications of obesity on the mother and her offspring. *British Journal of Obstetrics and Gynaecology, 113*, 1126–1133.

Chez, N. (1994). Helping the victim of domestic violence. *American Journal of Nursing, 94*(7), 32–37.

Connell, R. (1987). *Gender and power.* Stanford, CA: Stanford University Press.

Crandall, C. (1994). Prejudice against fat people: Ideology and self-interest. *Journal of Personality and Social Psychology, 66*(5), 882–894.

Crossley, M. (2005). Dimensions of equality in regulating assisted reproductive technologies. *University of Pittsburgh School of Law Working Paper Series,* paper 30.

Curry, M., Durham, L., Bullock, L., Bloom, T., & Davis, J. (2006). Nurse case management of pregnant women experiencing or at risk for abuse. *Journal of Obstetrical, Gynecological and Neonatal Nursing, 35*(2), 181–192.

Davies, D. (2001). *Genetic dilemmas: Reproductive technology, parental choices, and children's futures.* New York: Routledge.

Drury, C., & Louis, M. (2002). Exploring the association between body weight, stigma of obesity, and health care avoidance. *Journal of the American Academy of Nurse Practitioners, 14*(12), 554–561.

Emerson, R. (1981). Social exchange theory. In M. Rosenberg & R. Turner (Eds.), *Social psychology: Sociological perspectives* (pp. 30–65). New York: Basic Books.

Family Violence Prevention Fund. (2004). *National consensus guidelines on identifying and responding to domestic violence and victimization in health care settings.* San Francisco: Family Violence Prevention Fund.

Hertzig, K., Huynh, B., Gilbert, P., Danley, D., Jackson, R., & Gerbert, B. (2006). Comparing prenatal providers' approaches to four different risks: Alcohol, tobacco, drugs and domestic violence. *Women & Health, 43*(3), 83–101.

Johnson, M., & Ferraro, K. (2000). Research on domestic violence in the 1990's: Making distinctions. *Journal of Marriage and the Family, 62*(4), 948–963.

Kelly-Weeder, S., & O'Connor, A. (2006). Modifiable risk factors for impaired fertility in women: What nurse practitioners need to know. *A Journal of the American Academy of Nurse Practitioners, 18*(6), 268–276.

Lewis-O'Connor, A. (2004). "Dying to tell?" Do mandatory reporting laws benefit victims of domestic violence? *American Journal of Nursing, 104*(10), 75–79.

Lippman, A. (2001). Worrying—and worrying—about the geneticization of reproduction and health. In W. Teays & L. Purdy (Eds.), *Bioethics, justice and healthcare* (pp. 635–643). Belmont, CA: Wadsworth/Thomson Learning.

Marcellus, L. (2004). Feminist ethics must inform practice: Interventions with perinatal substance users. *Health Care for Women International, 25*, 730–742.

Mercer, R. (2004). Becoming a mother versus maternal role attainment. *Journal of Nursing Scholarship, 36*(3), 226–232.

Meyers, D. (2001). The rush to motherhood: Pronatalist discourse and women's autonomy. *Signs, 26*(3), 735–773.

Nelson, A. (2003). Transition to motherhood. *Journal of Gynecological, Obstetrical and Neonatal Nursing, 32*, 465–477.

Parks, J. (1999). On the use of IVF by post-menopausal women. *Hypatia, 14*(1), 77–96.

Pfeffer, N. (1987) Artificial insemination, in-vitro fertilization and the stigma of infertility. In: Stanworth, M., (Ed.), *Reproductive technologies*. Minneapolis: University of Minneapolis Press.

Pulerwitz, J., Amaro, H., De Jong, W., Gortmaker, L., & Rudd, R. (2002). Relationship power, condom use and HIV among women in the USA. *AIDS Care, 14*(6), 789–800.

Rubin, R. (1967). Attainment of the maternal role. Processes . . .part 1. *Nursing Research, 16,* 237.

Sandelowski, M. (1991). Compelled to try: The never-enough quality of conceptive technology. *Medical Anthropology Quarterly, 5*(1), 29–47.

Shanner, L. (1998). Pregnancy intervention and models of maternal-fetal relationship: Philosophical reflections on the Winnipeg C.F.S. dissent. *Alberta Law Review, 36,* 751–767.

Sherwin, S. (1992). *No longer patient: Feminist ethics and healthcare*. Philadelphia: Temple University Press.

Spinks, V., Andrews, J., & Boyle, J. (2000). Providing health care for lesbian clients. *Journal of Transcultural Nursing, 11*(2), 137–143.

Spriggs, M., & Charles, T. (2007). Should HIV discordant couples have access to assisted reproductive technologies? (HIV and assisted reproductive technologies). *Journal of Medical Ethics, 29*(6), 325–330.

Sullivan, C., & Hagen, L. (2005). Survivors' opinion about mandatory reporting of domestic violence and sexual assault by medical professionals. *Affilia Journal of Women and Social Work, 20*(3), 346–361.

Warshaw, C., & Ganley, A. (1996). *Improving the health care response to domestic violence: A resource manual for healthcare providers*. San Francisco: Family Violence Prevention Fund.

CHAPTER 10

Nursing Ethics and Advanced Practice: Adult Health

Jane Flanagan

The longest journey of any person is the journey inward.
Dag Hammarskjöld, 1961

INTRODUCTION

When I first began to write a chapter in this book on ethical issues for advanced practice nurses (APNs) in adult health nursing, I was excited knowing that this needs to be written. In my clinical practice as an adult health nurse practitioner (NP), I find that ethical rounds in hospitals focus far too much on one issue—decision making around the dying process at the very end of life. In fact, most problems for APNs are centered on determining what is good care on a daily basis and how to deliver it in the face of obstacles. Further, not all care provided by APNs is even in the acute care setting, but rather in primary care settings where the overall issue of good care is pressing and includes decision making around all aspects of health care. Although decision making at the very end of life is certainly an important issue, there are so many other ethical issues of concern for APNs.

The very title *advanced practice nurse in adult health* is problematic. How are the ethical issues of NPs and clinical nurse specialists (CNSs) different from other levels of nursing practice, and how are adult health nursing issues different from other specialty practices? I have never really agreed with the separation of adult versus family versus community in advanced practice. And despite being an APN in adult health, I was not really sure APNs could always articulate what was so different about their practice from that of non-APNs other than the fact that they "could do physicals and write prescriptions just like a doctor"—a fact friends, family, and other people outside nursing would remind me (and in doing so make me cringe).

Herein is my dilemma—to write a chapter about APNs in adult health when I neither agree with title or categorization of nursing in this way. To me, the idea that there are different levels of nurses is hierarchical and implies that issues that face APNs are somehow different from ones faced by other nurses, or that APNs have a greater depth and understanding of the discipline than do other nurses, which they then bring to their practice. I do not think

281

this is always so. Further, I agree with Northrup and Purkis (2001) in that the compartmentalization of specialties—adult, pediatric, gerontology, community, psychiatric, and so forth—causes nurses to lose sight of the philosophical and theoretical underpinnings of nursing. This results in that which is essentially *nursing* being forsaken by many APNs in the practice setting. For example, within the specialty of adult health nursing, both CNSs and NPs are often hired by institutions whose orientation and goals are disease and disease management. From a nursing disciplinary perspective, this focus on disease, cure, and the reliance on *efficiency models* (I question how efficient they are in fact) does not reflect my perspective of nursing. The actions APNs are encouraged to employ in the name of efficiency are not always directed at "good" nursing care from a nursing perspective.

What all APNs do have in common, however, is the fact that they all must take required core courses that provide them with greater contextual understanding of the nursing discipline than what they may have received in an undergraduate program; therefore, these courses may contribute to APNs being advanced in the discipline. The key here is whether these courses are (1) treated as nursing courses and taught from the disciplinary perspective, (2) regarded as perfunctory in which case the courses may not shape nurses' thinking of how they practice as APNs, or (3) integrated throughout the curriculum so that they do provide the APN with greater disciplinary perspective. If the preceding is true and the APN student has required courses in *nursing* ethics, research, role, and concepts that are later integrated into courses on adult health *nursing* theory, then it is possible that students are advanced in their thinking about *nursing care* of the adult population. Because nursing academics are also responsible for good care of persons, it is their moral responsibility to design curricula and provide education that results in good nurses who will practice in the discipline of nursing. Upon graduation, it is then crucial for APNs to find a role that allows them to practice in the way they were educated. But is the curriculum always created and integrated in this way, and is it always possible to find a position in which one can truly be advanced in the knowledge of the discipline? If it is not possible, then what should the APN do? Adding further confusion to this issue is the fact that state licensing bodies overseeing the regulatory issues of what defines an APN have in some cases decided *the* core curriculum courses for APNs are advanced health assessment, pharmacology, and pathophysiology. They have chosen to be silent about core courses in the disciplinary perspective of *advanced nursing practice*.

Contemporary forces affecting the nursing profession and consequently its ability to further its goals include (1) interdisciplinary research as a mandate from the National Institutes of Health, which provides the majority of funding for healthcare research, (2) issues around the initiation of a Doctorate in Nursing

Practice (which would require many additional courses in the curricula that are not nursing discipline specific—see discussion in Chapter 2), and (3) suggestions that transdisciplinary healthcare workers should be educated and could "fill in" for a variety of professionals.

All nurses, especially nurse educators and APNs, face a challenge (and the ethical responsibility, as argued in earlier chapters) to maintain nursing as a distinct and important discipline with a unique approach to patient care. (The idea of educational preparation affecting the practice of the APN is discussed in more detail later in the chapter.) With so many concurrent debates in health care directly affecting APNs, it is understandable that the focus of the nursing discipline can become murky. It is for precisely this reason that throughout these ongoing debates the imperative is for APNs to maintain their nursing focus.

This being said, the issues I have been asked to address include advocacy, health disparities, and health promotion. In earlier chapters, Grace provides a foundation for describing professional responsibility, disciplinary knowledge, and fiduciary relationships and has noted that the APNs who practice in an ethical way use disciplinary knowledge. Building on this foundation, this chapter first explores historical perspectives of the nursing discipline, nursing knowledge development, and other concepts that will provide background for the case studies that follow. As Grace has pointed out in the earlier sections of this book, it is imperative that APNs understand how the American Nurses Association (ANA, 2001) and the International Council of Nurses (ICN, 2006) Codes of Ethics serve to guide their unique role in caring for patients, families, and communities in the healthcare system. The adult health specialty in advanced practice encompasses all persons older than age 13 per the American Association of Colleges of Nursing (AACN) and the nursing-focused care directed toward them during periods of both health and illness. The level of nursing care addressed is relevant to all nurses but is specifically within the realm of the APN—both NPs and CNSs who practice in adult health nursing care.

The chapter utilizes both a reflective approach in that questions are posed throughout the chapter and a case-based exploration of ethical issues that confront APNs in adult health nursing care. The reflective questions are intended to help you pause to deliberate on the ideas and issues that are being reviewed. The cases are designed to stimulate discussion about how APNs in practice can maintain a nursing disciplinary perspective in their practice. Questions aim to provoke you to delineate the unique role of the APN from other healthcare workers. The cases address the topics of autonomy, health disparities, and health promotion. Questions raised can help NPs and CNSs begin to articulate their own individual position about who they are as an APN, what the role means to them, and how they meet (or do not meet) the needs of the public they serve. These discussions do not purport to answer the questions raised, but rather are meant to increase the self-awareness of APNs in practice so that they can recognize those constraints and issues in the healthcare system that affect practice. Further, APNs' responsibilities both to provide leadership and influence needed change within their environments of practice and the broader healthcare system, as discussed in earlier chapters.

More Notes on Nursing, the Discipline

To provide a foundation for the following discussion about how APNs use nursing disciplinary knowledge to guide their practice, I think it is important to highlight briefly some of the writings of nurse scholars who have grappled with the issues of what nursing is, what nurses do, and what knowledge is needed for practice. Nursing knowledge development—that is, knowledge needed for good nursing practice—occurred by borrowing ideas and theories from other disciplines such as anthropology, sociology, biology, and psychology to inform nursing's understanding of the human condition and human health needs and thus facilitate appropriate actions. From a historical perspective, Dickoff, James, and Wiedenbach (1968) proposed that nursing theory, practice, and research are all related and interdependent.

Nursing theory, which is the body of knowledge aimed at directing and supporting practice, is developed in a reciprocal fashion in that it is born from practice, tested in research, and brought back to practice for further theory/research progression. For example, an NP is working with a patient to educate him about care for diabetes. The NP begins by providing some general information about diabetes and basic information about what diet changes the patient must make until the NP is able to set up an appointment for him with a nutritionist. The NP uses a theoretical framework that includes stages of change as suggested by Prochaska and DiClemente (1983), but notes the patient is disengaged and that often this is the case with some of her newly diagnosed diabetic patients. Recognizing that the stages of change theory are not helpful in these situations, the NP begins to test a new intervention that allows patients to share their life stories. The NP recognizes that this leads the patients to feel known by and connected to the nurse and that this simple strategy allows patients some control over a situation in which they have little. The NP further tests this intervention, and in doing so further informs the original theory or develops another theory altogether. By virtue of the fact that nursing is a practice discipline, theories are intended for practice situations, and the testing and revising of theory is part of a natural and reciprocal process.

Dickoff and colleagues (1968) identified four kinds of theories that were in existence in the literature during the 1960s: (1) factor isolating; (2) factor relating; (3) situation relating; and (4) situation producing. They suggest that situation-producing theory is the highest level of theory construction. Situation-producing theory allows for the production of outcomes of a desired type that are in line with the goals of nursing theory such as improved health. Situation-producing theory is the most desirable for nursing if theory is to affect practice, but the perspective is paternalistic in that the patient's goal(s) or desired outcomes are not known but presumed. There are three essential ingredients of situation-producing theory: "a) goal-content specified as aim for activity; b) prescription for activity to realize the goal; c) a survey list to serve as a supplement to present prescription and as preparation for activity toward the goal content" (Dickoff et al., 1968, p. 421). Clearly, this approach stems from a medical model that is both paternalistic and prescriptive. It assumes that the provider knows what is best for the individual and all that is necessary for a desired outcome is the correct remedy to achieve the goal.

This prescriptive model of thinking was and is important to nursing. APNs are easily able to recount the things that they do *for* patients—listening to heart and lung sounds, taking a health history, teaching about disease and disease management, planning for a transition to another care environment. No doubt these activities are important, and often this is exactly what the public expects from APNs. But is it different from the approach of medicine? If this is true, how is it so?

It could be said that nurses utilize nursing theories to guide their practice. Historically, this is supported by the work of Johnson (1974), who suggests that nurses develop a theoretical body of knowledge from which practice emerges. She suggests that for nursing to develop as a profession, nurses must be able to engage in research activities that further develop and enhance the nursing discipline's theoretical body of knowledge. If a nurse engages in research about whether patients understand written hospital discharge information they receive and what impact adhering to the instructions has on the overall recovery experience, and a nursing theoretical framework guides the research, then this is nursing research that is intended to answer the questions of the discipline. Nursing conceptual models serve as a guide for this type of research.

Today it is often said and understood that there is a reciprocal relationship among nursing theory, research practice, and education—that is, the theory guides the research, but the results of the research may lead to the development of new concepts in the theory or practice changes. Donaldson and Crowley (1978) initially proposed this idea in their seminal work that synthesized the work of nursing science to date. Through their review of nursing research, they unveiled three themes that today serve as the essence of nursing:

1. Concern with principles and laws that govern life processes, well-being, and optimal functioning of human beings—sick or well.
2. Concern with the patterning of human behavior in interaction with the environment in critical life situations.
3. Concern with the processes by which positive changes in health status are affected (Donaldson & Crowley, 1978, p. 113).

These themes suggest that nurses are involved in more than just the things that they do. They are also involved in *being with* their patients in a dialogue and assisting in processing the goals of the patient. The work of Peplau (1952), Rogers (1970), and others is reflected in this perspective.

As theories of nursing have developed over the last four decades, the essence and goals of nursing, as discussed in Chapter 2, have essentially remained unchanged, and the notion of the relationship between nursing research, practice, and education as reciprocal remains supported today (Fawcett, 2005). Thus, we can see that nurse scholars and philosophers have traditionally been engaged in developing and clarifying ideas about nursing practice that reveal nursing to be distinguished from other healthcare practice professions by its holistic focus and interests as well as its knowledge development endeavors. This is important in light of the recent move of others in health care to claim holistic care and narrative inquiry as their specialty. Nursing has much to add to the discourse on transdisciplinary and interdisciplinary health care but needs to continue to anchor its endeavors in its own unique knowledge base.

As mentioned earlier, nursing science, which involves the research aimed at nursing knowledge development, has emerged by integrating ideas from other sciences. Pearson and Vaughn (1996) state that there are three major "borrowed" theories relevant to nursing models: (1) systems, (2) developmental, and (3) symbolic interactionism. Nursing models that have emerged from these theories agree on several concepts of importance that together are uniquely nursing related. They include assumptions of (1) health, (2) the holistic view of people, (3) the humanistic view of people, (4) the autonomy of patients, and (5) the need for a therapeutic relationship to develop between the nurse and those who are nursed. As a discipline, nursing remains focused on developing a specialized body of knowledge that uses these assumptions (Flanagan, in press). Attention to these concepts helps to distinguish nursing from other professions. A crucial idea drawn from these assumptions is that nurses seek to partner with patients. Within this relationship, the nurse openly explores possibilities with the patient and helps him or her make choices based on an understanding of personal life experiences and consequences of interventions related to that person's life. The focus of the discipline of nursing has been described as the partnership between the patient and nurse that seeks to understand the human health experience (Newman, Sime, & Corcoran-Perry, 1991; Parse, 1999).

Donaldson and Crowley suggested in 1978 that nursing theories have historically been directed at (1) practical aims to be utilized in practice; (2) prescriptive aims that seek to predict; and (3) descriptive aims that seek to know. If this has been so for 40 years, why do nurses still struggle to explain to the public (and each other) what this means, how it looks in practice, and how it is philosophically different from others in health care? How this partnership with the patient is actualized in a way that (1) the public recognizes and (2) expects from nursing is a challenge that remains true today. For example, in both my practice and my research, I often utilize the theoretical model of Newman (1994), who suggests nurses should draw out information from patients with questions like, "Tell me about the significant people and events in your life." In my dissertation work (Flanagan, in press), I studied nurses who used this methodological approach to "come to know" their patients, and the nurses often described that this question caught patients off guard because this was not something they expected a nurse to ask or viewed as the work of nursing.

In both my practice and in research I have completed since my dissertation, I have also used this methodological approach. Although some patients pause and then readily begin to share, I often am asked questions such as, "Are you a psychiatrist?" Clearly, these patients are not familiar with the nursing theoretical link to practice that suggests that I partner with my patient in a way that explores meaning and purpose. How is this in conflict with the ANA's (2003) *Social Policy Statement*, which suggests that nurses have a dynamic relationship with the public they serve? As a professional practice, nursing has a public it serves, and it is the actions nurses take that are the phenomena of concern, such as safe medication administration, provision of comfort, and alleviation of suffering. As a practice discipline, nursing is concerned with philosophical and theoretical knowledge, methodologies, and ethics. The discipline encompasses research, practice, and education. The process among the three is dynamic and reciprocal in that they inform each other, but all are ultimately concerned with facilitating the goals of the discipline with regard to the good of individuals and society.

Donaldson and Crowley (1978) conclude that nursing as a discipline and nursing as a profession are linked and influence each other, but the discipline of nursing must guide the practice rather than be defined by it. I wonder what practice it is guiding. That is, does the discipline guide the practice that is caught up in the things that I do, but to the point that the part of my practice in which I partner with my patients is devalued not only by other nurses but also the public because it is not what they expect of me?

Nursing—Is It So Unique?

In health care, professional practice disciplines have various styles of learning. In medicine, teaching/learning often occurs in groups during teaching rounds. The process is that the more experienced, "expert"-level physician questions the novice (not necessarily younger) in a series of questions that logically flow with the intent to flush out all the extraneous data and come to a conclusion or diagnostic evaluation. When a label does not fit, a cure is not effective, other anomalies arise, or something crucial is not known, and questions for research are generated. Many other disciplines in health care utilize this clinical decision-making model for teaching, learning, and generating new knowledge.

Nursing also uses this clinical decision-making model in caring for patients. Nursing, however, is unique among professional disciplines in that it also uses a self-reflective, intuitive model to examine patient care situations, ethics of good care, the nurse–patient dynamic, and gaps in nursing knowledge. This process allows both the individual nurse and the practice as a whole to question situations, raise other possible solutions to problems, advance ideas, generate new knowledge, and think in a way that encourages diversity of opinion. APNs do not toss aside medical and empirical evidence in patient care situations (or while conducting research) such as using an antihypertensive to control blood pressure. They also utilize an intuitive, reflective process and concurrently apply it while questioning the potential that one medical treatment such as a pill is the answer to the entirety of the person's health. APNs also consider the impact of a new diagnosis, the medical plan of action, the patient's story, and other life circumstances that contribute to the situation, as well as observe for aberrations from expected responses to therapeutic actions and partner with the patient to revise a plan of action or develop a new one.

Nursing as a discipline is also unique in that both practicing nurses and scholars are able to exemplify through their actions care that is often at the same time and in the same situation derived from several paradigmatic models: problem solving, process oriented, and aesthetic knowing (Roy & Jones, 2006). In the problem-solving approach, the nurse assesses the patient and discovers an issue, such as impaired mobility, and plans strategies to assist the patient. In the process approach for this same patient, the nurse recognizes that this person is unique and has a story to share not only about the overall change in physical status, but the patient's life as a whole. The nurse provides time for the patient to share the story of his life. The aesthetic approach suggests the nurse both uses intuition to act on a feeling that something more is going on than may initially appear and also allows the nurse to create ways for the patient to creatively express (for example, through poetry, art, music) what the experience has been like. Differences in these perspectives are addressed in the next section, but no one paradigm can be relied upon to resolve or answer all patient care dilemmas or questions for nursing.

From a nursing point of view, people are unique and complex; thus, one type of solution, or a solution to one type of problem, will not fit all cases. For example, even if a treatment does work, this doesn't necessarily mean that a person's quality of life is improved. Thus, an even more important question for nurses is what defines quality of life for that individual? Many people may in fact benefit from a treatment, but it is just as likely that patients may choose not to take the treatment, or that this treatment may cause hardship or simply not work. It is these unique situations that are phenomena of concern for nursing.

From a philosophical perspective, nurses do not see people from a viewpoint that reduces people to parts and solitary functions only, but from one that includes holism. This is not to say that nurses cannot or will not treat the particulars or use the deductive process to inform their decisions, but rather it is not the only process used—it is part of what is necessary to get the whole picture. Nurses will, for example, provide the patient with and educate about how to use a medication that best evidence suggests will work for a particular problem. However, nurses will use the context of the patient's life in choosing the medicine that best fits the patient's lifestyle and needs. Further, this holistic perspective may cause the nurse to ask pertinent questions such as: "Can this person afford the medication once discharged?" "Will he or she be able to get to a pharmacy?" "Can the person see well enough to distinguish this medication from the one that looks like it but that is taken on a different schedule?" "Does this person even have a desire to treat the problem in a way that is recommended?"

Changes in Health Care and the APN

Rapid changes have been occurring in health care over the past two decades that have greatly affected patient care delivery for all healthcare providers. A healthcare system emphasis on economic concerns has led to (1) shortened time for all primary care visits with providers, (2) early discharge from acute care settings post procedure or event, and (3) less follow-up by nurses as patients transition to home care. As a result, more questions are raised for nursing to address: Do nurses in general, and APNs in particular, really practice holistically? Are there really differences in the care delivered between nurse providers and other healthcare providers? Is care adequate to meet a patient's real needs in either case? Do nurses on all levels, more realistically, adapt to a system that collectively has silenced the voice and perspective of nursing? If this is so, are nurses practicing nursing or some modification of it? Have the lines between what is a nurse and what is another type of healthcare provider become blurred?

If so, is there a need for nursing to exist as its own unique entity? The discipline's self-reflection and the reflection of individual practitioners and scholars allow nursing to question its current purpose, its knowledge development, and its future. Ultimately, this is necessary to continue to meet the needs of patients related to health and well-being.

NURSING KNOWLEDGE AND NURSING PRACTICE

Nursing Practice, Philosophical Perspectives, and Theory-Guided Practice

As mentioned previously, nursing is both a practice profession and a practice discipline (Northrup et al., 2004). Nursing knowledge development is derived from three different perspectives: problem-solving, process-oriented, and cosmic imperative (Roy & Jones, 2006). Although each perspective is unique, nurses in practice often use all three approaches with patients in an effort to come to know patients as unique, complex beings. Knowing the patient as a contextual and relational individual has been identified as essential to nursing practice (Radwin, 1995). How nurses come to know their patients (through problem-solving, process-oriented, or cosmic imperative approaches) can vary, but ideally it is always done within a nursing disciplinary perspective. The next section describes the various approaches to nursing knowledge development and knowing the patient from a nursing disciplinary perspective.

The Problem-Solving Approach

A very rudimentary explanation of the problem-solving approach to knowledge development is that problems exist that need to be solved and that scientific inquiry, including research, is aimed at doing so. For APNs who see problem solving in this way, the approach to care of the patient is problem oriented. From a nursing perspective, a systematic approach using a functional health pattern (FHP) assessment, which is composed of 11 areas of concern, is reviewed with the patient to determine the presence or absence of problems (Gordon, 1994). NPs, though, often forgo the FHP and utilize a medical model to assess patients. This is a system model that focuses on bodily functions and disturbances. In either case, parts of a person are separated out and evaluated individually. The APN, using either method, seeks to understand the person through knowing how each part of that person functions or does not function and what requires assistance or fixing. Once the problem is understood, a plan is formulated that is aimed at correcting the situation.

In describing the problem-solving approach and its relationship to nursing, Rodgers (2007) suggests that this does not mean that this attempt to "solve the problem" is as simplistic as it may initially seem (or as many nurses have been taught or think that they were taught to approach it). Rodgers counters that the values, philosophy, and various approaches of nursing cannot be ignored by a nurse using disciplinary knowledge and are therefore inherent in the problem-solving approach. An underlying assumption of the problem-solving approach is not exclusive of the disciplinary perspective, which is that people are whole beings with physical, emotional, spiritual, and social dimensions. Rodgers suggests that to come to know and understand the patient or the problem, a nurse must use multiple ways of knowing—for example, aesthetic, personal, and scientific.

This willingness to use not only the hard objective data from the patient or personal experiences but also subjective information and perception to formulate ideas about what is a problem and how to intervene and measure the outcome of interventions is unique to nursing knowledge development. Classifying and grouping problems into phenomena of concern is a goal of groups concerned with nursing language development such as the North American Nursing Diagnosis Association (NANDA). Rodgers (2007) suggests this work is important in that it identifies nursing problems as specifically nursing related and delineates how nurses think to improve or stabilize a problem.

The Process-Oriented Approach

Knowledge as process in nursing involves the nurse engaging over time with the patient in an open, nondirected dialogue about meaning and purpose. Philosophically, knowledge as process in nursing has roots in a school of thought that rejected the idea of postmodernism and poststructural feminism as discussed in Chapter 1, that is, empirical science is the only way to know truth. From a nursing disciplinary perspective, Rogers (1970) first describes human beings as irreducible in terms of essence in that they cannot be broken down into parts for the purpose of addressing their health problems. Another underlying assumption of this perspective is that definitions of health or disease are arbitrary, value laden, and culturally infused and that any perception of disease or ill health is inseparable from the person as a whole. The process-oriented approach to nursing knowledge development can be focused on the individual or, from a poststructural feminist perspective, on groups, particularly oppressed groups.

The focus of the process approach to knowledge is that nurses come to know patients within their experiences of health and illness. There are several approaches described in the nursing literature, but in each the nurse mutually dialogues with the person (or if the person is unable to communicate, his or her designee) in a nondirected fashion. The approaches, generally qualitative in nature, also assume openness to the potential of what may be and the possibility of transformation. Some approaches to the nurse–patient relationship include narrative analysis, reflective nursing practice, and aesthetic approaches such as storytelling, art, and music (Jones, 2006).

Cosmic Knowing

A third perspective on nursing knowledge development is the cosmic imperative of Roy (2006). There are three characteristics of this perspective: unity, purposefulness, and promise. Based on principles from quantum physics, unity suggests that as humans, we are one with the universe and our being is a microcosm of the cosmos. That is, the particular—individual human beings—are made up of the same materials as the universe, so it is reasonable to conclude that there is unity or oneness with that universe. Purposefulness within this perspective implies that there is creative yet intentional and increasingly complex unfolding of the universe through which a higher power is revealed. Last, promise evokes the ideas of timelessness and expansiveness of the universe within the context of a convergence of one point, the omega point, in which human meaning is rooted. The underlying assumption of the cosmic imperative is that the principles of unity, purposefulness, and promise compel nurses to practice well.

Blurring of Lines in the APN Role: The Good APN

Each approach to knowledge development as discussed previously has methods applicable for nursing research and theories applicable in nursing practice. For example, the FHP assessment is appropriate to use in the problem-solving style, and a narrative analysis such as Newman's (1994) is appropriate in the process approach. Often, many nurses utilize a combination of approaches to come to know their patient. But APNs too often describe they have "no time" to do this work. This begs the question, what type of nursing are they practicing? Earlier in this book, Grace identifies several components of good care, which include drawing on previous experiences, utilizing nursing knowledge including ethics, an ability to reflect and clarify, and personal characteristics.

As discussed earlier, there are several reasons many practicing APNs do not practice nursing from the disciplinary perspective espoused by the scholars. Because nurses enter the profession at different levels of educational preparation, many APNs have never been acquainted with the philosophical and theoretical foundations of their discipline. Even when academic programs in nursing require courses or modules in nursing theory and nursing ethics, there are differences in knowledge about, or depth of commitment to, these goals on the part of instructors. This can result in students not understanding the basis of their practice in nursing theory and nursing goals. As a result, many nurses have a cursory grasp of nursing theory and do not understand its relevance to practice, research, or even their own education.

Nursing education on both the undergraduate and graduate levels is often focused on tasks and skill acquisition. Basic sciences predominate the initial curriculum, often followed by courses that are disease focused with emphasis on tasks and clinical reasoning with theory and research as additional courses separated from patient care situations. Early in the career process, nurses complete nursing assessments, develop plans of care, and determine the effectiveness of outcomes, but this is when things begin to blur. The AACN (American Association of Colleges of Nursing, 1995) delineates a "doer" role—the nurse who does things for the patient—from the "insider" role—the nurse who knows the human health experience. The AACN task force suggests nurses on all levels be accountable for both dimensions and acknowledges a need to balance "doing" with "being with." But this suggests a dualism that is uncomfortable to me and I am sure to many nurses who philosophically engage in an ethic of caring and being with patients in a mutual, intentional process.

To me, it suggests that the things I do, the tasks, are performed adeptly and proficiently, and that the standard of measuring this is to have done the actual procedure correctly. To be considered competent, a nurse must be able to perform the tasks. This type of caring by doing permits an easily measured outcome—either the nurse can safely do the task or not.

Measuring a nurse's ability to care in the sense of "being with" includes compassion, intentionality, but measuring this is more nebulous, and by virtue of the fact that they chose to enter a "caring" profession, it is often assumed that nurses are able to be caring in this way. If conducted in a task-oriented way, care that does not consider the person in a holistic way is done without attention paid to "caring for and with" the patient (DeRaeve, 2002). This type of care may include carrying out tasks with great attention paid to the details of the task—such as changing a dressing and using good sterile technique—but with no attention paid to the person and what it may mean to her to have a wound. Care that is merely task-oriented does not assess for or necessarily address the contextual contingencies of a patient's situation. Thus, a person may not be willing to follow what is suggested as a plan for health or well-being. So, although the nurse's stated goal may be to assist and care for a person through a process of restoring wellness, maintaining health, actualizing the person's potential, or alleviating suffering, the process is limited and "tunes out" other ways to come to know and care for the patient.

As Christensen and Hewlett-Taylor (2006) suggest, such patient care is lacking in expertise. They point out that expertise does not equate with experience. An experienced nurse may be caught up in the ritual of the act of doing or performing a skill in a proficient way rather than being an expert nurse who mutually engages and interacts with the patient while in the process of completing a task. The expert nurse uses the theoretical knowledge that defines and facilitates expert nursing care and in the process attends to all of the patient's needs. That is, the nurse provides care that is both proficient and completed in such a way that includes intuitive knowledge. Do APNs ever practice in a way that is proficient, yet lacking in care? If so, how would their performance appraisal differ from an APN who took time to talk to the patient about the overall care experience? Would his or her work be valued equally by an administrator?

Too often the distinction between what makes a "good" APN (depending on one's definition of *good*) and what makes a proficient APN is based not on nursing knowledge but on skills, ability to work with fast patient turnover rates, and modeling of physician language and assessment skills (Rashotte & Carnevale, 2004). For example, when I have attended NP conferences, the presentations are often given by physicians, and the topics are oriented to diagnosis and treatment of disease and to efficiency models. As noted earlier, although this is an important skill and necessary for good holistic care, it is inadequate (necessary but not sufficient for good care). Although some attention paid to this may be important, the question is, who benefits from nurse functioning in this "mini doc" capacity? How is the NP practice different from that of a physician? At these NP conferences, there is little to no attention paid to functional health patterns and certainly none to health in the human experience. But when an APN functions from a pure medical model, as is often encouraged by employers, physicians, and other APNs, it is at the risk of abandoning the professional responsibility entrusted to that APN, who is a nurse first and foremost.

The education and the practice environment of the nurse both influence a nurse's ability to practice good nursing. But nurses who understand the bases of their professional responsibilities in nursing are more able to resist becoming indoctrinated into some other discipline's practice model. As discussed earlier, not all nurses are educated in core courses that reflect the essence of the discipline, and as a result there is a tendency in practice to devalue that which is nursing. Educational preparation and the environment of the practice setting are, of course, not the only influences on good nursing care; personal knowing, an ability to be reflective, and professional accountability are some other factors that are equally important. As argued earlier in the book and in this chapter, APNs are nurses and their practice should reflect that. A blurring of the lines of distinction among healthcare professions is dangerous to the development of nursing knowledge, the profession, and thereby the public that nursing serves.

A good APN has a capacity for self-reflection, is able to reflect on practice, and is willing to raise questions about what is good nursing care (Christensen & Hewlett-Taylor, 2006; Hardingham, 2004; Tarlier, 2004). Benner, Tanner, and Chelsea (1996) maintain that the ability and willingness to reflect are what distinguishes an expert-level nurse from peers. Reflection is a more complicated idea, though, than it may initially seem. Even a nurse who is able to reflect on a practice situation and envision what good practice requires may be confronted with situations that he or she has no idea how to process and where mentorship or other resources are not readily available. She may sense that something is wrong, but raising either personal awareness or group awareness can come at great cost because it may be seen as challenging the status quo. In other situations, a nurse may not be mature enough as a person, in the sense of having life experiences that have challenged personal knowing, to recognize the ethical content of a particular situation.

That is, a variety of factors can obstruct good practice even when the APN understands the holistic nature of nursing practice and possesses the knowledge, skills, and characteristics necessary for good care. In these situations, the nurse's accurate perception of the issue, ethical decision-making capacity, and/or motivation for action may all fall short. This problem is explored further in the case studies later. First, however, it is important to address autonomy in practice and bring clarity to the issue. This awareness and discussion may help to initiate improvements in practice at all levels but especially in advanced roles. The next section highlights some of the problems for nursing in fulfilling professional goals.

THREATS TO AUTONOMY

In this section, autonomy is discussed on two levels: personal and professional. Personal autonomy and professional autonomy are in one sense two very different things, but in reality they are intrinsically linked. As described in Chapter 1 by Grace, *autonomy* is a word that has many meanings, but for the purpose of this discussion personal autonomy is defined as an individual's right to self-determine his or her own actions. Professional autonomy is discussed in terms of nursing as a profession and focuses on the fiduciary relationship between nursing and the public.

Nursing, a Trusted Professional Discipline

Academically, nursing is a young discipline, but it is generally accepted that nursing is a professional and practice discipline that has a unique body of knowledge and perspective that shapes practice, research, and education (Northrup et al., 2004; O'Shea, 2001). Both the ANA (2001) and ICN (2006) Codes of Ethics for nurses suggest that as a professional discipline, nursing is both responsible and accountable to the society it serves. The ANA's (2003) *Social Policy Statement* suggests that this relationship between nursing and the public is intended to be dynamic and that there is dialogue between the public and nursing as an organization. Grace (1998) discusses the fact that because the profession is responsive to societal changes and needs, the goals and the good of the public are reflected in the formulation of the ANA Code of Ethics, but the reality is that the public is only indirectly involved in this dialogue. Further, Neale (2001) suggests that without knowing and understanding the public, nurses are not directing care at patient-sensitive outcomes.

Although it has been argued that many in the public are unclear about what nurses do, in surveys nurses consistently rank highly as trusted professionals (DeRaeve, 2002; O'Shea, 2001). Practicing nurses may agree with the idea that nursing is a discipline unique from other healthcare disciplines and may take pride in and agree that, as a profession, nurses are trusted. They may, however, not be able to say what underlies this trust, or why it is even relevant to their everyday practice. What is worse is that many will more readily point to times of moral distress or times when they felt their voice was not heard than agree that they can be trusted to fulfill professional goals in the face of environmental barriers. Of course, the implication is that nurses should not be trusted because they do not have the knowledge or power to do what is needed to fulfill professional goals. A further implication is that nurses could be held accountable for professional promises if the code was readily accessible to the public (Grace, 1998, 2001). No doubt the inability of many nurses to articulate the perspective of the discipline is a result of varying educational preparation, the failure of some academic curricula, and current healthcare economics (O'Shea, 2001). Traditionally nurses have been for the most part employed by and therefore embedded in a system with a historical tradition that values nurses for the tasks that they do to support the functioning of that system rather than for the questions they raise or the perspective they contribute. Nurses are paid by this system, and it is therefore at great personal risk that nurses counter this system (Grace, 2001).

This reality is contrasted with the notion that nurses are trusted by the public to collaborate with peers and to be advocates of patients in a shared decision-making process that permits a patient's real needs to be uncovered and addressed. Because, however, what nurses really do is unknown to most consumers of health care, and because many nurses report moral distress resulting from conflicts of varying sorts, questions can be raised about the professional responsibility of the nurse and how the public is both served and informed by nursing (Corley, 2002; Corley, Minick, Elswick, & Jacobs, 2005;

Jameton, 1984). This situation is more complex in light of advanced practice nursing. This is especially true when CNSs and NPs are not educated about and/or do not value the particular disciplinary perspective of nursing. For this reason, many either do not understand what is, or find it difficult to practice, good nursing care. The result is that they practice in a blended capacity, that is, a medical model with a few undertones of nursing. As a result of this type of care, the public often suffers from nurses who do not understand what nursing is. A core value of good nursing practice is the ability to be reflective, and as Grace has pointed out earlier in this book, this process allows nurses to consider ways that practice can be improved.

Therefore, this book and especially this chapter highlights questions that can and should be raised about APNs' professional responsibilities and the nature, scope, and limits of APNs' capacity as a group to advocate for patients within the current healthcare system or effectively work at the societal level to change inadequacies in the system. For example, patients who undergo procedures are increasingly rushed through a given institutional system and sent home inadequately prepared to care for themselves during their recovery and without transitional homecare.

Further complicating this picture is the fact that many procedures could have been avoided altogether had the appropriate preventive nursing care been incorporated into the care delivery model. Additionally, perhaps there would be a decrease in complications from the procedure or recidivism if nurses were part of a transition model caring for patients at home. So, if nurses are really to serve as trusted advocates for the public, nurses must understand their own disciplinary perspective so that the voices of nursing and those who are served by nursing are heard.

Tarlier (2004) suggests that respect, trust, and mutuality are key elements of the process needed for nurses to form responsive relationships with their patients. She describes trust as being founded on personal morals and relates it to the ability of the nurse to be competent, skilled, and qualified. Prerequisites to trust are sincerity, genuineness, and acceptance. Implicit in this is a two-way dynamic of nurses being genuine, competent, and caring and patients trusting in nurses enough that they feel free to be open, honest, and trusting. This two-way dynamic is essential because patients spend a great deal of time with nurses while hospitalized and while in vulnerable situations (Grace, 2004). DeRaeve (2002) suggests that patients do not automatically place blind trust in individual nurses or in nursing actions. That is, they do not rely on us to do certain things such as advocate for them, primarily because they do not know what it is that we do and assume the role is limited to completing a series of tasks. Individual relationships developed between patients and nurses set the stage for therapeutic relationships to emerge. Implicit in this dynamic though is whether or not nurses can and do control whether a therapeutic relationship will occur in the nurse–patient relationship. For example, if a nurse is too busy to form this relationship, patient care may suffer—not only because the patient is unknown in a unique way, but also because the patient is in a susceptible position and unable to address the feeling of being neglected without potential consequences. Further, if a nurse does not value being genuine, caring, *and* competent, the patient may be known and cared for in a way that is not consistent with the values of what it means to be a nurse. Patients, however, do place trust in nurses as a group. This type of trustworthiness has a moral dimension and obligation and suggests that nurses must talk openly and honestly with patients about nursing's competing agendas, such as unsafe staffing levels that may interfere with patient care.

Autonomy

Professional Autonomy

Recently, the *New York Times* featured a piece titled "In the Hospital, a Degrading Shift from Person to Patient" (Carey, 2005) about several individual hospitalized patients and their hospital experience. Overall, the patients described their experiences as "degrading." At first, when I read the article I really wanted to believe that everyone else involved in the patients' care were the cause of these horrible experiences and that somehow nurses came to the rescue and made it all better. Sadly, what I read, though, resonated with me. I know from my own research (Flanagan, 2005, 2006, in press) and from personal experiences of both family and friends that nursing on all levels does not equal care or caring.

The article suggests that nurses do not "know" their patients very well. In the article, one patient describes having no idea who her nurses were, and she did not know any of their names. Another patient describes how she unhooked her own intravenous line and got dressed to go across the street to have lunch—all without her nurse even knowing or realizing that she was missing. This patient wanted to feel more human, but the mere fact that she could carry out these activities unnoticed, be absent for so long, and not be missed is alarming. As I read the article, I realized that not only were nurses not the heroes, but they were also part of the problem. I also began to grasp the idea that this was true but only a glimpse of the problem: patients are often left feeling lonely and abandoned in the process of being "cared for" in today's industrialized healthcare system. This occurs throughout the lifespan care of any one person—from seeing a primary provider to episodic care including recovery. My previous research on surgical patients (Flanagan, 2005, 2006, in press) suggests this is so of "the system," but somehow I still hoped that nursing would be viewed differently in the eyes of patients.

Patients spend more time with nurses than they do with any other healthcare provider. But in reality do nurses actually spend time with patients; or rather do they work on the patients' paperwork for discharge, teaching and referrals, and overall documenting? Is the time spent coming to know the patient in a problem-solving, process-oriented, or cosmic knowing sort of way? Or is it time spent filling out required paperwork, which can make nurses feel disjointed from the science of what nursing is? Are nurses prepared educationally and/or emotionally to actually care for patients on the level suggested by theorists and other scholars of the discipline?

Patient Autonomy

The Patient Self-Determination Act of 1991 (PSDA) provides patients with the right to decide what, if any, treatments they would like to have in the course of care. Personal autonomy suggests that a patient has the ability to process the information provided and has the freedom to make choices (Grace & McLaughlin, 2005). According to Faden and Beauchamp (2003), for consent to be considered voluntary several conditions must be satisfied: (1) the patient must have a considerable understanding of the procedure, (2) the patient must experience substantial absence of control by others, and (3) the patient must provide intentional authorization that allows the professional to carry out the intervention. For the APN to determine if the patient is able or at a point when he is ready to make informed decisions about his health care, I add to the preceding list the fact that the APN must come to know the patient from a nursing disciplinary perspective.

Another article in the *New York Times* titled "Awash in Information, Patients Face a Lonely, Uncertain Road" (Hoffman, 2005) suggests that patients today are so inundated with medical information and choices that they are in fact in some ways less informed (and therefore less autonomous) than patients were a generation ago. In fact, some ethicists have called this abandoning patients to their autonomy (Loewy, 1989, 2005; Smith, 1996). Hoffman (2005) interviewed patients and physicians. (My premise is that APNs often practice within the medical model, so they could also be included; in this section, although Hoffman describes physicians, I use the term *healthcare provider*.) The article describes the many sources of medical information, which in the end overwhelm people who attempt to make an informed decision. The Internet, radio, television, newspapers, and healthcare providers bombard patients with all the options, but with few conclusions or decisions. Often, "informed" patients will come to a healthcare provider asking for tests they heard about via the media. Hoffman describes healthcare providers who feel they should provide patients with a "maddening litany of medical correctness." In other words, they feel they must provide all the choices but avoid suggesting a preferred treatment in the name of autonomy. Additionally, Hoffman describes that because of time constraints healthcare providers do not "know" their patients and therefore practice defensive medicine and resort to increased testing, which requires further interpretation or medical language that is incomprehensible to most laypeople.

Patients too often are previously unknown to their healthcare provider, have no one coordinating their care, are left to gather information where they can, must arrange for their own consultations, or are left to their own devices in interpreting medical jargon. Thus, they may well make decisions about their care that may or may not be the best choice for them.

The purpose of emphasizing the importance of autonomy as patient rights to self-determination is because in the past medical paternalism denied patients any involvement in deciding what was best for their individual and particular needs. However, today the pendulum may have swung too far in the opposite direction. Although in general people should be considered capable of self-determination, if they meet the criteria for being able to process information, to exercise their right to self-determination, they must possess the appropriate information, couched in understandable language and tailored to their particular needs. This all too often does not happen. As said by one patient Hoffman interviewed, at age 57 it was a little late for him to return to medical school so that he could understand the medical language being used in his care.

The following case studies exemplify the points made in this *New York Times* series of articles. They are drawn from my practice and are based on real patient experiences (identifying characteristics have been changed to preserve anonymity).

CASE STUDY

Barbara N. is a new graduate of a master's program in nursing. Her prior nursing experiences were gained in various acute care settings. Most recently, she had worked on a surgical unit that specialized in orthopedics, oncology, and general surgery while at the same time undertaking part-time studies that culminated in a Master of Science in Nursing degree and prepared her for the role of Adult Health Nurse Practitioner. The university she attended had the reputation for graduating NPs who were "really strong" clinical nurses.

She has just assumed her first NP position in a busy surgical oncology office. In this office, which is run by physician oncologists, visits are limited to 15 minutes per case. Most of her work involves seeing patients for any or all of the following purposes: consultation for surgical intervention for an oncology problem prior to surgery, testing, or procedures; postrecovery teaching; and obtaining presurgical consent. Barbara created templates for obtaining and documenting all of her patients' histories so that she could be more efficient. Her patient workup includes ascertaining the following: chief complaint, history of present illness, past medical history, a review of pertinent systems, and a focused physical exam.

Mr. S. is a patient who was referred to the clinic by his primary doctor for consultation. Mr. S. understands this visit to be related to the fact that he has an unresolved problem on his x-ray that could be either an infection or something more serious. He has arrived at the clinic with his wife and two sons. He is a 76-year-old Anglo-Saxon male.

From what she can tell from her schedule, Barbara notes that he has a new diagnosis of lung cancer that has yet to be staged. Barbara, who is already running behind schedule, assumes Mr. S. is aware of the reason for his visit and calls out his name at which point both Mr. S. and his entire family respond and ask if they can be present during the visit. Barbara is at first a little taken aback. She does not want to appear cold, so she invites them all to come in and join the exam.

While obtaining the history of present illness and past medical history, she realizes Mr. S. is very quiet and that he defers all questions to his son who is a dentist. The son answers each question intended for his father. His other son interrupts his brother periodically to clarify dates or share further details. Both Mr. S. and his wife sit quietly and offer very little information. From the information she has gathered, Barbara understands that Mr. S. is a nonsmoker and otherwise has been healthy. Because Mr. S. had a past chest x-ray and unresolved symptoms related to pneumonia, he was referred by his primary care doctor to this clinic for consultation. Again, she assumes he has been notified by his primary that there is a question of lung cancer, and it is obvious to Barbara that the son who is a dentist is knowledgeable about the diagnosis. The history takes Barbara much longer than she planned, and Barbara becomes anxious that she is not moving along her patient schedule quickly enough and fears being reprimanded by her program director for being too slow. Although she does so calmly and pleasantly, she asks the family to sit back in the waiting area, hoping that she can proceed more quickly while she examines Mr. S. alone. She assumes Mr. S. will provide her with quicker, more direct answers and that this will not only speed up the visit but will allow her to get to know him without all the interference.

Barbara begins the physical exam and asks Mr. S. some questions, but he barely speaks and appears to be angry. Again, taken aback by this, Barbara asks if he would like the family to rejoin them so that she can explain the available options, obtain an informed consent for a lung biopsy, and discuss various potential outcomes and options as well as other testing that will be required for staging the tumor. Mr. S. appears confused about all that Barbara has discussed, and he says that he would like to have his family present.

They rejoin Mr. S., but now they also appear angry and Barbara is not quite sure what she did wrong but proceeds to explain various options and various procedures that are required for Mr. S. She then decides to check the scheduling program to determine options for dates for the biopsy. Because she must leave the room to do so, she decides that it would be good for the oncology nurse to come in and see Mr. S. and his family to provide teaching about the oncology center and services available.

The oncology nurse introduces herself to each member of the family. She then provides them with information about rides to chemotherapy, social work availability, nutrition services, support groups, and so on. The entire family is pleasant to the nurse, but they have no idea why she is providing them with this information. The family is still only aware that a chest x-ray and symptoms related to pneumonia were unresolved. The son who is the dentist suspects it is cancer, but no one has told them that in fact this is the actual or most likely diagnosis. No one has mentioned the word *cancer*. Having services described is perplexing, but they assume the nurse was sent into their room to stall for time.

Barbara has made and continues to make the assumption that the family is fully aware of the diagnosis, although she herself only mentioned that the biopsy "would provide more information as to why this spot on his chest x-ray has not cleared." Barbara then returns to the room and provides Mr. S. with a variety of options that are possible once the cancer has been confirmed and staged by biopsy, including "watchful waiting," surgery, chemotherapy and radiation, or a combination of these. She then mentions a variety of tests he "could choose to undergo so that he can find out a more accurate diagnosis." These tests include a lung biopsy, CAT and PET scans along with further blood work; that is, if he chooses to have any at all.

Mr. S. is surprised to learn that he must undergo more tests and, potentially, surgery, but more important, he does not understand why he has not been told exactly what is wrong and exactly which option is best for him. He looks to his sons for advice, and they suggest he get the biopsy. Barbara describes a procedure that will require anesthesia so that biopsies can be obtained and a litany of other tests to "see if anything else is going on." He admits later that he "never heard a word" Barbara said after agreeing to this, but he signed the informed consent anyway because he knew his sons thought he should. Mr. S. signs the consents and quietly the entire family walks away.

Let's pause here and reflect on this case:

1. What information do you think the primary provider may have given Mr. S. or his family? How is continuity from the time of primary care through to homecare after treatment been ensured in the healthcare system?
2. What assumptions has Barbara made about Mr. S. and his family? Has Barbara made assumptions about the sons' knowledge and what information they may have shared with the parents? In the interest of time, have you ever felt rushed to "get through the visit"? What has this been like for you? How has Barbara come to know her patient? Has she utilized disciplinary knowledge?
3. Do you believe all patients understand why they are referred to specialists? How does Mr. S.'s care reflect shared decision making? How do APNs in practice ensure that continuity of care is assured? Do you think this type of efficient care is valued by Barbara's practice?
4. What would you do differently if you were Barbara? What nursing knowledge would guide your thinking? How does the APN in this role distinguish what it is

that she brings to this patient encounter that is different from other healthcare providers?

5. Have you ever heard patients describe this sort of experience? Because APNs have a social mandate with the public they serve, how can APNs assure the public that they are advocates for them through this sort of system of care?
6. What burden has been placed on the sons, especially the one who may have some sense of what is happening but who is certainly not an expert in this type of problem/care?

In this particular case, the primary provider had told Mr. S. only that he was concerned about Mr. S.'s pneumonia not resolving and wanted this other doctor to look at the results. Mr. S. had no idea that there was any question of cancer and thought the referral was for an unresolved pneumonia, not cancer. His son, Michael (the dentist), knew they were being referred to an oncology practice and shared this information with his brother. Michael was still unclear if the diagnosis was definitive and assumed that if it was, the primary provider and/or oncologist either explained or would explain the diagnosis. Barbara assumed Mr. S. and the entire family knew why he was there and that the primary provider had explained the situation. The note from the primary provider mentioned only that a referral was made and did not mention any discussion with the patient, but this is typical. Barbara and the primary provider never spoke to each other about the case.

Mr. S. now suspects more is going on than he was initially led to believe, but he has not yet been told he has cancer. Moving ahead in this case, Mr. S. goes for all his testing, and the diagnosis is confirmed that this is an early stage lung tumor. It can be treated by surgery alone and no further treatment is necessary. Throughout follow-up visits, the healthcare team, including Barbara, now use the word *cancer* and tell Mr. S. how lucky he is to have such a treatable type of cancer. He goes through presurgery testing in a haze because he is so stunned with this new diagnosis, but he continues to hear he is "lucky." He is scheduled for surgery, the CNS of the unit he will go to is notified, and she promises to make sure things are coordinated for him. But, in reality, staffing is poor and the unit is going through a huge turnover period. The CNS is very busy orienting new staff to the unit and making sure the sickest of the patients are getting the best care possible.

Mr. S. is not nearly as sick as other patients on the unit, so his son and other family members make themselves more available to care for him throughout the hospitalization. They do this because other patients' family members on the unit tell them that this is the only way to ensure that Mr. S. is cared for during his stay. Mr. S.'s recovery is smooth, but he remains surprised at the diagnosis and is unable to integrate this new illness into his personhood. He describes feeling alone and abandoned while in the hospital. His sons have tried to explain the diagnosis and treatment, but their father remains too overwhelmed to comprehend this information. They are at a loss to explain it further. Mr. S. now considers himself a very sick person and worries constantly about a recurrence of cancer, which seems warranted given the repeat scans that are required over the next year. From a purely medical perspective of cure, Mr. S. is a success story, but from a nursing perspective of care, Mr. S.'s story is a dismal failure.

Let's pause again for further reflective questions.

1. Has Mr. S. been abandoned by the medical system, medicine, or nursing? What is a goal of nursing care in the human health experience? Has this goal been met on any level for Mr. S. or his family?
2. The CNS agrees to coordinate things for Mr. S. but in reality is unable to because there are other more pressing issues on the unit. How do these issues factor into the reality of practice? How do they interfere with the CNS being able to function in the capacity of the role?
3. How has Mr. S.'s experience been reflective or not of "good nursing care"? What nursing intervention or strategy would you suggest for Mr. S. and his family to help them through the transitions that have occurred?

A more recent *New York Times* article, "Cancer Patients: Lost in a Maze of Uneven Care" (Grady, 2007), describes patients as having to fend for themselves and "patch" information together. Patients interviewed for this feature described their experience as having no one healthcare professional who understood their whole story. Although each healthcare provider they saw knew his or her own role well, there was a lack of coordination of care. Further, patients were often left to their own devices to find what care they needed.

Several years ago I read about and was impressed by a nursing model of care used in Arizona at St. Mary's Hospital (Michaels, 1992). In the case management model of care, primary nurses were assigned to patients at the time they chose a primary physician in the healthcare plan. Utilizing a Newman (1994) framework, the nurses came to know their patients and followed them over time. In doing so, they were responsible for and able to appropriately coordinate care and obtain necessary consultations for patients. This model of case management truly fosters the idea of nurses helping patients navigate the healthcare system, and it resulted in increased patient satisfaction and decreased healthcare expenditure.

In my research, I describe a model of care that includes nurses being mentored on incorporating nursing theory into practice. In addition, reflective rounds were incorporated into the practice setting to allow nurses to think not only about what did not go well in their patient/family interactions, but also what they could do to improve the individual situations and/or overall care environment (Flanagan, in press).

Unfortunately, to my knowledge, there has not been further expansion of either of these models, but if the series in the *New York Times* are any indication of public opinion, I think these types of models need to be more broadly implemented. But at issue with this within nursing is the fact that funding sources such as the National Institutes for Nursing Research do not support these types of bold initiatives such as patients having a primary nurse along with a primary physician when they sign on for health insurance. Rather, the focus tends to be on an acute care medical model of treatment and prevention of disease—especially complex diseases. Although helping patients manage disease is certainly an interest of nursing, having most of funding directed at this level of care does not address all persons. It seems that at this time we need more rigorous studies of patient experiences to provide us with the tools necessary to change practice. First, nursing funding on the federal level must allocate money for this type of research to occur. Some smaller nursing organizations have provided financial support to conduct these studies, but to date this has not allowed for rigorous investigations. (See Chapter 4 to review other political strategies for implementing change.)

HEALTH PROMOTION

Nurses as members of a profession are concerned with the core concepts underlying professional practice. These core concepts include health, holism, environment, person, and partnership. The question could be raised, however, whether nurses are unique in this perspective. Isn't it true also that a doctor who listens to a patient and encourages that person to share his or her concerns is also partnering with the patient to provide good care? Isn't this same doctor also concerned with the whole person? Many physicians would argue that they are concerned with understanding the person as a person and have a holistic approach to care. This raises anew the question of what is so unique about nursing. As Grace suggests in Chapter 1, different professions do share the same goals, but it is the knowledge of the discipline that shapes how the goal may be achieved or how outcomes related to the goal will be measured.

Nursing is unique from other disciplines in the way that nurses work together with the patient to set goals and measure the outcomes related to those goals. However, not all nurses are aware of or choose to acknowledge that their disciplinary knowledge base is important and should underlie all patient care endeavors. The profession of nursing purports to have a unique focus on health, holism, and the nurse–patient relationship. If this is so, then nursing must develop and expand its own body of knowledge focused on health, holism, and the nurse–patient relationship to further enhance the quality of life of each individual and be true to the goals set forth by scholars of the discipline (Allan & Hall, 1988; Fawcett, 2005).

Health promotion has always been a key component of the NP role, and until the addition of acute care NP roles, it was a primary focus. CNSs tend also to focus on health and healing and use a holistic approach to care. CNSs have been instrumental in the development of screening, health promotion, and classes designed to educate and motivate people to improve their health. For example, they developed smoking cessation programs both for inpatients and for outpatients. It is important to recognize that health promotion is not limited to prevention of problems such as diabetes, obesity, and smoking-related issues, but rather is far more expansive. Health promotion also includes a nursing focus on the current situation the patient faces and partnering with the patient throughout the care journey—health in the human experience. Promoting health in this realm requires nurses to come to know their patients more fully than most standard nursing assessments or physical assessments allow. The next case study serves as an illustration.

CASE STUDY

J.S. is a 44-year-old female patient who presents to a preoperative clinic to be evaluated prior to surgery. J.S. is having surgery for a brain tumor. She has previously had radiation to shrink the tumor, and it is hoped that by having the surgery, much of the tumor can be removed, but it is doubtful that the surgeons will be able to remove it entirely. Her prognosis is uncertain.

In the clinic, she sees an anesthesiologist, who determines which anesthesia is most appropriate for the surgery and provides teaching according to the plan; a nurse, who performs a nursing assessment and provides pre- and postoperative teaching; and an NP, who provides the perfunctory presurgery history and physical. In this particular clinic, the CNS has successfully implemented a nursing model of care for patients who are seen by the nurse, although it is not integrated into the NPs' practice. The model includes interviewing patients using the praxis methodology of Newman (1994). In this method, patients are asked to discuss the significant people and events in their life. In addition to being interviewed, patients are also offered therapeutic touch, meditation, and/or other relaxation techniques while they are in the clinic and throughout the hospitalization recovery process.

The first provider that J.S. sees is the anesthesiologist, who carefully reviews her previous history and discusses the anesthesia plan. J.S. finds talking with the anesthesiologist comforting. The anesthesiologist takes time to explain everything that will happen prior to and after surgery from the anesthesia perspective. Additionally, this anesthesiologist has gone through the spirituality fellowship at the hospital and has integrated this type of care into her practice. On ascertaining J.S.'s desire for this, she offers to pray with J.S., who agrees and is thankful for this opportunity. The anesthesiologist promises to follow up with J.S. on the day of surgery because coincidentally she will be scheduled for the neurology cases that day.

The next provider J.S. sees is the NP, Debbie, who appears quite harried. Debbie comes out to the waiting area to call J.S. and then asks her to have a seat in her office. Debbie then steps outside the office to complain to the other NPs about how busy she is and how distressed she is by the heavy schedule she has this day. Debbie sticks her head back in the room and states that she will be right back because she needs to discuss the case with the anesthesiologist. Debbie leaves the room for 25 minutes, and during this time, J.S. hears other people calling her name for more testing, so she steps out to let them know that she is in Debbie's office. Debbie returns to her office and finds J.S. gone because the lab technician has decided to take her from Debbie's room to draw her blood. Debbie sees this and gets angry and says to J.S., "I don't know if I can see you now. You might just have to wait until I am ready now."

J.S., not sure of what to say, asks if Debbie had a chance to talk to the anesthesiologist. At this point, J.S. is just trying to calm Debbie down because she sees that she is angry. Debbie responds: "No, I can't find her anywhere either. Today is just one awful day." Debbie then turns around and says, "Well, I'm off, I've got other things to do."

After her blood is drawn, J.S. goes back to the waiting area, but after waiting a long time, she wonders if she was supposed to just walk back to Debbie's office, so she goes to Debbie's office. Debbie is on the phone and says to J.S., "What, are you checking up on me now?" J.S. apologizes and returns to the waiting area. Eventually, Debbie takes her to her office and does a focused physical exam that takes about 10 minutes in total. Debbie barely speaks to her the entire time, and J.S. is feeling very vulnerable, so says nothing either. Finally, Debbie says to J.S., "You are all set for surgery," and sends her back to the waiting area. At this point, J.S. is holding back tears.

I would like to be able to say that no NP would act like this, but I can assure you that this behavior is not uncommon. You might also question whether an anesthesiologist could be so "caring," but I can attest that these cases come from my practice or research. I do know some anesthesiologists that practice in this way. Let's pause here for some questions.

1. As a nurse, how would you say you care? Would this care be different from the care provided by the anesthesiologist? How would this look or be different from the anesthesiologist in this case?
2. Have you seen nurses act in the manner that Debbie did? What have you done when you have seen this behavior? If nothing, what has caused you not to deal with it? If you have dealt with this, did it make a difference? Were you supported? By whom?
3. The way Debbie acted was certainly not "health promoting." Do you think that the public would know what to do if they had a nurse who acted in this way? Is there in fact a way for them to deal with this behavior? What impact do you think Debbie had on J.S.?

The next person to see J.S. is in fact the CNS, Ann. One of the technicians saw J.S. crying and thought Ann would be the best person to see her, given how upset she is. Ann calls J.S. into her office, which has soft lighting, plants, and a waterfall that makes soothing, musical noises. In addition, serene artwork adorns the wall. Immediately, J.S. senses something different, but she is still quite upset. Ann suggests that J.S. relax by taking some deep breaths, and J.S. does so. Ann begins to ask a few questions that are part of the standard nursing assessment: previous hospitalizations, medications, allergies, living situation, pain and anxiety levels. Ann continues to address these perfunctory questions, but instinctively knows that more in-depth questions need to be asked. She waits, though, until J.S. seems more relaxed, and then asks: "Tell me about you. Who are the significant people in your life? What are the significant events?"

J.S. begins with her childhood and describes it as an overall happy one until her mother died when she was 14 years of age. Her mother died of ovarian cancer, and J.S., who was the oldest daughter and child, began to care for her younger siblings. While her mother was ill, her father worked long hours, so J.S. essentially was the primary caregiver for her mother through her dying experience. J.S. lived at home during college so that she could continue to care for her siblings. She then described moving away from that life, getting married, and loving the first few years of marriage because "it was the first time I could just be free." She had children, an experience she thoroughly enjoyed, but gradually she and her husband drifted apart. They are now divorced. She has two children, 15 and 13, and her biggest fears and concerns are around how they will handle her illness. J.S. describes, "I am not so afraid of death, but I am afraid for them. I know what it is like to care for someone who has cancer, I know what it is like to be left alone."

Ann and J.S. continue to dialogue about meaningful events and experiences. Ann is fully attentive to J.S. and engaged in her story. Ann is completely open, allowing J.S. to provide the details as she chooses and carefully listens without interrupting, yet shares ideas, thoughts, and reflections. Ann offers J.S. therapeutic touch and says that she can visit her in her hospital room postoperatively. J.S. is grateful for this.

Her recovery goes smoothly, but her prognosis remains uncertain. Over the course of the next year, she continues "to check in with Ann" and share with her what is happening in her life. J.S. has made several changes, including incorporating yoga and a healthful diet into her regime. She has moved to a smaller, more manageable home and has planted a garden. She has found a new job that is less stressful, participates in a theater group with her two children, and has reconnected with old friends. J.S. describes the experience of meeting Ann as "a gift that was meant to be." Ann is gracious but says that this story is not unusual for her now that she practices nursing "in a way it was meant to be." Ann says that she loves her work, that it gives her life great meaning, and through connecting with her patients in this way, she too gains from the experience.

Here are some further questions for discussion:

1. Would you describe the care Ann has provided as health promoting?
2. How is this different or not from your original ideas about health promotion?
3. Do you think it is possible for nurses to practice in this way?
4. What would be the deterrents to such a practice?
5. What or who would be the support for such a practice?
6. If this is true nursing care from a disciplinary perspective and yet it is unusual because of constraints placed on nurses in practice, how do we as nurses address this as part of our commitment to the public as outlined in our *Social Policy Statement* (ANA, 2003)?

ACCESS TO CARE

The issue of access to care is of utmost importance to nurses. Although many see access to care as an issue of the underserved and those without insurance, being poor and uninsured are not the only factors that relate to access to care. I take the issue to be broader in scope, at least in the United States, and it includes those who do have insurance, too. My perspective is informed by the fact that I have practiced in what is increasingly a profit-driven or economically focused healthcare system. I have already discussed the problem of patients who are left to their own devices to navigate the healthcare system or to inform themselves about available choices. To me, this is, along with the plight of the poor and underserved, another aspect of poor access to appropriate care. The problems associated with a profit-driven healthcare system and what this means both for patient care and preventive care is the second issue that I consider under the umbrella of access to care.

In an economically driven healthcare system, emphasis is primarily on economic concerns and not primarily on trying to meet patients' needs, so it is important to discuss the implications of access to care in such a profit-driven system. Understanding this issue permits APNs to collaborate with others such as the public, lawmakers, and other healthcare providers in the interests of good patient care.

The numbers of short-stay surgeries and procedures continue to increase for several reasons, including improved anesthesia care, improved surgical technologies, and an aging population who have more health problems. Also, however, these procedures are highly profitable. Some surgeries and procedures that are increasingly used include bariatric, plastic, orthopedic, cardiac, and vascular. As a nurse, this is concerning to me on many levels. Most of these procedures require patients to spend little or no time on an inpatient unit. Inpatient care is, of course, expensive and can drive up the costs of procedures. But this also means that patients spend less time with nurses. Thus, the care that nurses provide such as partnering with the patient through the experience, teaching, and health promotion is missing.

The institutional emphasis becomes shifted toward providing those procedures and interventions that are likely to be profitable. This means the system rewards those physicians who do a large number of these types of procedures. Further, nurses who work within this system are paid by this system, which can raise conflicts of interest. The complexity of the system with the competitive nature of healthcare insurance companies and the fragmentation of services all tend to shift the emphasis of healthcare services away from attention to other types of care and the need to look at social conditions that lead to health disparities. Thus, health promotion, public health, and the health needs of the underinsured and underserved populations tend to be neglected.

Also, the idea of health promotion has fallen so far out of favor as a result of profit-driven care that I no longer even see this issue as a major focus of most care within this system. If you have a problem and you have insurance, there is a procedure to fix it. Are you obese? Have gastric bypass surgery. Are you aging? Many plastic surgery options are available. Are you stressed? Have a procedure and take legitimate time off from work. I know this may seem extreme, but again, my perspective is from within the profit-driven system. I do not see nurses partnering with patients to explore purpose and meaning so that they can understand the person in the human health experience. They are caught up in this system of high productivity and turnover and do not have the time to provide "nursing" care.

I have personally witnessed surgeons being pressured to keep up the actual numbers of surgeries that they perform. Performance indicators for them are around the number of surgeries booked as well as their ability to "turn over" an operating room or procedure room rapidly. Physicians, who are able to respond to this message with increased numbers and faster turnaround times, are rewarded with prime operating schedules; those who do not respond, lose time. If you have ever worked in a procedure-oriented area, you are well aware that some surgeons book ghost cases—that is, they leave the room booked so that they can have the time "just in case." Clearly, given the cost of running an operating room efficiently, this behavior had to be addressed, but to take it to the extreme just described is also problematic.

Putting pressure on surgeons to do surgery places an unfair burden on them, and on patients and the nurses who in theory are trusted professionals who advocate on patients' behalf. Elective surgery or procedures are just that—*elective*—and important things to consider include but are not limited to the following: (1) Is this the best option available to this patient? (2) Will the patient in fact benefit from this surgery? (3) What is the patient's overall health status and how will it be affected by the surgery? (4) Does the patient have the resources in place to enhance recovery from surgery? (5) What if the surgery is not successful? (6) Is there another option, perhaps one that is nursing oriented, that is less costly overall and that will help this person instead of surgery?

In my research (Flanagan, 2005, 2006, in press), I raise the issue of patients not fully understanding that they have a choice of whether or not to have surgery. I also describe cases in which patients describe surgery and the recovery time as a chance to get a break because they feel they just could not take time off work or be away from their daily obligations otherwise as recovering from surgery would allow. So, although surgery is an expensive, risky way for people to take time for themselves, it is an allowable way—both according to society's norms and healthcare reimbursement. Surgery does not, however, address the underlying problem—a need for a less stressed lifestyle.

Perhaps, for example, as nurses look at the issues related to aging—people living healthier, longer lives and wanting to contribute later in life to the workforce—in addition to considering lack of planning for retirement and concerns about skyrocketing healthcare costs, one solution could be to offer working people adequate breaks or sabbaticals every 5 or so years. This would allow people to take time off while raising a family, pursuing advanced degrees, caring for elderly parents, or just to take a vacation, pursue interests, and rejuvenate. It would also allow for people who would like to work later in life to do so, perhaps in roles as mentors and advisors to the younger workforce. Nurses, particularly APNs who see the myriad of health-related consequences and huge costs associated with not caring for individuals throughout various life stresses, must work through their professional organizations such as the ANA to create, lobby, and implement innovative policies that affect the health of society. Policies that make this option available to people will take overhauling current health strategies and creativity to implement, but an option like this that really allows people time away from a harried lifestyle could have an enormous impact on the overall health and well-being of individuals and society as a whole. Situations such as the one described previously—taking time off by having surgery—left nurses confounded. How on earth do they begin to address this? The following is a case study that exemplifies this situation.

CASE STUDY

W.D. is a 52-year-old man who presents to the office for a medical clearance for laparoscopic surgery. He had a gallbladder attack 6 months ago but has changed his diet so that he consumes much less fat. Since then, he has not had another gallbladder attack. While in your office, W.D. mentions that he also plans to have an arthroscopy of his knee that has "been bothering me forever." He is a teacher in a major urban school system and reveals that he has been under a lot of stress recently, both at work and at home. He has a second job working as an auto mechanic. As you talk further with him, he reveals that the principal of the school is after every teacher to improve standardized testing scores in the classroom. W.D. has always been interested in teaching the students with social and personal challenges and fears that this new mandate compromises his values as a teacher. Further, he has been caring for his wife, who has been quite ill with breast cancer, and although she is now doing well, he remains worried about her.

As you talk, and as more and more of his story is revealed to you, you begin to recognize that W.D. is completely stressed. He describes being unable to sleep, has been losing weight without trying (20 pounds in 6 months), and complains of feeling a constant knot in his stomach along with constant stomach irritation. Later, he shares, "I need a break, so I'm just going to have this surgery and when I get better from that, I will have the other. I don't know what else to do." W.D. does have problems that may benefit from surgery, but these surgical procedures are not risk free. In addition, his stress is not being addressed. Consider these questions:

1. What do you do in this situation?
2. What biases do we as healthcare providers bring to this type of situation?
3. Although it is true that he may have underlying problems that could require surgical intervention, is it necessary for him to have these surgeries to correct the problems?

4. When considering access to care as described earlier, how does a case like this contribute to the problem?
5. How is the public informed about unnecessary surgery without violating the trust they have in the system?
6. How would you begin to address the stigma of a patient like W.D. taking time off to address the real problem of stress as opposed to the perceived legitimate time off that recovery from surgery allows?

There are many other issues relevant to access to care that are related to underserved populations, but I think the overwhelming (and increasingly so) underlying issue is a healthcare system that does not work. One reason for the malfunctioning system is the emphasis on profits or cost savings and no attention paid to the real health needs of individuals and society (Mechanic, 2006). And although there may be some good things that result from this system, it is inherently unfair. It is unfair, for example, that members of the U.S. Congress have unlimited access to a universal-type health plan while millions go without even basic health care. It is unfair to have a system that pressures surgeons to produce and turn over cases or lose surgical privileges. It is unfair for nurses to be either so blinded by the system that exists or aware but silenced. And it is an apoplectic situation for patients to be so trusting of the system and the providers, including nurses, that they never question if in fact we have their best interest first and foremost in mind in the way we deliver care.

CONCLUSION

The purpose of this chapter is to review ethical issues that confront adult health APNs in daily practice. Discussing these issues in light of the disciplinary perspective and knowledge development can provide context. All the case studies were derived from my practice. They are not exaggerations—although as I wrote them and reflected on them, I wished they had been. I also wondered what I would do in those situations. Would it be enough? Should I have done more? If so, how? Grace points out in earlier sections that speaking up is not without risk, and no one person should stand alone. This does not mean that situations should be overlooked, and sometimes situations are more successfully addressed one person to another.

In reality, though, most of these issues are too big for one person to tackle and address alone. Hopefully, you are part of a hospital system that has a nursing ethics team or rounds. If so, bring these sorts of issues to the table for discussion. If your hospital does not have such a group, check out local colleges with schools of nursing and make alliances there. Join and actively participate in nursing organizations that address these issues of concern. Self-reflection on both the individual level and organizational level is unique to nursing, and it is imperative that APNs

(1) are aware of the issues, (2) recognize how situations that may seem normal or routine conflict with the disciplinary perspective, and (3) are able to raise the questions that the public expects of nursing—a most trusted profession.

REFERENCES

Allan, J., & Hall, B. (1988). Challenging the focus on technology: A critique of the medical model in a changing health care system. *Advances in Nursing Science, 10*(3), 22–34.

American Association of Colleges of Nursing, American Organization of Nurse Executives, & National Association of Associate Degree Nursing. (1995). *A model for differentiated practice.* Washington, DC: American Association of Colleges of Nursing.

American Nurses Association. (2001). *Code of ethics for nurses with interpretive statements.* Washington, DC: Author.

American Nurses Association. (2003). *Social policy statement.* Washington, DC: Author.

Benner, P., Tanner, C. A., & Chelsea, C. A. (1996). *Expertise in nursing practice: Caring, clinical judgment and ethics.* New York: Springer.

Carey, B. (2005). In the hospital, a degrading shift from person to patient. *New York Times*, August 16, 2005.

Christensen, M., & Hewlett-Taylor, J. (2006). From expert to tasks, expert nursing practice redefined? *Journal of Clinical Nursing, 15*, 1531–1539.

Corley, M. C. (2002). Nurses' moral distress: A proposed theory and research agenda. *Nursing Ethics, 9*(6), 636–650.

Corley, M. C., Minick, P., Elswick, R. K., & Jacobs, M. (2005). Nurse moral distress and ethical work environment. *Nursing Ethics, 12*(4), 381–390.

DeRaeve, L. (2002). Trust and trustworthiness in nurse-patient relationships. *Nursing Philosophy, 3*, 152–162.

Dickoff, J., James, P., & Wiedenbach, E. (1968). Theory in a practice discipline, part one: Practice oriented theory. *Nursing Research, 17*(5), 415–435.

Donaldson, S. K., & Crowley, D. M. (1978). The discipline of nursing. *Nursing Outlook, 26*(2), 113–120.

Faden, R., & Beauchamp, T. (2003). The concept of informed consent. In T. Beauchamp & W. LeRoy (Eds.), *Contemporary issues in bioethics* (6th ed.) (pp. 145–149). Belmont, CA: Wadsworth.

Fawcett, J. (2005). Integrating nursing models, theories, research, and practice. In J. Fawcett (Ed.), *Contemporary nursing knowledge: Analysis and evaluation of nursing models and theories* (2nd ed.) (pp. 589–599). Philadelphia: F. A. Davis.

Flanagan, J. (2005). Creating a healing environment for staff and patients in a pre-surgery clinic. In C. Picard & D. Jones (Eds.), *Giving voice to what we know: Margaret Newman's theory of health as expanding consciousness in nursing practice, research and education* (pp. 53–63). Sudbury, MA: Jones and Bartlett.

Flanagan, J. (2006). The nursing theory and practice link: Creating a healing environment within the pre-admission nursing practice—an exemplar. In C. Roy & D. Jones (Eds.), *Nursing knowledge development and clinical practice* (pp. 275–286). New York: Springer.

Flanagan, J. (In press). Patient and nurse experiences of theory-based care. *Nursing Science Quarterly.*

Gordon, M. (1994). *Nursing diagnosis: Process and application.* Philadelphia: Mosby.

Grace, P. J. (1998). *A philosophical analysis of the concept "advocacy": Implications for professional-patient relationships.* Unpublished Dissertation. University of Tennessee Knoxville. Available at http://proquest.umi.com. Publication number AAT9923287, Proquest Document ID No. 734421751.

Grace, P. J. (2001). Professional advocacy: Widening the scope of accountability. *Nursing Philosophy, 2*(2), 151–162.

Grace, P. J. (2004). Patient safety and the limits of confidentiality. *American Journal of Nursing, 104*(11), 33, 35–37.

Grace, P. J., & McLaughlin, M. (2005). When consent isn't informed enough: What's the nurse's role when a patient has given consent but doesn't fully understand the risks? *American Journal of Nursing, 105*(4), 79–84.

Grady, D. (2007). Cancer patients, lost in a maze of uneven care. *New York Times,* July 29, 2007.

Hardingham, L. (2004). Integrity and moral residue: Nurses as participants in a moral community. *Nursing Philosophy, 5,* 127–134.

Hoffman, J. (2005). Awash in information, patients face a lonely, uncertain road. *New York Times,* August 15, 2005.

International Council of Nurses. (2006). *Code of Ethics for Nurses.* Geneva, Switzerland: Author. Retrieved May 28, 2007, from http://www.icn.ch/icncode.pdf.

Jameton, A. (1984). *Nursing practice: The ethical issues.* Upper Saddle River, NJ: Prentice Hall.

Johnson, D. E. (1974). Development of theory: A requisite for nursing as a primary health profession. *Nursing Research, 23*(5), 372–376.

Jones, D. (2006). A synthesis of philosophical perspectives for knowledge development. In C. Roy & D. Jones (Eds.), *Nursing knowledge development and clinical practice* (pp. 164–180). New York: Springer.

Loewy, E. (1989). *Textbook of medical ethics.* New York: Plenum Medical Book Company.

Loewy, E. (2005). In defense of paternalism. *Theoretical Medicine, 26*(6), 445–468.

Mechanic, D. (2006). *The truth about health care: Why reform is not working in America.* Piscataway, NJ: Rutgers University.

Michaels, C. (1992). Carondelet St. Mary's nursing enterprise. *Nursing Clinics of North America, 24*(1), 77–85.

Neale, J. (2001). Patient outcomes: A matter of perspective. *Nursing Outlook, 49,* 93–99.

Newman, M., Sime, A. M., & Corcoran-Perry, S. (1991). The focus of the discipline of nursing. *Advances in Nursing Science, 14*(1), 20–24.

Newman, M. A. (1994). *Health as expanding consciousness* (2nd ed.). New York: National League for Nursing.

Northrup, D. T., Coby L. T., Olynyk, V. G., Schick Makaroff, K. L., Szabo, J., & Biasio, H. A. (2004). Nursing: Whose discipline is it anyway? *Nursing Science Quarterly, 17,* 55–62.

Northrup, D.T., & Purkis, M.E. (2001). Building the science of health promotion practice from a human science perspective. *Nursing Philosophy, 2*(1), 62–71.

O'Shea, H. (2001). The state of the discipline in nursing: Science, technology, and culture have stirred rapid change. Accessed May 7, 2008 from http://www.emory.edu/ACAD_EXCHANGE/newinquiriescc.html.

Parse, R. R. (1999). Nursing: The discipline and the profession. *Nursing Science Quarterly, 12,* 275.

Pearson, A., & Vaughn, B. (1996). Common characteristics of nursing models—the patient or client. In: A., Pearson M., Fitzgerald & B. Vaughn *Nursing models for practice.* (pp. 39–55) Oxford: Butterworth Heinemann.

Peplau, H. E. (1952). *Interpersonal relations in nursing.* New York: G. P. Putnam's Sons.

Prochaska, J. O., & DiClemente, C. C. (1983). Stages and processes of self-change of smoking: Toward an integrative model of change. *Journal of Consulting and Clinical Psychology, 51,* 390–395.

Radwin, L. E. (1995). Knowing the patient: A process model for individualized interventions. *Nursing Research, 44*(6), 364–370.

Rashotte, J., & Carnevale, F. A. (2004). Medical and nursing clinical decision-making: A comparative epistemological analysis. *Nursing Philosophy, 5,* 160–174.

Rodgers, B. (2007). Knowledge as problem solving. In C. Roy & D. Jones (Eds.), Nursing *knowledge development and clinical practice* (pp. 107–118). New York: Springer.

Rogers, M. E. (1970). *An introduction to the theoretical basis of nursing.* Philadelphia: F. A. Davis.

Roy, C. (2006). Unity, diversity, conformism, and chaos: Applications of Roy's epistemology of the universal cosmic imperative In C. Roy & D. Jones (Eds.), *Nursing knowledge development and clinical practice* (pp. 307–314). New York: Springer.

Roy, C. & Jones, D. (2006). *Nursing knowledge development and clinical practice.* New York: Springer.

Smith, G. (1996). *Legal and healthcare ethics for the elderly.* Washington, DC: Taylor & Francis.

Tarlier, D. (2004). Beyond caring: The moral and ethical bases of responsive nurse-patient relationships. *Nursing Philosophy, 5,* 230–241.

CHAPTER 11

Nursing Ethics and Advanced Practice: Psychiatric and Mental Health Issues

Pamela J. Grace and Pamela A. Terreri

There was a change in Boldwood's exterior from its former impassibleness; and his face showed that he was now living outside his defences for the first time, and with a fearful sense of exposure.

Thomas Hardy, *Far from the Madding Crowd*

INTRODUCTION

The authors of this chapter collaborated on the content. One of us has expertise in ethics and adult health advanced practice, and the other is an experienced advanced practice mental health nurse, psychotherapist, and educator. We worked together to make the content as relevant and helpful as possible in the limited space available. The aim of this chapter is to provide the basis and resources for advanced practice psychiatric mental health nurses (APPMHNs) to gain confidence in their ethical decision making. However, topics explored within this chapter have salience for all nurses and advanced practice nurses (APNs). We are sure that there are many areas of specific concern that have not been addressed here. However, resources and strategies are provided throughout this chapter to help provide a basis for understanding the nature of professional responsibility in this specialty area and direction for action in difficult situations.

All specialty practice nurses benefit from collaboration and consultation with thoughtful and knowledgeable colleagues. Of course, it is best if one has assistance during the development of a problem, but confidence in ethical decision making is also built by after-the-fact analysis of cases with peers, allied professionals, and when possible an ethics expert. Maintaining patient confidentiality is, of course, a crucially important aspect of psychiatric and mental health care, including during the process of collaboration and supervision. There are few exceptions to this rule because of the harm that can be caused to patients by the careless exposure of their history. When exceptions are necessary, for example, when the patient or others are at serious risk of harm as a result of their uncontrolled behavior, a judicious sharing of only necessary information is warranted. Additionally, it is necessary to try to ameliorate any damage to the trust relationship that may be caused by this information sharing.

As has become the convention, we take the term *psychiatric* to mean associated with a mental illness perspective and *mental health* to mean concerned with restoring a person's sense of well-being and integration. Thus, the advanced practice of psychiatric–mental health nursing utilizes "a wide range of explanatory theories and research on human behavior as its science and the purposeful use of the self as its art" (Kneisl, Wilson, & Trigoboff, 2004, p. xix) in promoting the mental stability or well-being of persons or in reducing their suffering.

We understand that the current nature of the healthcare delivery system, its associated economic problems, and the structure of the mental health care system cause some of the more difficult issues for APPMHNs. Addressing such problems requires the action of all professions and professional groups whose patient populations are negatively affected. Chapter 4 provides further resources and suggestions for addressing broader healthcare delivery or policy issues that are unjust. This chapter concentrates on analyzing and clarifying the nature of problems faced in direct practice.

Good Psychiatric Advanced Nursing Practice

Foundations

The warrant for psychiatric advanced nursing practice, like other nursing specialties, issues from the goals and objectives of the nursing profession. These objectives are to provide a good for individuals and society related to their health or well-being, as described earlier. They require a focus on persons as unique individuals, deserving of dignity and of equal moral worth with others (see Table 2-2 from the ANA *Code of Ethics for Nurses*). Historically, patients suffering from mental illness have been especially stigmatized. *Stigma* can be defined as a negative image held by society or groups within a society toward those who are perceived as different from the majority in some way. The problem with stigma is that it facilitates the poor treatment of such people by others—they are treated as less than fully human or less worthy of moral concern. Another problem with stigma is that it can prevent people from seeking mental health care. Some researchers have pointed out that it is not only those suffering from mental illness that are likely to be stigmatized but also associated others such as relatives and even psychiatric–mental health professionals themselves (Halter, 2008). Thus, the responsibility exists for APPMHNs both to treat each patient as an individual equally worthy of dignity with other individuals and to address the stigmatizing attitudes of others through raising public consciousness.

Difficulties

Decisions about which actions are appropriate often must be made under conditions of extreme uncertainty that add to the difficulty of providing good care. Additionally, APPMHNs may face pressures from colleagues, employers, or funding sources to abandon their professional goals for the purposes of expediency or of meeting institutional or practice needs. Conflicts of interest are prevalent in psychiatric and mental health settings as they are elsewhere, but the particular nature of mental health practice—concerned as it is with people who are made especially vulnerable by perceptual and reasoning difficulties—gives these problems their own particular nuances.

A firm understanding of what good nursing practice is in psychiatric and mental health care settings is crucial both for resisting pressures to make choices that are not ethically supported and for articulating reasons for one's actions and decisions to others. The next section provides background on the nurse–patient relationship and its importance in advanced practice psychiatric and mental health settings.

Nurse–Patient Relationship: History

The process of knowledge development for nursing practice was discussed in earlier chapters. However, it is important to note that several early nursing philosophers and theorists derived their understanding of what nursing is and what it does from their practice in psychiatric settings. Hildegard Peplau (1952), Ida Orlando (1961), and Joyce Travelbee (1966) all practiced at one point in their careers as psychiatric nurses. Their writings and theoretical explanations of nursing and the work nurses do emphasize the therapeutic importance of the nurse–patient relationship in recognizing and identifying a person's needs and thus promoting that person's well-being or relieving suffering. Their insights were recognized as important for all areas of nursing practice, not just for practice in psychiatric settings.

The implications of therapeutic nurse–patient relationships applied and apply to all patients in need of nursing services. Their understanding of persons, nursing, environment, and health—nursing's *metaparadigm* concepts as elucidated by Fawcett (1984)—is congruent with the nursing discipline's focus on persons as complex and integrated wholes. Because human beings are understood as being integrated wholes, a breakdown or threat of breakdown in any area of life—physical, psychological, or social—could negatively affect an individual's experience of well-being.

Disruptions in well-being can occur in multiple ways. The insights of these scholars, along with those of other nursing philosophers and theorists, have ensured a nursing perspective that, regardless of area of specialty practice, views persons as unique and contextual. This perspective necessitates engaged interaction with the person in question for the purposes of ascertaining that person's needs.

Current Trends

Some commentators note that there is a trend away from this traditional focus of psychiatric advanced practice nursing on the importance of the nurse–patient relationship. Perraud and colleagues (2006) attribute the "sweeping changes in mental health delivery" (p. 216) along with the inception of the psychiatric nurse practitioner role as being instrumental in diluting the "profession's core identity" (p. 216). Although biological and theoretical knowledge developments along with an understanding of societal needs can provide an ever stronger base for practice, they can also shift the emphasis of care away from the therapeutic alliance. Perraud and associates (2006) note that "under the paradigm shift ushered in by the decade of the brain" (p. 216), neurobiological advances and a firming up of core curricula for psychiatric mental health nursing at the advanced practice levels, a new emphasis emerged. "PMH graduate programs began teaching the primary care trio of physical assessment, pathophysiology, and pharmacology" (Perraud et al., 2006, p. 216), and these innovations may have accidentally served to lessen the perceived importance of nursing practice as being founded in the nurse–patient relationship. They argue that a shift back to the primacy of the nurse–patient relationship need not exclude the development of knowledge and skills related to pathophysiological/neurobiological advances.

Thus, it can be argued that APPMHNs can be differentiated from nurses in other specialties not by goal but rather by substance. They acquire, via theoretical knowledge and experience, an in-depth understanding of factors that influence mental health. This knowledge may come from within or outside of the nursing discipline. Knowledge from other disciplines such as psychology, biology, and the cognitive sciences when used in nursing practice is necessarily filtered through the lens of nursing goals. These are asserted in the Preamble to the International Council of Nurses *Code of Ethics* as being "to promote health, to prevent illness, to restore health and to alleviate suffering" (International Council of Nurses, 2005) and are rooted in the ideal that the nurse–patient relationship is of primary importance in practice with individuals. The ethic of care as discussed in Chapter 1 is a good way to conceptualize the APPMHN's relationship to individual patients.

Psychiatric and Mental Health Ethics: Importance for All APNs

APPMHNs become experienced in applying knowledge gained in their education and experience, via clinical judgment, to ameliorate a given patient's problem or suffering. However, the ethical issues that face advanced practice psychiatric nurses are not isolated to psychiatric settings and may well confront other nurses and APNs working in a variety of settings. For example, APNs who practice in emergency departments, in primary care practices, or with children are all liable to care for patients with concomitant mental health issues, whose physical symptoms have implications for their mental health, or whose mental health issues pose a threat to their physical well-being. Moreover, the complex and interwoven nature of human beings is such that any one of us can be susceptible to integrity disruptions that threaten our mental and physical well-being. Thus, all nurses benefit from understanding what constitutes ethical practice for those experiencing disturbances in health, whether this manifests in physical ways or in perceptual changes or some combination of both.

As discussed in Chapter 5, collaboration and sharing expertise are responsibilities of advanced practice. APPMHNs may well be called upon to collaborate with, educate, or assist colleagues in situations that require their expert knowledge. Additionally, advisory supervision is accepted practice both for novice and experienced psychotherapists and has been proposed as important in other settings where difficult cases are encountered. Those working in large institutions often have access to an ethics expert or resource for assistance in resolving dilemmas or difficult issues—those in primary care or smaller practices may have to develop their own discussion groups or resources.

The discussion, cases, and analyses that follow focus on either especially difficult or frequently encountered problems in psychiatric settings; they can be helpful for other healthcare professionals as they attempt to provide good care under uncertain, dangerous, or difficult circumstances. The cases are presented and explored with the aim of separating out important aspects and providing some clarity. Pertinent strategies and resources for resolving problems are offered. Before moving on to the cases, though, some themes prevalent in psychiatric settings and those that historically have been seen as related to the particular nature of mental health problems are discussed for the purposes of comprehending why decision making and action are sometimes so tricky.

PSYCHIATRY AND MENTAL ILLNESS: GOALS AND ETHICAL PRINCIPLES

The Relationship of Goals of Nursing to Goals of Mental Health Care

The Good of the Individual

The goals of nursing apply to advanced practice psychiatric nursing care no less than they do in other environments of nursing care. Disorders or disturbances of mental health, whatever the underlying cause, have effects that occur along a continuum: they can be relatively mild, causing slight altered experiences of health, perspective, or mood, to severe, causing distortions of reality that can be dangerous for the person or others in range of that person's destructive behavior. However, even mild mental health problems affect people in complex ways, altering their relationship to their environment and the contexts of their daily lives. In the absence of a risk of harm to others from the person in question, the focus of therapy or the therapeutic relationship is to provide a good for the individual, to help him or her restore the prior sense of well-being or improve it. Although achieving this goal may be difficult given all sorts of constraints placed upon the APN by the healthcare environment and the status of contemporary knowledge, locating the idea of professional responsibility in the goals of the profession provides guidance about what constitutes ethical action.

Mental Illness: Avoiding Harm from Misunderstanding

Based on historical accounts, pervasive misunderstandings about mental illness have resulted in terrible atrocities. In ancient times, mental symptoms were taken as signs that the person was possessed by an evil spirit. In the Middle Ages, people showing signs of mental illness were imprisoned in mental asylums and often treated as animals, ridiculed, and even exhibited as entertainment. More recently, mental illness was viewed as a genetic problem curable by eliminating from the breeding population those who showed signs of imbalance or retardation (Kelves, 1999). To give one extreme example, the Nazi "euthanasia" programs of the 1930s were responsible for the deaths of thousands of mentally ill persons (Kelves, 1999). Nurses were among those who were complicit in these programs (Benedict, 2003). Ongoing studies in moral development, the cognitive and behavioral sciences, and psychology have provided explanations why and under what conditions human beings may not follow the moral course of action. This knowledge permits professionals to develop a mindfulness that resists succumbing to pressures not to do the right thing for patients.

Despite advances in understanding the complexity of mental illness, contributing factors and their interrelationships, stigma persists, and not infrequently those with mental illness are perceived as being or are held partially responsible for their illness (Halter, 2008). Moreover, from culture to culture mental illness is viewed very differently. Some societies do not recognize the concept of mental disorder at all, and some critics in Western countries, where providing mental health services is an accepted practice, have called into question the purpose of the label "mental disorder" (Wakefield, 1992). It is beyond the purpose of this chapter to provide a philosophical discussion of the nature of mental illness. Controversies continue to be the subject of debate within mental health and philosophy circles. The interested reader is referred to Green and Bloch's (2006) collection of essays and articles for further information about these historical and ongoing debates.

The important point is that conditions continue to be ripe for misunderstandings about the nature of mental illness, which in turn cause further suffering for persons. APPMHNs are well positioned to inform policy making and public discussions related to this problem for the purposes of promoting good patient care and the provision of adequate and appropriate services. Additionally, they understand the implications for patients of lapses in confidentiality given that negative attitudes about mental illness persist.

Ethical Principles Plus the Goals of Nursing: Providing Direction

Ethical principles and considerations that have special salience in psychiatric/mental health settings broadly include autonomy, beneficence, and nonmaleficence. Justice is also an important factor because it provides the basis for addressing issues of needed change at the social or institutional policy level. That is, the principle of justice as fairness is important in helping us to see problems related to the inadequate or inappropriate healthcare service provision related to the population's need for access to mental health services. However, see Chapter 4 for a more in-depth discussion of professional responsibility for social action.

Each of these principles (autonomy, beneficence, and nonmaleficence) has important implications for the safety and well-being of persons experiencing mental health problems and places responsibilities upon professional providers of care. Although an in-depth discussion of these principles and their applications was given in Chapter 1 and later chapters, their particular implications for mental health are discussed here. As stressed previously, the principles are useful only insofar as they provide clarity. The main focus of ethical decision making is primarily about trying to achieve a good for the patient and in the process prevent harm to that person or others.

Perhaps the most problematic aspects of mental health disturbances are that they cloud judgment or alter persons' perception of the nature or meaning of their lives, which in turn renders voluntary informed decision making difficult, if not impossible. This particular problem presents APPMHNs and other psychiatric mental health professionals with some of their most difficult challenges. Aligned with this issue is the problem that impaired judgments can lead to personal harm for the patient, harm to significant others or innocent bystanders, and sometimes harm to the professional. A further issue described by Sadler (2007) is that associated with the conception of "personal self." He notes that "the personal self is a Western common-sense concept which is characterized by five aspects: agency, identity, trajectory, history and perspective . . . the personal self has considerable psychiatric significance in moral, professional, research, and existential realms" (p. 113). The idea of a personal self is very much bound up with the idea of autonomy in ethical psychiatric mental health practice.

Autonomy

Limits and Problems

In the discussion of autonomy earlier in the book, the question was raised, "Is anyone ever really capable of autonomous action?" The suggestion was made that we are all susceptible to subtle and not-so-subtle influences of various sorts; thus, no one is truly autonomous. Moreover, physiological influences also cause disruptions in cognition and perception. Diseases or conditions that alter cerebral perfusion, biological changes that alter neurological functioning, and chemicals including pharmaceuticals can all contribute to perceptual or information-processing problems.

Conditioning influences resulting from one's previous life experiences and culture give rise to certain beliefs and values. These may change over time and with education, exposure to other viewpoints, and other life experiences. Some influences are external and derive from the expectations of those around us, the need to earn a living, the legal system, and so on. That is, we all have conscious and unconscious drives that cause us not always to know what is in our best interests. Even if we know what is in our best interests, we do not always know what actions are most likely to further these. Stated another way, our actions often do not have the effects we desire or expect even when we think that we have accounted for everything in our decision-making process.

Given that this is true, there are several questions to answer. If we all have flawed decision-making processes, why would we think that certain people might make better decisions (those that are in line with their personal best interests) than others do? If we can answer this satisfactorily, we can then ask, "Is it ever permissible for a person to make a decision on behalf of another in the absence of that person's permission?"

Harm to Self or Others

Generally, it is accepted that if a person's actions are unlikely to cause significant harm to self or others, interfering on behalf of that person is not warranted. A person is expected to know what is best for him- or herself. Even if this knowledge, as noted earlier, is somewhat imperfect, it is still probably better than an outsider's knowledge of that person—as long as the subject is in possession of pertinent information. When significant harms to the person or others are certain or highly likely, then a more stringent evaluation is warranted and a responsibility to intervene may exist. The purpose of intervening when harm to the person is likely is to restore the person to his or her previous ability to exercise autonomy. For example, we would stop someone from jumping off a high bridge because this would result in certain death—and, thus, no further opportunities for the person to exercise autonomy exist.

Some of the following cases exemplify conditions of uncertainty where significant harm is possible. They are explored using points from the discussion here. Criteria for judging the ability of people to make their own informed decisions were given in Chapters 1 and 4 and include the ability to process relevant information, articulate how personal goals are likely to be met by given specified courses of action, and discuss the risks and provide reasoned explanations about why these risks are acceptable.

Buchanan and Brock's (1989) comprehensive look at decision making for those with impaired cognition has provided helpful insights in psychiatric–mental health settings. They note that decision-making abilities should be judged relative to a given task. In psychiatric–mental health settings, tasks might include such things as refusing medicines or accepting or refusing other therapies. Limits placed on a patient's freedom to make his or her own decisions are based either on that person's best interests (using what is known about the patient when possible) or on the likelihood that another will be significantly harmed by the person's actions.

So, a person's right to autonomy in choice of action may be limited because of lack of decision-making capacity and should be judged according to the degree of risk to self that is present. But a person's right to autonomous action may also be limited when that person presents a significant threat of harm to others. (This idea is discussed later in the chapter.) The serious and imminent threat of harm to others serves as a valid reason to limit a person's autonomy. When persons are prevented from following self-chosen courses of action because of worries that they may cause harm to themselves, the term used to justify the restriction is *paternalism.*

Paternalism

Paternalism is often used as a somewhat derogatory term to describe the imposition of the will of one person on another less powerful person. In healthcare ethics, the term *paternalism* is derived from the doctrine of *parens patriae* in medieval English Common Law and represents the responsibility of governments and states to protect those who cannot protect themselves (Payton, 1992). The intent of paternalistic actions is to ensure the safety and well-being of the vulnerable such as children and the cognitively impaired. Paternalism also captures the idea that when a person's decision-making capacity is impaired such that the person may not be able to protect him- or herself from harm, efforts should be made to decide appropriate actions. *Appropriate actions* are those that are in line with what is known about that person's beliefs, values, and previous life trajectory. That is, the chosen action is not based on what the proxy decision maker would want for him- or herself, but rather what the impaired individual would want for him- or herself.

Only when nothing is known about the individual in question is a best-interest or reasonable person standard used as the next best option. The reasonable person standard is self-explanatory: a decision is ethically warranted if it is what a reasonable person would want. Sometimes, of course, it is hard to determine what a reasonable person would want, but the standard does provide some guidance for action when it is not knowable what the person him- or herself would wish. Although paternalism does permit the conceptualization of actions that are likely to further the specific interests of an incapacitated person, it is obviously not as good as being able to follow the person's own articulated directions. For such reasons, and as a result of ethics debates and discussions, the idea of having psychiatric advance directives arose in the 1980s (Green & Bloch, 2006).

Psychiatric Advance Directives

Many psychiatric illnesses cause fluctuations in a person's ability to make reasoned or informed decisions about acceptable care and therapeutics. Sometimes a person has decision-making capacity, and sometimes while experiencing a relapse, he or she does not. Examples of such problems are schizophrenia and bipolar disorders. In the 1980s, a revolutionary idea was proposed to help patients diagnosed with relapsing psychiatric illnesses retain control over what treatment would be acceptable to them in the event of decision-making incapacity (Culver & Gert, 1982; Green & Bloch, 2006; Howell, Diamond, & Wikler, 1982; Lavin, 1986; Winston, Winston, Appelbaum, & Rhoden, 1982). These are variously named psychiatric *advance directive*s, *Ulysses contracts*, *self-binding contracts*, and *advanced treatment authorizations* (Green & Bloch, 2006, p. 183). The advance directive can be either instructional or be realized by way of appointing a trusted proxy decision maker. For written directives, a discussion involving the person and his or her psychiatric–mental health provider occurs in which possible scenarios are articulated and acceptable treatments and interventions are agreed upon. The limitations of this are that not all possibilities can be anticipated. The appointment of a proxy can resolve this problem to a certain extent, although then the patient may need to be assisted in identifying a trustworthy and capable proxy. The combination of written instructions and an appointed proxy may be even more effective in providing what the patient would want. As you will have noticed, psychiatric advance directives resemble advance directives as used in the broader healthcare setting; they differ only in that they are specific to the mental health needs of the patient. APPMHNs who work with such patients have an important role in assisting patients who are willing to prepare their own advance directives. This requires a careful process of decision making and information sharing.

Nonmaleficence

The principle of nonmaleficence as discussed in Chapter 1 and later chapters captures the idea of a power imbalance in healthcare provider–patient relationships. The principle cautions us to avoid doing harm in the course of our professional endeavors. In psychiatric mental health settings, harm to the patient can be caused in a variety of ways. A person can be harmed as a result of his or her illness-related actions, vulnerability to the condition, lack of knowledge about therapeutics and their aims, unethical practitioners, limits on freedom, or any combination of these. Some specific examples of particular harms include inappropriate referrals, misdiagnosis, boundary violations, restrictions on freedom, abandonment (Gutheil & Simon, 2003), and inappropriate dissemination of information gained in the course of the therapeutic relationship. Maintaining a focus on the fiduciary aspects of the nurse–patient relationship is important. As noted in earlier chapters, the fiduciary relationship is based on trust. The patient should be able to trust that the healthcare provider maintains the patient's best interest as his or her primary concern.

When the problem is that the patient poses a risk to others, the trust versus safety issue presents tension for the APPMHN. The principle of nonmaleficence imposes a responsibility to lessen the harm that results from the necessary breech in confidentiality that results from the need to protect others from the patient's actions.

Breaking Confidentiality

Although the principle of autonomy underlies the idea that maintaining confidentiality is crucially important in healthcare settings, it is not an absolute value as discussed in Chapter 1. Limits to respecting a person's autonomy occur when a person's action might cause danger to self or others. The idea behind confidentiality is that the person has a right to say what can be done with his or her information and who can have access to it. However, when information that has implications for the well-being of another person is shared with a healthcare provider, that provider is faced with the task of determining the likelihood and severity of the risk and making a judgment about whether that information should be shared and with whom.

At one time, the provider–patient privilege was understood to be as binding as that of the clergy or advocate. *Privilege* means that it is "shielded from exposure to the legal system" (Grace, 2005, p. 114). Several landmark legal cases changed ideas about provider responsibility to break confidentiality and under which sorts of conditions they must do so. Healthcare providers have duties to warn others

> who are unknowingly endangered. This duty was highlighted by the . . . *Tarasoff* case. On October 27, 1969, Prosenjit Poddar killed Tatiana Tarasoff. Poddar was receiving psychiatric care during this period. He had informed his therapist two weeks earlier that he was going to kill a certain girl, easily identifiable as Tarasoff, on her return from Brazil. At the time his therapist tried to have him committed. The police detained Poddar briefly but decided he was rational so released him. No one warned Tatiana of the danger and Poddar killed her. (Grace, 2005, p. 115)

The courts concluded that "once a therapist does in fact determine, or under applicable professional standards reasonably should have determined, that a person poses a serious danger of violence to others, he bears a duty to exercise reasonable care to protect the foreseeable victim of that danger" (*Tarasoff v. Regents of University of California*, 1976).

But nonmaleficence also warns us to limit the harms that can be caused by a possible loss of trust in the therapist, which in turn has implications for the patient's well-being. Loss of trust may mean that a patient holds back important information that can lead to effective interventions. Trust is also lost when a decision is made to hospitalize a patient against that person's will or without that person's permission. Additionally, while hospitalized (voluntarily or involuntarily), a decision may be made to use chemical or physical restraints to control a person's harmful behavior. Both the principles of nonmaleficence and beneficence apply to decisions to involuntarily hospitalize patients or to use restraints to control behavior.

Beneficence

Involuntary Hospitalization and Chemical and Physical Restraints

Harm can also be caused in the course of trying to provide a good for the patient when the patient needs to be restrained to prevent harm to self or others. Beneficence, the ethical principle that best captures the healthcare provider's duties to provide a good for persons, is also relevant to the discussion related to behavior control. (The principle of beneficence is described in more detail in Chapter 1.)

Chodoff's (1976/1999) carefully argued defense both of the need for involuntary hospitalization and the criteria that should be applied to such decisions remains pertinent today. He presents a series of cases, and then makes an argument that the nature of mental illness is such that we are warranted in involuntary hospitalization in certain instances on the grounds that it will further the person's good (note that this is not the issue of dangerousness to others as discussed earlier but is concentrated on the likelihood of personal harm). He argues that involuntary hospitalization may be warranted if "obvious disturbances that are both intrapsychic [for example, the suffering of severe depression] and interpersonal [for example, withdrawal from others because of depression]" (p. 108) exist. The criteria for such hospitalizations are that the institution has treatment available, there is a focus on the patient regaining control rather than on controlling the patient, and adequate surveillance exists. In the absence of the possibility of cure, the amelioration of suffering is the goal (Chodoff, 1976/1999).

SUMMARY

The preceding discussion is far from a complete account of issues encountered in psychiatric and mental health care environments or in society in general. Other contemporary issues worthy of further discussion relate to managed care funding issues, parity in healthcare coverage by insurance companies, problems caused by profit-motive health care and the pharmaceutical industry, direct-to-consumer marketing of drugs and treatments, and even the development of new diseases for which new drugs can then be developed and prescribed. Such topics can be given as class assignments to explore further. The next section presents cases with associated discussion and questions to stimulate further thought. The cases are composites and details have been altered to maintain confidentiality.

CASE 1: INADEQUATE CARE

Andrew is a graduate student in psychiatric nursing and has a clinical placement at a crisis intervention center of a local mental health clinic. Martha Adams presents for an evaluation and states that she has not been able to contact her psychiatrist, who practices at a well-known teaching hospital and that she is in need of a renewal of her antidepressant medication. In fact, she took her last dose of paroxetine 3 days ago and has been questioning whether paroxetine is the right medication for her. She has experienced a number of side effects that include a 30-pound weight gain and a decreased libido. Martha sees her psychiatrist once every 6 months for 10-minute visits during which her doctor always seems rushed and more focused on other office issues. Martha has not felt that her doctor listens to her concerns, and after meeting with Andrew and his preceptor, she asks if there is another medication to try and if she could possibly return and be followed here at this clinic where she feels her concerns are heard.

Andrew notes Martha's symptoms of decreased concentration, lethargy, and lack of motivation coupled with her desire to quit smoking, and he thinks that a change of medication possibly to bupropion would be beneficial to the patient because it is helpful in smoking cessation. In addition, he discusses the need for Martha to be in ongoing therapy to help with her self-esteem issues and depressed thoughts. When he reviews his plan with his preceptor prior to presenting it to the client, Andrew's preceptor instructs him that they will renew the paroxetine that she has been already prescribed and will call and leave a message for the psychiatrist. The preceptor is very aware of the need to maintain a positive rapport with the psychiatrist who is a well-known lecturer in psychopharmacology. Andrew feels that this is letting the patient down because they have already heard from the patient her desire to seek more active treatment. He is mindful of the need to be an advocate for the patient in her efforts to obtain quality care.

Discussion

As a result of Andrew's advanced practice educational process and his previous nursing experiences, he knows that the primary goals of care for Martha are to establish a therapeutic relationship and use sound clinical judgment (Table 4-1) in assisting her to receive the care she needs. His holistic approach to her care has already unearthed some of the complexities of her case, including weight gain, libido problems, and the desire to stop smoking. If Andrew were the primary provider in this instance, he could use his judgment about how to address the issue of appropriate care. Various strategies could be tried, depending upon the patient's needs and Andrew's knowledge of the psychiatrist in question. For example, Martha could be empowered to decide for herself whether to change providers and how to go about this. Additionally, Andrew could persist in trying to contact the psychiatrist to discuss his concerns, including the fact that Martha stopped taking paroxetine and that he would like to try something that would work for both the depression and the smoking cessation.

Although there is a responsibility not to undercut a patient's trust in another provider, when we are sure that the other provider's care is not serving the patient well we have a responsibility to help the patient figure out how she can get her needs met. For U.S. nurses, the American Nurses Association *Code of Ethics for Nurses with Interpretive Statements* (2001) provides guidance related to the practice of other professionals. Provision 3.5 clearly affirms that the nurse's "primary responsibility is to the health, well-being and safety of the patient" and this preempts loyalties to other professionals who are not serving the patient's interests.

Abrupt withdrawal from antidepressants also has negative consequences, and renewing the paroxetine is no guarantee that Martha will take it. In fact, when she has clearly stated her issues with it, persisting with the prescription is likely to undermine her trust both in Andrew, who has developed a rapport with her, and in his preceptor, who would presumably be the one to have an ongoing relationship with her. Thus, there is the possibility of harm to Martha both from the withdrawal from the antidepressant in the absence of a substitute and perhaps even more important from the loss of trust in providers.

However, Andrew is not the primary provider in this instance. He is faced with the tricky issue of working with a preceptor and as such being a "guest" in that environment. Preceptors often give their time with no obvious rewards except the fact that they are contributing to the discipline and think that they can have a positive influence on the development of good practitioners. So, Andrew does not have the power to override his preceptor's decision, and he must have strong rationale for his point of view; he should be willing to hear his preceptor and accept a reasonable decision. Failing this, he can try to articulate his concerns and find a middle ground that serves the patient's best interests while maintaining a rapport with his preceptor. If, however, Andrew has other concerns about his preceptor's philosophy of practice, then his next step is to talk to his supervising faculty about the possibility of a more suitable clinical placement.

CASE 2: SPLIT TREATMENT AND ALICE'S WELL-BEING

Alice is a 20-year-old single woman currently in her third year of college. She has struggled with symptoms of major depression and anxiety since early adolescence. At age 13, she began individual therapy with a social worker specializing in child psychiatry and a child psychiatrist who prescribed medications. She attended a therapeutic high school and during the last half of her senior year made an unsuccessful suicide attempt. She was admitted to a psychiatric hospital against her will.

When it came time for discharge planning, the hospital staff in consultation with her outpatient therapist began to form a treatment team of clinicians specializing in care of adults that could follow Alice over the long term. She was referred to an art therapist (AT) named Amy Bowen for individual therapy and to a clinical nurse specialist (CNS), Lynn Arnold, who would monitor her response to medications and her overall well-being. At that time, her diagnoses were Bipolar I Disorder—her most recent episode of this was severe and she exhibited psychotic features—and Attention Deficit Disorder Hyperactive (ADDH) type. As graduation approached, Amy Bowen, Lynn Arnold, and the social worker met with Alice to plan for her transition from therapeutic high school to college. This meeting offered Alice and all present the message that her treatment was a team effort.

Two years into Alice's college experience, Amy (the AT) reluctantly withdrew her services due to a family crisis that had ongoing sequelae that resulted in her closing her clinical practice. After consulting with Lynn Arnold, Amy informed Alice of the reasons for her decision and referred Alice to another AT, who unbeknownst to Amy did not share Amy's willingness to collaborate treatment with a prescribing clinician. Lynn attempted to leave messages for the new therapist after each visit with Alice but never received return calls. Alice reported feeling very comfortable with her new therapist and indicated the presence of a strong alliance, albeit not the same as the one she experienced with Amy.

Alice began to miss follow-up appointments with Lynn and does not return calls. Attempts to reach the new therapist go unanswered. Only when Alice's prescriptions run out does Lynn hear from Alice. Lynn has been seeing Alice for 3 years at this point but is now concerned that she is participating in a treatment protocol that is inadequate and that the possibility of harm exists related to Lynn's limited ability to evaluate Alice's overall health status and thus anticipate problems and provide appropriate care.

Discussion

This case raises several issues. First, when a referral or replacement for one's services is needed, the provider has a professional responsibility to try to ensure that the replacement is appropriate based on knowledge of the patient's needs and that the philosophy of care of the replacement fits in with the established team. Expectations of the collaborative relationship need to be articulated openly. All parties must understand their respective role and reach agreement with other members. In this case, this arrangement is most likely to serve Alice's needs and permit anticipation of emerging problems. In view of the problem encountered in this case, it is probably also prudent for the team to talk about how a change of therapist will be handled by the group. Because team relationships are inevitably altered as members change, it might be prudent to have a group meeting to discuss roles and role responsibilities. At that meeting, an important aspect to be discussed is how a breakdown in communication among the members of the team will be handled. That is, besides serving Alice's current needs, future issues are anticipated. This kind of planning could also be called preventive ethics. *Preventive ethics* tries to anticipate future problems and put into place a structure to deal with them. Because of the seriousness of

Alice's mental health issues, optimal care for her warrants egalitarian collaborative relationships where all members can expect to have their perspective heard.

However, this current situation has gone beyond the stage when preventive ethics could play a role. Now a new avenue must be explored. As an important part of the team, the AT has some crucial information that needs to be shared for Alice's health to be optimized. Alice's CNS, Lynn Arnold, is in the best position to evaluate Alice's ongoing needs. She has the knowledge and expertise to understand the interplay of physical, chemical, and psychosocial aspects of care and how disruptions in any one of these may lead to a deterioration of Alice's health. But she can plan appropriate care and therapeutics only if she has adequate information to do this. It is unclear what Lynn's relationship with Alice is, but if a rapport has been built up, then Lynn could explore with Alice the need for, or the possibility of, a group meeting to ensure that the plan of care continues to meet her needs. She could try to discover how Alice usually contacts the AT when she has to cancel appointments. A concern here might be that Lynn's frustration with her inability to contact the new therapist and uncertainty about Alice's health might cause an inadvertent break in the alliance that Alice has formed with the new therapist, which could be harmful (breaching the principle of nonmaleficence). Lynn must be careful not to communicate negative feelings about the AT, which might make Alice feel that she has to choose between the two.

Perhaps the AT prefers a mode of communication other than the telephone. One option for Lynn might be to write her concerns in a letter to the AT, describing the original arrangement, why it was deemed important, and why ongoing communication is important to Alice's health. Sending the letter by certified mail would permit verification that the letter was received. Lynn could also try to discover if others have had similar problems and how these have been resolved. Resolution of such issues depends on the nature of the problem and clinical judgment about the patient's good and what is required to further this. Keeping the focus on the patient's needs rather than one's own frustration is most likely to lead to appropriate and sound actions.

CASE 3: THE LIMITS OF RESPONSIBILITY

Megan was referred to Beverly Sweeney, APRN, BC, by her college health service during her first semester of school. Megan presented with symptoms of major depression that included difficulty concentrating, sleep disturbance, anhedonia, increased irritability, and recurring thoughts of harming herself. A treatment plan was established that included weekly individual psychotherapy sessions and medication management. Megan had a positive response to treatment and eventually saw Ms. Sweeney every 2 weeks to work on her negative cognitions and low self-esteem. Her treatment included a prescription for a daily dose of 40 mg citalopram, an antidepressant.

As graduation approached, it was clear that Megan would be moving out of state to pursue job opportunities and thus therapy with Beverly would need to be terminated. As a result, Ms. Sweeney encouraged Megan to use the remaining few weeks before her move to review her experiences of therapy. Megan was able to articulate her ambivalence in saying goodbye to Ms. Sweeney. This ambivalence is understood to be a normal response to the ending of a therapeutic relationship, whether this is because treatment is no longer needed or a transfer to another therapist is needed. Megan and Beverly spent the last few sessions discussing the need for follow-up care and how to find an appropriate provider after relocating. Because Megan felt that she needed to continue on the prescribed antidepressants, a new provider who could evaluate her progress was essential.

During their last session, Ms. Sweeney gave Megan a 1-month prescription for citalopram with three refills. They agreed that this would get Megan through the initial period of getting settled in a new area. Besides the psychological impact that a relocation can have, it takes time to find a place to live, a job, new health insurance, and new healthcare providers. Thus, a 3-month supply seemed appropriate. They parted toward the end of July with the acknowledgment that the therapy had been successful but more follow-up would benefit Megan as she went through the stress of relocating.

Toward the end of November, Ms. Sweeney received a phone message from Megan stating that she was about to run out of her citalopram because she had only three pills left. She left a pharmacy phone number along with her cell phone number and asked whether Ms. Sweeney could please call in a prescription to her new pharmacy. Beverly is alarmed at her own emotional reaction to this situation. She feels an intense irritation and wonders what the root cause of it is.

Discussion

This case raises several questions. We do not know whether Megan is seeing a new therapist who does not have prescription privileges or if she has other reasons for not following through on the suggested interim therapy. Is this a type of boundary issue as described by Gutheil and Gabbard (1993/2006)? Is Megan is suffering from the psychological effects of withdrawal from her therapist that has been worsened by the stress of trying to adapt to new circumstances? Gutheil and Gabbard note that "almost all patients who enter into a psychotherapeutic process struggle with the unconscious wish to view the therapist as the ideal parent" (p. 61). Thus, Megan may be acting out her insecurity by returning to a reliance on, or a demand for, the attention of Beverly. More information is needed before an ethical course of action can be determined.

Initially, on hearing the phone message Ms. Sweeney had viewed this problem as a dilemma. Having not seen Megan in several months, and thus not being able to evaluate her mental health status on a face-to-face basis, she wondered whether she should call in a prescription or not. She felt somewhat irritated that Megan had not acted responsibly. On the other hand, she was worried that if she did not fill the prescription, Megan might suffer withdrawal symptoms. Nevertheless, she was reluctant to fill the prescription knowing that Megan was not being monitored appropriately.

On further reflection, Beverly felt that she had explained in great detail to Megan during a couple of their therapy sessions the unpleasant and sometimes harmful effects that abrupt withdrawal from this type of drug could have and that if she decided she didn't need it anymore the dosage must be slowly tapered. She began to realize that in fact this current situation did not constitute a true dilemma and that several alternative options were open to her.

She could talk to Megan on the phone and discuss with Megan her status and what her options are. If it turned out that Megan has been receiving care from a therapist who does not have prescription authority, then Megan should be encouraged to talk to her current therapist about how he or she normally handles a case where pharmaceutical intervention is seen as a necessary adjunct to therapy. Most nonprescribing clinicians have collaborative relationships. If Megan is not having therapy, does she need it? If it is apparent that she does, perhaps a contract with Megan can be made. Beverly could help Megan identify resources in her area and give a modified (perhaps a week's supply) prescription with the understanding she be notified when an appointment has been made. Given that we are reasonably sure Megan is capable of making her own decisions (has decision-making capacity) and that she is able to appreciate the implications of her actions for her own goals and values, responsibility for the current situation properly resides with her. In fact, to come to her rescue may not be therapeutic. It could be the equivalent of failing to respect her autonomy and may undermine the previous work done with her related to developing her self-esteem and confidence.

On reflecting about her own irritated reaction, Beverly realizes that she has mixed feelings about Megan's behavior. One of her concerns is that her therapy with Megan was unsuccessful. She had hoped that Megan would take responsibility for her ongoing mental health by seeking out appropriate care. It is important that Ms. Sweeney sort out and understand the source and nature of her own reactions to formulate an ethical response to Megan's request, one that will maximize Megan's well-being and reduce the possibility of harm.

Complicating Ms Sweeney's reaction is the issue of compensation because she does not get paid for her time or expertise unless she sees the patient in the office. This can be a boundary issue related to the therapeutic contract—that is, the issue of holding patients responsible for their agreed part of a contracted service agreement. Alternatively, it could be a system problem related to fair reimbursement by insurance companies, which depends for its resolution on health policy changes. This discussion is beyond the scope of the current chapter but is addressed in Chapters 2 and 4 and elsewhere in the book.

Conclusion

The nature of psychiatric–mental health advanced practice can present the clinician with a wide variety of difficult and ambiguous situations. Although a focus on professional goals, an understanding of ethical language and pertinent principles, and experienced clinical judgment is most likely to lead to a sound course of action, elements of uncertainty will often persist. In such cases, and where time permits, consultation with another professional or an ethics expert may be helpful. The following case is posed for class exploration and discussion or for discussion with colleagues.

CASE 4: THE ANGRY SON

Mr. A., a 23-year-old single man employed full time as a city sanitation worker, seeks help for what he describes as unbearable anxiety and depression. In his words: "I can't stand the way I feel. Every morning I wake up and ask, 'Why me? What did I do to deserve this?'" He contacts a psychiatric CNS who has a private counseling practice. As is her usual practice, Ms. P. reviews with Mr. A. policies that she follows, including the fact that personal information divulged in therapy is confidential by law and that Ms. P. cannot share this information without his permission. She notes that the only exception to this would be if she has good reason to believe that he is in serious and imminent danger of hurting himself or someone else. Mr. A. has no intention or plan of killing himself at this time and he agrees to call if his feelings change or if he feels in any danger of hurting himself. They agree on an initial treatment contract that includes meeting for four sessions to evaluate the best course of treatment, which may or may not include medication to help with his anxiety and depression.

Despite Mr. A's obvious discomfort and anxiety, he settles into a fairly comfortable rapport with Ms. P. and seems calmed by the fact of having made the decision to get help. His initial mental status exam offers no evidence of thought disorder, and although he had experienced past substance abuse with alcohol and cocaine, it has been more than a year since he has used either of these substances. He denies having any active problems with these substances.

During a therapy session, Mr. A. reveals that he is the youngest of five children and the only boy born to a couple of Italian descent. His mother worked as a court stenographer, and his father was a firefighter who left the family when Mr. A. was 5 years old. Mr. A. has no memory of his father being in the house when he was growing up and states that his father was an alcoholic. After his parents' divorce, Mr. A. continued to have little attention from his father despite the fact that his father lived nearby. Mr. A.'s mother "disciplined" him by using ridicule. On many occasions, his sisters joined in the ridicule, commenting that he was "a sissy." He shares a particularly painful memory of having his older sister making fun of him for crying and calling him "a girl."

Three days after the session in which this was revealed, Mr. A. calls Ms. P. by phone and states, in a slurred voice, that he has a weapon and is going to kill his father. Ms. P. attempts to calm Mr. A., but he remains agitated, yelling into the phone, "My father should pay for running out on me and leaving me to be raised by women. . . . I feel like I am less than a man." Ms. P. manages to establish the fact that Mr. A., is in his home alone. She does not have the father's address and is convinced that Mr. A., in his intoxicated state, is a threat to his father and possibly to himself. Ms. P. tells Mr. A. that she is very concerned about him and does not want him to act on his feelings, adding that it is her job to do whatever she can to keep him safe. Mr. A. screams some unintelligible words into the phone and hangs up.

Ms. P. is very concerned both about the safety of Mr. A.'s father and the harm that will accrue to Mr. A. if he acts on his impulse (jail, remorse, and so forth). She decides to inform the police, telling the dispatcher that Mr. A. is a psychotherapy patient in her private practice who is threatening to kill his father. She adds that Mr. A. has only just begun to acknowledge some painful memories and that he is primarily depressed and anxious. Although Mr. A. states he has a weapon, Ms. P. does not know for certain that this is the case. What prompts immediate concern is that he is very depressed, agitated, and intoxicated and thus may not be able to control his impulses as he might when sober.

DISCUSSION QUESTIONS

1. Using the decision-making framework from Chapter 2 and the information in this chapter, analyze this case. What ethical principles are important and why? Did Ms. P. have any alternative courses of action? Take into account the following concerns and describe the part they play in your analysis of the case.

    a. Under what sorts of conditions is a breach in confidentiality warranted?
    b. How might trust be reestablished after the danger has resolved?
    c. What are the implications of alerting the police about Mr. A.'s threats if he has experienced failure in past treatment attempts?

2. You have a patient, Mr. Benson, who suffers from bipolar disorder. When he experiences a manic phase, he refuses to take his medicine. He typically goes on buying sprees and puts himself and his family (wife and one child) at economic risk. Last time this happened they were evicted for nonpayment of rent. His sister has taken them in several times when this happened but says she will not do it again. When his disorder is managed, he experiences remorse and regret about his risky behavior. As his long-term psychotherapist, you have decided to talk to him about a psychiatric advance directive. How would you go about discussing this with him?

REFERENCES

American Nurses Association. (2001). *Code of ethics for nurses with interpretive statements.* Washington, DC: Author.

Benedict, S. (2003). Killing while caring: The nurses of Hadamar. *Issues in Mental Health Nursing, 24*(1), 59–79.

Buchanan, A., & Brock, D. (1989). *Deciding for others: The ethics of surrogate decision-making.* New York: Cambridge University Press.

Chodoff, P. (1999). The case for involuntary hospitalization of the mentally ill. In T. Beauchamp & L. Walters (Eds.), *Contemporary issues in bioethics* (pp. 105–115). Belmont, CA: Wadsworth. (original work published in 1976, *American Journal of Psychiatry, 133*, 496–501).

Culver, C., & Gert, B. (1982). *Philosophy in medicine. Conceptual and ethical issues in medicine and psychiatry.* New York: Oxford University Press.

Fawcett, J. (1984). The metaparadigm of nursing: Present status and future refinements . . . for theory development. *Image, 16*(3), 84–87.

Grace, P. (2005). Ethical issues relevant to health promotion. In C. Edelman & C. L. Mandle (Eds.), *Health promotion throughout the lifespan* (6th ed., Chapter 5, pp. 100–125). St. Louis, MO: Elsevier/Mosby.

Green, S., & Bloch, S. (2006). *An anthology of psychiatric ethics.* New York: Oxford University Press.

Gutheil, T., & Gabbard, G. (2006). The concept of boundaries in clinical practice: Theoretical and risk-management dimensions. In S. Green & S. Bloch (Eds.), *An anthology of psychiatric ethics* (pp. 60–66). New York: Oxford University Press. (Reprinted from *American Journal of Psychiatry, 150*, 1993, 188–196.)

Gutheil, T., & Simon, R. (2003). Abandonment of patients in split treatment. *Harvard Review of Psychiatry, 11*, 175–179.

Halter, M. (2008). Perceived characteristics of psychiatric nurses: Stigma by association. *Archives of Psychiatric Nursing, 22*(1), 20–26.

Howell, T., Diamond, J., & Wikler, D. (1982). Is there a case for voluntary commitment? In T. L. Beauchamp & L. R. Walters (Eds.), *Contemporary issues in bioethics* (2nd ed., pp. 163–168). Belmont, CA: Wadsworth.

International Council of Nurses. (2005). *Code of ethics for nurses.* Geneva: Author. Retrieved January 19, 2008, from http://www.icn.ch/icncode.pdf.

Kelves, D. (1999). Eugenics and human rights. *British Medical Journal, 319*, 435–438.

Kneisl, C., Wilson, H., & Trigoboff, E. (2004). *Contemporary psychiatric-mental health nursing.* Upper Saddle River, NJ: Pearson/Prentice Hall.

Lavin, M. (1986). Ulysses contracts. *Journal of Applied Philosophy, 3*, 89–101.

Orlando, I. (1961). *The dynamic nurse-patient relationship: Function, process, and principles.* New York: Putnam.

Payton, S. (1992). The concept of the person in the Parens Patriae jurisdiction over previously competent persons. *Journal of Medicine and Philosophy, 17*(6), 605–645.

Peplau, H. (1952). *Interpersonal relations in nursing.* New York: Putnam.

Perraud, S., Delaney, K., Carlson-Sabelli, L., Johnson, M., Shephard, R., & Paun, O. (2006). Advanced practice psychiatric mental health nursing, finding our core: The therapeutic relationship in 21st Century. *Perspectives in Psychiatric Care, 42*(4), 215–226.

Sadler, J. (2007). The psychiatric significance of the personal self. *Psychiatry, 70*(2), 113–129.

Tarasoff v. Regents of University of California. (1976, July 1). California Supreme Court 131. *California Reporter,* 14.

Travelbee, J. (1966). *Interpersonal aspects of nursing.* Philadelphia: F. A. Davis.

Wakefield, J. (1992). The concept of mental disorder: On the boundary between biological facts and social values. *American Psychologist, 47*, 373–388.

Winston, M., Winston, S., Appelbaum, P., & Rhoden, N. (1982). Case studies: Can a subject consent to a "Ulysses Contract"? *Hastings Center Report, 12*(4), 26–28.

CHAPTER 12

Nursing Ethics and Nurse Anesthesia Practice

Gregory Sheedy

Don't be afraid. Remember I'm here. The noise in the street will soon disappear. When the soft eyes of mercy are blinded by the dark. I will stay with eyes open, stay here with eyes open, to watch over you and take away the sadness and the fear. I'll be here.
The October Project, 1993

INTRODUCTION

Certified registered nurse anesthetists (CRNAs) are faced with complex and critical decision making as a normal part of their practice of providing anesthesia care to patients. Many of these decisions must be made before a patient enters the operating room (OR) suite, and they involve some of the most difficult life issues. For example, CRNAs may have to help patients understand that they have the right to refuse life-sustaining treatment and what that means in the context of surgery and anesthesia delivery; assist a patient in deciding whether to participate in controversial procedures; determine if a patient is capable of giving consent for a procedure; and protect patients from incompetent or dangerous healthcare providers. *Timing* is a key concept that lends a particular urgent quality to ethical decision making in anesthesia practice.

Consider that the decision for a patient to have a surgical procedure is most often determined before the anesthesia provider is introduced to the patient. In many of these cases, the nurse anesthetist is asked to rapidly assess the patient and proceed to surgery with minimal delay. Some of these cases involve patients whose likelihood of survival, or of sustaining a reasonable quality of life, after surgery is in doubt, yet no code status has been established, nor have discussions of medical futility occurred. CRNAs are faced with problems caused by communication failures earlier in the patient's evaluation or treatment process and by the patient's lack of knowledge about the anesthesia process or about his or her medical problems.

Production pressure and moving patients through the OR in as little time as possible are realities of current-day delivery of surgical services, at least in the United States. Patients are sometimes treated as if they were commodities,

339

where patients become products instead of being the focus of personalized surgical care. This creates an environment where any anesthesia care provider may be requested to participate in activities that conflict with personal and professional beliefs about what constitutes good care and their understood primary ethical obligations to the patient. Conflicts among the surgical care team members, colleagues, and surgeons develop as a result of different perspectives on what is the appropriate ethical treatment of patients requiring surgery.

Ethical conflicts in the context of anesthesia practice may also involve other parties beside the anesthesia provider, the surgeon, and the patient. Primary care physicians, nurse practitioners, perioperative nurses, family members, legal counsel, patient proxies, legal guardians, and other consulting health-care providers may also have a stake in the patient's operative and anesthesia course. Imagine the difficulty in resolving a disagreement between an appointed guardian of an incompetent patient who insists on surgery for his client, the primary care physician who insists that surgery is not consistent with the plan for comfort care, and the surgeon who has a small window of opportunity to perform the surgery because of a busy schedule. The nurse anesthetist is placed under enormous pressure to fulfill the wishes of multiple parties while trying to advocate that the patient receive appropriate care.

Ethical dilemmas and problems arise with such frequency in the clinical practice of nurse anesthetists that becoming familiar with facets of the ethical decision-making process is essential for facilitating good care of the patient. Additionally, because of the everyday nature of many of the barriers to good (ethical) anesthesia care, overcoming obstacles and resolving problems are inescapable professional responsibilities of all CRNA practice and cannot be left to the ethics experts. Although ethics experts and resources can provide expertise in especially difficult cases, the nurse anesthetist knows what constitutes good anesthesia practice for a given patient. For this reason, it is important for all CRNAs to develop confidence in their ethical decision making. See Chapter 2 for a discussion of professional responsibility and ethical decision making in nursing practice in general.

Ethical Theory and Problem Solving

The ethical principles of autonomy, beneficence, nonmaleficence, and distributive justice are commonly utilized in analyzing ethical dilemmas in health-care settings. As discussed in Chapter 1, they help provide clarity and reveal underlying assumptions that are being made. For each situation, however, the relevance and value of each principle must be weighed (Boudreaux, 2001). As noted in Chapter 2, because nursing goals are usually to promote the good of a particular patient, they guide which principles are either relevant or the priority in a given case. Beneficence is the obligation to perform an intervention or provide for the benefit, or good, of a patient, where benefits are weighed against the risks of a proposed intervention. Nonmaleficence is the obligation to prevent harm to a patient, and the principle of autonomy refers to respecting one's right to make one's own decisions without the overriding influence of medical authority (Boudreaux, 2001). Distributive justice is the principle that guides the decisions by which healthcare resources are fairly distributed to patients. These principles were discussed in detail in Chapter 1 and are discussed further in this chapter as they are introduced related to the specific topic or case.

Principle-Based Ethics

Principle-based ethics as an approach to decision making, as noted previously, is based in Western values as these have developed over time. Consideration of each principle offers the freedom to examine every ethical conflict or situation in its own context. Not every principle will be relevant in every case. Problems arise when principles give conflicting direction or seem to hold equal weight in a particular decision-making context. One example of this is the conflict between the provider's professional understanding of a critical need to transfuse blood (beneficence) to a patient whose religion is Jehovah's Witness, and the patient, who as a result of his beliefs would rather die than receive blood (autonomy). Deciding which principle is more important to honor in a given case depends on viewpoints of the involved parties, as discussed in Chapter 1. For this reason, principle-based ethics alone cannot solve most problems in anesthesia practice. Ultimately, the resolution of a problem is for the benefit of a particular patient or patients. Thus, a focus on the patient good is pivotal in decision making.

Case-Based Ethics

Case-based ethics is a more practical method of ethical problem solving that has been used in health care as well as legal settings. This method, also called *casuistry*, takes the facts of a case and organizes them in an orderly fashion, and then compares them to the facts in other similar cases where a resolution of a conflict has been achieved (Jonsen, Siegler, & Winslade, 1998). In the legal system, previous cases set a legal precedence for successive cases having relevantly similar characteristics (Boudreaux, 2001). This method, although helpful for teaching, has several drawbacks. There is a relative lack of freedom to judge each case in its own context. Additionally, several decision makers may have or think they all have a stake in the outcome of the ethical conflict or problem. The perspectives of these diverse parties cannot always be accounted for by a casuist approach. Further, casuistry does not necessarily identify which problems are recurring and thus doesn't facilitate needed changes in institutional policy.

The subsequent sections of this chapter explore ethical issues of particular concern to CRNA practice. Each section makes use of a key ethical principle and discusses the interplay of other ethical principles. In addition to presenting a case study to illustrate an ethical dilemma, problem, or topic of particular concern in anesthesia practice, the case is analyzed, relevant ethical elements discussed, and questions raised. This method is designed both to provide practice in ethical analysis and to assist the CRNA in developing confidence in his or her own knowledge and abilities related to ethical issues in practice.

DO-NOT-RESUSCITATE ORDERS DURING SURGERY

DNR and the Principle of Autonomy

Do-not-resuscitate orders, or DNR orders, as they are commonly called, are an apparatus by which patients are spared unwanted heroic measures in the event of a cardiac or cardiopulmonary arrest (Margolis et al., 1995). I suspect that many of the readers of this text assume that a patient's DNR "doesn't count" or is "not valid" when a patient is having surgery. This is because many of the anesthesia processes commonly used affect the respiratory and circulatory systems, requiring respiratory and circulatory support—the very interventions that a DNR exists to prevent. Although there is increasing awareness that DNR orders can cause problems of interpretation in the OR, and that patients have rights to make their own decisions about what medical care they will or will not accept, much confusion remains about this particular issue. Anesthesia providers often don't understand what their role should be in advising patients, and patients often don't have an appropriate understanding of what is at stake. The ethical principle of autonomy is at the forefront of ethical discussions and policy formation around the topic of honoring DNR orders during surgery and anesthesia. The ethical content of this frequently encountered issue is a conflict between the obligation to honor a patient's self-determination (autonomy) and the obligation to prevent harm (nonmaleficence) to the patient and provide beneficial care. The main questions are, What is beneficial care in each case, and what is its relationship to a patient's autonomous choice of action?

The ethical principle of autonomy, as discussed in more detail in Chapter 1, essentially argues that a patient is free to make his or her own decisions according to his or her own will and without undue influence from others (Beauchamp & Childress, 2001). Two conditions are almost universally agreed upon for autonomy to exist: first, the independence of controlling forces, and second, the capacity to make independent choices (Beauchamp & Childress, 2001).

For individuals to make an autonomous decision, then, they must not be coerced into their decision or experience other factors that limit their liberty to make a decision, such as being imprisoned or serving in the armed forces. Additionally, as noted earlier, a person with a severe mental handicap or a person with physical or cognitive impediments to the adequate processing of information cannot make informed decisions (see Chapter 3) because the person lacks the necessary capacity for intentional action (Beauchamp & Childress, 2001). However, even patients who are deemed incompetent or those who lack the mental capacity to make mature and meaningful decisions about complex healthcare issues do make autonomous decisions for less critical matters, such as what to eat or what to wear (Beauchamp & Childress, 2001) and may be allowed to make decisions that, even if not adequately processed, are unlikely to cause harm.

There are also people who would not be deemed incompetent and who clearly have the necessary intellect to make informed, autonomous decisions, yet who appear to lack an understanding of the implications involved in a proposed course of action, perhaps because of situational stressors affecting their ability to reason or deeply rooted ideas that are not easily amenable to change. Responsibilities to identify and address this problem also fall to the CRNA charged with providing anesthesia for the patient.

DNR and Patient Self-Determination Act

Chapter 3 discusses the Patient Self-Determination Act (PSDA) in more detail; however, it is also pertinent here. The PSDA became law in 1991. It mandated that all hospitals accepting Medicare funding offer written information concerning patients' rights to make decisions concerning their health care and their right to consent to or refuse medical treatment (Smith, 2000). This act did stimulate increased interest as evidenced in the upsurge in medical and nursing literature concerning a patient's right to self-determination with special attention to advance directives and DNR status (Margolis et al., 1995), although many forces still work against the reality of patients' wishes being adequately informed or accounted for (see Chapter 3).

Advance directives are instructions created by an adult patient used to direct physicians, nurses, and healthcare workers as to what kind of care that patient would want to receive in the event he or she cannot make decisions or is unlikely to participate effectively in decision making in the future. DNR orders are a specific type of advance directive used during the event of a cardiopulmonary arrest. This section deals particularly with the advance directive of DNR orders in the patient receiving anesthesia.

DNR and Policy

Professional associations are among those who have addressed this topic and formulated policy statements accordingly. Such policy statements are designed to ensure that proper attention be given to a patient's needs for information so that the patient is facilitated in making choices for care that fit his or her values and beliefs rather than those of providers. Policy statements are meant to provide guidance to professionals about acceptable standards and expectations of behavior.

The American Association of Nurse Anesthetists (AANA) adopted a policy in 1994 that rejects the notion of automatically suspending DNR orders during surgery and instead recommends that the DNR status of the patient be readdressed before proceeding to surgery (American Association of Nurse Anesthetists [AANA], 2004). In essence, AANA recommends that the patient, or proxy, be allowed to discuss the specific aspects of the DNR order. It advises accurate documentation in the patient's chart of all agreed-upon interventions, including those that are to be withheld, and suggests provider–patient discussions during which specific circumstances under which interventions will be performed or withheld are determined. Additionally, the point at which DNR orders are to be reinstated postoperatively is defined (AANA, 2004).

The American Society of Anesthesiologists (ASA) also has a policy for requiring that DNR orders be readdressed instead of automatically suspended when proceeding with surgery (Palmer & Jackson, 2003). The ASA offers three alternatives to the DNR order during the perioperative period: first is full suspension of code status intraoperatively and in the immediate postoperative period; second, only certain procedures may be carried out that are deemed essential to the success of the procedure; and third, the anesthesia provider uses his or her judgment about what constitutes appropriate interventions during the intra- and postoperative period while the patient is receiving anesthesia intraoperatively and in the postoperative period based on an informed understanding of the patient's wishes (American Society of Anesthesiologists, 2001).

The Association of Perioperative Registered Nurses (AORN) has issued a statement similar to the preceding ones, except that the AORN declares in its position statement that each nurse has the right to withdraw from participating in a situation where the reconsideration of DNR orders is in moral conflict with his or her beliefs. However, the responsibility of that nurse to ensure the availability of a replacement is highlighted (Association of Perioperative Registered Nurses, 2004).

DNR and Required Reconsideration

A term used frequently while addressing the matter of DNR orders in the OR is *required reconsideration*, which essentially means that although a DNR order is a legitimate order and must be honored as such, there are circumstances, such as undergoing a surgical procedure and anesthesia, that require a reexamination of this order to ensure that the patient's wishes about and need for care are met and the caregiver is not placed in any ethically compromising positions (Cohen & Cohen, 1991).

Despite the increased attention to, and body of literature addressing DNR during surgery, many institutions still suspend DNR orders during surgery and do not have a policy of required reconsideration or any clear strategies to ensure that a patient's right to self-determination be sustained (Fallat & Deshpande, 2004). Indeed, a dilemma almost inevitably arises in the absence of guidelines because certain types of anesthesia cause autonomic and metabolic suppression, requiring what would in nonanesthesia settings be considered resuscitative efforts. This fact of anesthetic agents is not reconcilable with an order that is created to prevent resuscitative interventions. Many patients do not understand this paradox because they don't have an adequate understanding of what is entailed by using anesthesia. It is counterintuitive to insist that someone not be resuscitated during general anesthesia when general anesthesia causes a state where a patient must be mechanically ventilated to sustain oxygenation (Margolis et al., 1995). This question of compatibility between a DNR request and the nature of traditional anesthetic practice has been a source of confusion and misunderstanding for both the healthcare provider and patients who do not wish to be resuscitated but who require surgery that necessitates general anesthesia.

The principle of autonomy declares that individuals have the right to determine what will be done with their bodies and to base this determination upon their own set of beliefs and values (Fry & Veatch, 2000). Based on this principle, the nurse anesthetist is obligated to recognize the validity of any request to withhold any intervention that is life saving or life sustaining, whether or not the CRNA agrees with a patient's reasoning, given a competent adult patient or a proxy whose decision is informed by the patient's values. This reflects a modern approach to ethical standards and a movement away from a more paternalistic style where a healthcare professional would ultimately influence the decisions made concerning a patient's health care (Roberts, Geppert, Warner, Green Hammond, & Lamberton, 2005).

However, should we consider every decision made by a patient as worthy of honoring simply because it was "self-determined"? How strict should the criteria be for self-determination? After all, advanced practice nurses (APNs) have advanced training, education, and often years of clinical experience. Using sound clinical judgment, they often make difficult clinical decisions that a layperson would lack the knowledge to make. Therefore, we might reasonably ask: Is this current trend away from paternalistic health care warranted? Is a patient's healthcare decision-making ability comparable to that of an advanced healthcare professional? A strict believer in the principle of autonomy might be inclined to support the seemingly autonomous decision of a patient without making a concerted effort to ensure that the patient understands that the course of action agreed upon cannot meet his or her real needs. The nurse anesthetist is therefore obligated to undertake special efforts to ensure that patients and their families understand the purpose of a DNR order and the reason that they have such an order and must seek to clarify any misconceptions surrounding such an order. This will become salient with the discussion in the first case study presented. See Chapter 1 for a more in-depth discussion of autonomy and its requirements.

This first case illustrates a conflict related to honoring patient autonomy. In this case, the obligation of nonmaleficence (preventing or doing no harm) seems to be in conflict with the responsibility to provide a beneficial treatment for the patient.

CASE STUDY 1: DNR IN A HEALTHY PATIENT

Tina is a 37-year-old woman who is employed at an unspecified type of healthcare facility. She arrives at the hospital's operating department to have a gynecological procedure done under laparoscopy. This procedure requires general anesthesia with an endotracheal tube. Tina has a past medical history of asthma as a child with no recurrences in many years, takes only oral contraceptives and multivitamins, and has never received general anesthesia before. Tina has a DNR order signed by her and her primary care MD, which lists the prohibition of cardiopulmonary resuscitation (CPR), vasoactive drugs, and airway intubation in the event of a cardiopulmonary arrest. Tina has no known cardiac abnormalities and has never had a cardiac event. There seems to be no medical data to support her decision to be a DNR patient.

Karen is the nurse anesthetist assigned to do this case and discusses this DNR order with Tina prior to surgery. Tina requests that Karen perform some form of anesthesia other than general anesthesia with an endotracheal tube because she "under no circumstances wants to be intubated." Karen instructs Tina that general anesthesia with an endotracheal tube is the common accepted practice for delivering a safe anesthetic during a laparascopic procedure and there are no realistic options supported by evidence-based practice that favor performing a regional technique safely for this procedure. Tina reluctantly agrees to be intubated for her surgery but insists on not changing any of the conditions of her DNR order and does not want to spend the rest of her life "on a breathing machine." Efforts by Karen to discuss the use of resuscitative drugs and other measures during the unlikely event of a cardiopulmonary arrest are unsuccessful in persuading Tina to amend her DNR status for her surgery. Karen tries to differentiate between vasoactive medications used for treating transient hypotension during anesthesia and the drugs and doses that are used during a cardiac arrest, with the intention of being clear about what Tina's requests are for her anesthesia care. Tina insists that she sees no difference and repeats her demand that her DNR be honored as it is. Karen is unable to resolve this conflict between honoring Tina's request and her (Karen's) duty to provide safe anesthesia. Karen declines to participate in Tina's surgery, and the case is ultimately canceled.

QUESTIONS

1. Is Karen justified in refusing to participate in this case?
2. Is Tina's DNR order valid, and should it be honored here?
3. How could this situation be resolved with both Karen's and Tina's autonomy respected?
4. Do CRNAs, as a group, have a responsibility to educate primary care healthcare practitioners about how to advise their patients related to DNR orders and anesthesia?

DISCUSSION

This case seems to demonstrate a conflict between the autonomy of the patient and the judgment of the practitioner. But, as we shall see, this misplaces the problem. Moreover, even if we recognize that a person such as Tina has the innate right to determine her own actions as discussed in Chapter 1, this right is constrained by the fact that individuals are at times placed in a position where they are dependent on others to carry out their wishes (Veatch & Fry, 2005). This is especially true in healthcare settings. Patients are dependent upon providers to perform procedures that patients cannot carry out themselves. We suppose that Tina needs the surgery. The question arises, Do we know enough to determine whether Tina's request can really be considered autonomous? What criteria would it have to meet? What are Karen's responsibilities here? What alternatives or strategies might resolve the situation?

Tina has a right to expect that her best interests would be the primary concern of the CRNA (see Chapter 4 for a discussion of rights). We are assuming that Tina does need the laparoscopy. However, she may not need it urgently, which would give Karen time to work with her. There is no obvious reason to believe, given Tina's health history, that a general anesthetic would be directly harmful to her. However, there seems to be more to this story than meets the eye. Did Karen violate her obligation to "do good" here by refusing to administer her anesthesia?

Perhaps Karen was focusing primarily on "avoiding harm" by refusing to be an agent of a possible, however unlikely, morbid outcome while being constrained by an order not to intervene in a proper manner. But the direct result was that the surgery was not performed, whether because of a shortage of willing anesthesia personnel or because of a busy OR schedule, and Tina will either have to reconsider her DNR status during surgery or find a willing participant to accept her conditions as they are.

Alternatively, we could devise a plan to discover what Tina's fears are. It is unlikely that these could be addressed in the short window of time available. Tina is not the type of patient who commonly presents with a DNR order. Usually, DNR orders are written for patients with a terminal illness or a health status tenuous enough that heroic measures of any kind could result in irreversible limitations to a patient's quality of living. However, in either case, when a patient makes a decision concerning his own health care, including anesthesia care, that appears to be based on fear, bias, or a deficit in medical knowledge, even though he may otherwise be considered competent, the nurse anesthetist is faced with making a judgment about the validity and efficacy of the decision and what to do next.

Clear communication with the patient and consideration of all the ethical elements of such situations are critical before proceeding with cases like this. As mentioned previously, the CRNA is obligated to clarify misunderstandings surrounding a patient's DNR order before proceeding with surgery. Indeed, the nurse anesthetist is obligated to assist a patient or the patient's family member to understand the DNR order, especially when it appears some knowledge deficit resulting from a communication problem or a lack of knowledge concerning DNR orders is present. At some point, Tina's reasons for making herself a DNR patient despite her good health will have to be addressed or this issue is likely to repeat itself with no foreseeable resolution.

Indeed many patients with a DNR order have morbidities and prognoses that are consistent with such an order. This group of patients is increasingly having surgery for palliative treatment or other procedures that are meant to improve or sustain quality of life, rather than as a curative intervention (Margolis et al., 1995). In fact, it is estimated that 15% of patients with active DNR orders undergo surgical procedures (Margolis et al., 1995). The risk of morbidity during surgery for these patients is obviously much higher than for the collective population, but the benefit of maintaining some quality of life outweighs the risk of death. The next case is an example of honoring a patient's autonomy when the risk of morbidity is high.

CASE STUDY 2: RECONSIDERATION OF A DNR ORDER IN A HIGH-RISK PATIENT

Dan is a 91-year-old man with extensive cardiac, vascular, and pulmonary disease, who comes to the ambulatory surgery center to have a cataract removed from his right eye. Dan has suffered two myocardial infarctions, the last one 18 months ago, which occurred postoperatively after he had an endovascular repair of an abdominal aortic aneurysm (AAA). Presently, Dan is very limited in his activities and spends a majority of his time lying or sitting. He is able to ambulate only for short periods in his house before becoming short of breath. His most recent development is an intraluminal leak in his endovascular repair of his AAA, which has drastically increased the size of his aneurysm, and the risk of rupture has been deemed "imminent" by his vascular surgeon, "if not immediately repaired."

Dan has refused surgery to his AAA and has an advance directive consisting of a DNR order in the event of a cardiac and respiratory arrest that states that he likely would not survive another surgery and that he has "had enough." Dan is consenting to have this cataract surgery because he is having trouble reading the newspaper, and his wife affirms that he "lives to read about his favorite sports teams." Dan was a coach of a high school baseball and football team for more than 40 years, and he states that he lives for sports.

The anesthesia interventions that were discussed with him during his preoperative screening are intravenous (IV) sedation in addition to a nerve block using local anesthetic that will be instilled into the retrobulbar region of his eye. The retrobulbar block is to be performed by the surgeon in this case, but, the anesthesia provider, in many cases, performs it. Dan has refused to amend any of the conditions of his DNR order for surgery.

Ben is a nurse anesthetist who is being supervised by an attending anesthesiologist, Dr. Glen, who recommends that the anesthesia department should not get involved in this case. Ben is worried because he believes that a member of the anesthesia department would be best equipped to provide support in this case. Dr. Glen contacted Dan's vascular surgeon concerning the status of his aortic aneurysm and was told by the vascular surgeon that Dan is a very high-risk patient and that an aortic rupture is very likely without treatment. Dr. Glen suggests that the surgeon performing the cataract surgery administer the local anesthetic without sedation and proceed without the assistance of anesthesia personnel. He argues that there would be limited benefit from anesthesia because the injection of even small doses of sedating medications may be an unnecessary risk compared to their benefit and that this intervention is occasionally done without any anesthesia in other settings.

Ben disagrees with Dr. Glen and believes that allaying any pain or anxiety during the injection of local anesthetic and during surgery would be beneficial to the patient and may even prevent an ischemic cardiac event. Dr. Glen elects not to participate in this case and is replaced by a different anesthesiologist, Dr. Stuart, who agrees with Ben's position. IV sedation is administered during the retrobulbar block, and Dan's requirement for further sedatives during his operation is minimal. Dan is transferred to the recovery room after his procedure breathing room air spontaneously and he was discharged to home 1 hour later.

QUESTIONS

1. Did Ben's decision to give Dan anesthesia comply with the conditions of Dan's DNR order?
2. Under what conditions might Ben's position be justifiable/unjustifiable?
3. Was Dr. Glen justified in his decision to withdraw from the case?
4. What conditions could you change to make Dr. Glen's position justifiable/ unjustifiable?
5. Would Ben be justified in administering CPR or other resuscitative drugs and measures, such as mechanical ventilation, against the expressed will of Dan in the event of an accidental overdose of sedating medication?
6. What is Ben's obligation to ensure that Dan fully understands the consequences of refusing resuscitative treatment during this procedure?

DISCUSSION

Unlike the patient in Case 1, Dan's decision to have a DNR order written is not in question given his health status, his understanding of what would be involved, and his goals. However, Dan's risk is infinitely higher as compared to that of the previous patient. Thus, Ben's decision to participate in Dan's case is difficult because the likelihood of a morbid outcome is so much greater than in the Case 1 example. However, a focus on Dan's considered goals and the professional goals of nurse anesthesia practice (facilitating Dan's good) in this case justifies Ben's participation and could even be considered a moral responsibility of good practice.

All goes well with the case, but even if it had not, Ben's decision is justified because Dan understands the risks and is willing to assume them to get a better quality of life. Ben's clinical judgment is that he could provide a *beneficial* intervention that would lower the risk that an increased cardiac output, caused by the pain and anxiety of the procedure, would cause cardiac ischemia, infarction, or rupture of the aneurysm.

What is Dr. Glen's professional responsibility? Is he acting unethically in refusing to take part? Interestingly, whereas the American Medical Association (2001) code of medical ethics provision VI states, "A physician shall, in the provision of appropriate patient care, except in emergencies, be free to choose whom to serve, with whom to associate, and the environment in which to provide medical care," the American Nurses Association's (ANA) code of ethics for nurses does not support a nurse's freedom to choose whom to serve.

Alternatively, perhaps Dr. Glen's refusal is based on a conscientious objection to causing physical harm. Would this be warranted in Dan's case (see Chapter 3)? Is Dr. Glen unjustified in suggesting that the patient should not receive any additional anesthesia after the surgeon provides the retrobulbar block? Dr. Glen seems to be trying to avoid harm to Dan by withholding an intervention that poses some physical risk, which in this case is IV sedation. However, Dr. Glen may be more concerned with his own well being than the patient's. He might be fearful of being "linked" to a risky procedure—retrobulbar block poses a risk of bradycardia, which may be catastrophic to a patient like Dan if not immediately treated—rather than raising a conscientious objection to it (Morgan, Mikhail, & Murray, 2002).

It could possibly be argued that Ben's decision to proceed is careless or negligent because of the risks involved with IV sedation in an elderly patient. Because Ben is the experienced healthcare professional, his responsibility is to ascertain what Dan knows and what measures he would agree to in the event of a problem. Then, Dan's DNR order would reflect this discussion and the agreed-upon interventions should an episode of bradycardia or even apnea occur (Morgan et al., 2002).

We see here another example of the constraints in honoring a patient's right to make decisions concerning his own health care. Dan likely possesses little or no knowledge of the complications of a retrobulbar block, and he appears not to be interested in hearing them at the time of his surgery. However, it could be argued that poor timing is at fault. These possibilities should be introduced when the patient has time to process the information. Ben has to determine if Dan actually understood the possible complication of this surgery and anesthetic, or if Dan was simply being recalcitrant out of fear that his wishes would not be honored if he agrees to compromise his DNR order or because of the feeling that he couldn't trust the providers. The manner in which patients are addressed or engaged in discussion frequently makes a difference in their willingness or ability to process the information and make an informed decision (Chapter 3).

DNR Orders with Incompetent Patients

Some of our patients do not have the capacity to decide for themselves whether they want DNR orders to be instated and what the specifics of these orders should be (see Chapter 3 for a fuller discussion of decision-making capacity). These patients are deemed to be mentally incompetent, whether from a chronic mental illness, an acute traumatic brain injury, a progressive mental illness, or because the patient is a child with a terminal illness. In these cases, a competent surrogate or parent must represent the patient's interests. Sometimes what these interests are can be ascertained by understanding the previous beliefs, values, and goals of the patient; for other persons there may be no available knowledge.

The related principles used for decision making are similar to those employed when dealing with patients who are able to make competent decisions concerning their health care, but the circumstances may make the decision-making process much more complex. Problems can arise when what the surrogate proposes conflicts with what are perceived to be the patient's likely wishes, and/or a caregiver objects to what the surrogate proposes, or the healthcare team does not feel that what is proposed is likely to benefit the patient and may cause harm. In these situations, it may be necessary to involve authorities who are not immediately involved in the issue and who have the skills to provide a balanced perspective. Institutions often have an ethics resource or committee that can be helpful. But in other cases when a resolution can't be achieved and there is significant risk to the patient's interests, the legal system may be needed to provide advice or mediation.

DNR Orders in Pediatric Patients

The matter of DNR in the pediatric patient deserves further mention here. The PSDA, which requires hospitals to recognize patients' rights to make their own decisions with their health care, does not address the needs of the pediatric patient (Fallat & Deshpande, 2004). A recent survey of anesthesiologists and surgeons revealed that less than half of those surveyed collectively felt that the institutions where they worked had effective policies in place for pediatric patients whose medical status requires a DNR order (Fallat & Deshpande, 2004).

The purpose of a DNR order for a pediatric patient undergoing surgery is to prevent resuscitative measures that would provide no clear benefit to the patient and possibly prolong a poor quality of life (Fallat & Deshpande, 2004). This is under the assumption that a cardiopulmonary arrest is the direct result of a terminal illness. However, as mentioned earlier, like the surgery itself, the anesthesia process may place an additional strain on the pediatric patient, and an arrest can be precipitated in the course of anesthesia induction. Some anesthesia providers view DNR orders in a pediatric patient as a breach of the obligation of nonmaleficence (doing no harm) because it prevents intervention in the event death occurs. Others, however, take it to be harmful to prolong a child's poor quality of life by attempting to prolong it with heroic measures (Fallat & Deshpande, 2004). The basis for either perspective needs to be justified in terms of what definitions of suffering and harms are being used by the parties, and who should be the ultimate decision maker.

It is easy to see here that the sensitivity inherent in dealing with the pediatric population and their families necessitates special attention to such issues. In these situations, the DNR status, as it relates to the pediatric patient having surgery, would be better addressed at the time of its activation rather than readdressed or "reconsidered" at the time of surgery. This would allow more time for the family to discuss with providers what constitutes resuscitative efforts during anesthesia and surgery and to consider what treatments, if any, can reasonably be withheld during the perioperative period. This would also allow family the time to access other sources of advice or information so that they can be comfortable with their decision.

As with adults, the importance of discussing in detail the goals of the family and the patient as they relate to the patient's illness and surgery cannot be overstated. However, it may be more useful with pediatric patients to have a more procedure-directed focus to avoid any ambiguity (Fallat & Deshpande, 2004). The parent or surrogate of the pediatric patient should be provided with a detailed list of interventions that are commonly utilized during anesthesia and those that are utilized during a cardiopulmonary arrest. Perhaps a good strategy is to offer booklets for parents and guardians that show some of the more common or likely anesthesia protocols. The purpose is to show the crossover of interventions between what can be considered common medical and airway techniques to achieve stable hemodynamics during anesthesia and those that are used under more emergent circumstances. Such interventions could include endotracheal intubation or reintubation, tracheostomy, vasoactive medications, chest compressions, IV fluid therapy, blood transfusions, IV colloid therapy, and electrical countershock (Waisel, Jackson, & Fine, 2003). The parent and child should also be assured that in the event of a full suspension of DNR orders during surgery, such orders may be reinstated in the event of a full cardiopulmonary arrest or when it becomes clear that resuscitative efforts would be ineffective at producing any benefit to the child (Fallat & Deshpande, 2004).

THE JEHOVAH'S WITNESS PATIENT

Doctrine on Blood Transfusions

Members of the Jehovah's Witness religion pose a particular challenge to the nurse anesthetist because of their belief concerning the receiving of blood products. These are forbidden under any circumstances, including in cases of emergency. Jehovah's Witnesses are in many cases willing to accept death as a result of blood loss or hypovolemia rather than receive blood products (McNeil, 1997). This becomes an important concern for anesthesia providers because they are almost always responsible for transfusing any required blood during and after surgery, and 50% of the nation's blood supply is given by anesthesia providers (Doyle, 2005).

Jehovah's Witness is a Christian religion whose doctrine prohibits consumption, storage, and the transfusion of blood (Doyle, 2002).The patient's right to refuse medical treatment and the obligation of healthcare professionals to honor such refusal from competent adults has been upheld by court decisions in Canada and the United States (Doyle, 2005). Nevertheless, this gives rise to a potentially troubling issue for anesthesia providers.

The idea that a healthy individual could accept and risk death that is avoidable by a common, low-risk intervention because of religious beliefs seems to run counter to the belief that we, as health professionals, have an obligation to prevent harm and provide beneficial care to the individual. The right of a Jehovah's Witness to refuse blood transfusions under any circumstances is justifiable under the precepts of the principle of autonomy, which (given the person meets the voluntariness criteria) declares that competent individuals must be free to decide for themselves what actions they may take or actions they would receive concerning their health (Beauchamp & Childress, 2001).

Informed Consent with the Jehovah's Witness Patient

The ethical dilemmas involved with the Jehovah's Witness patient's refusal of blood products are similar to those encountered during the management of the patient with DNR orders where a patient's autonomy may seem to conflict with the caregiver's obligation to uphold the principles of beneficence and nonmaleficence. In each case, we are obligated to accept certain decisions that we view as being of questionable benefit to the patient. But, what if the patient's decision is based on inaccurate or false information? For example, what would your obligation to the patient be if the patient refused all narcotics before, during, and after surgery because she believes such substances would make her mentally ill? Controlling the patient's hemodynamic response to pain during surgery and pain management after surgery would hardly be possible if such a refusal was honored so strictly. The practitioner would have to assess the nature of such a request and determine if educating the patient on the use of intraoperative narcotics and their effects on body systems would influence the patient's decision. If it is determined that the patient is not able to process this information adequately (see Chapter 3 for informed consent criteria), then we cannot say that the patient's decision is autonomous—the decision does not meet the criteria for voluntariness. We see here that autonomy is constrained by the informed consent process because informed consent is a necessary condition of autonomy, and an individual can make autonomous decisions only if that person has necessary decision-making capacity (Van Norman, 1999).

The next case introduces a problem of informed consent in anesthesia practice and a person's capacity to receive and understand relevant information. Although, as previously mentioned, a Jehovah's Witness is prohibited from receiving a transfusion of allogenic blood, which includes red cells, white cells, platelets, or plasma, or a transfusion of autologous blood, there are medical procedures involving blood that are not prohibited by their doctrine, such as cell saver or blood salvage, albumin, erythropoetin, epidural blood patch, and fractionated clotting factors (Doyle, 2002). Followers of this faith believe that the Bible clearly states in passages from Acts 15:29, Genesis 9:4, and Leviticus 17:12–14 that eating of the blood, which is interpreted as accepting of blood, is strictly forbidden by God (Doyle, 2002). Transfusion of blood products for medical purposes is also interpreted as accepting of blood and is therefore forbidden under the Jehovah's Witness doctrine.

Because of the complexity related to what constitutes a "blood transfusion" and is not permissible versus what in the way of blood products is permissible for Jehovah's Witnesses to accept, there is a great potential for anxiety and confusion about Jehovah's Witness patients who are trying to make the right decision. When the nurse anesthetist is not sure that a patient is adequately informed about what is allowed by the religion, aspects of the surgery, or potential side effects, and these side effects are both likely and serious, this further complicates decision making. With this in mind, it is highly beneficial for nurse anesthetists to familiarize themselves with policies of allowable and prohibited blood transfusion therapies and ways to minimize blood loss, and to consider providing written information for Jehovah's Witnesses as they are evaluated during the prescreening process. Here are two additional Internet Web addresses that may be of assistance to the anesthesia provider caring for the Jehovah's Witness patient:

Associated Jehovah's Witnesses for Reform on Blood: http://www.ajwrb.org

Tower to Truth Ministries: http://www.towertotruth.net/Articles/blood_transfusions.htm

CASE STUDY 3: A JEHOVAH'S WITNESS PATIENT'S QUESTIONABLE CAPACITY TO CONSENT

Mick is a 29-year-old Jehovah's Witness who is brought to the surgical department for repair of bilateral multiple leg fractures following a motor vehicle collision. Mick is accompanied by two police officers, and he is handcuffed to his hospital bedrail. Mick is under arrest for fleeing a crime scene, drug possession, theft, and other related infractions, and his car accident is a result of fleeing from police. Mick will require general anesthesia for surgery, and the potential for blood loss is serious given the extent of his injuries.

Tom is a nurse anesthetist who is assigned to Mick's case and begins to discuss the anesthesia plan with Mick. Mick does not acknowledge Tom directly and avoids eye contact while Tom is discussing his plan of care. Tom is aware of this and asks Mick to repeat what Tom has said. Mick grows angry and insists he is listening. When Tom addresses the topic of blood transfusion, Mick interrupts him by stating, "I don't want blood." Tom then asks that if there is a chance of Mick dying, would Mick still refuse blood transfusions. Mick says, "Look, I told everyone downstairs [emergency department], I told the doctor, I told the nurses, and now I'm telling you, I don't want blood put into my body, OK!"

Tom then tries to clarify his request by listing some of the medical interventions that many previous Jehovah's Witness patients have accepted, such as blood salvage, albumin, and fractionated clotting factors, only to be met with more angry resistance from Mick. Mick then says, "I don't even know why I talk to you people when you're just going to do what you damn well please anyhow." Tom tries to continue the conversation, but Mick does not acknowledge Tom and stays silent. Tom is unsure why Mick is so resistant to communicate with him, and Tom is unaware of any recent circumstance or encounter with healthcare personnel that would cause such resistance.

The OR is ready, and Tom starts to bring Mick in for surgery when Mick asks for pain medication because he is in "incredible pain." Tom assures Mick that his pain relief will be a priority during and after surgery because of his extensive injuries. Surgery begins, and as predicted, Mick steadily begins to lose blood. Tom informs the surgeon that a prolonged case would place the patient at risk for hypoxemia resulting from poor oxygen-carrying capacity because of blood loss, and the surgeon tells him to "do whatever you can."

QUESTIONS

1. Did Mick demonstrate a capacity to understand the implications of a decision not to receive blood?
2. How is Mick's capacity to make decisions compromised? How is his autonomy limited here?
3. Is Tom obligated to honor Mick's request to refuse blood products? Why or why not?
4. Should Tom decide for himself, or with his care team, to give those interventions that are not explicitly prohibited by Jehovah's Witness doctrine? What options exist?
5. What is Tom's obligation related to determining Mick's capacity to understand the consequences of his decision? Could this provider–patient interaction have gone better?
6. If it is determined that Mick lacks decision-making capacity, what should happen?

DISCUSSION

Mick's ability to make an informed decision is in question. Mick is in "incredible pain." Mick is angry. He expresses distrust in his care team, and he is under arrest with physical restraint (handcuffs). There is a question of him being under the influence of drugs or alcohol. At best, he has shown poor judgment (running away from police and so forth). There is no evidence to suggest that Mick is incompetent in the legal sense or of marginal intelligence, although either of these factors could preclude a person from being able to make an informed decision, but he does have situational influences that may hinder him from choosing wisely.

Mick's pain may cause him to be too distracted and irritated to answer any more of the same questions, especially questions that force him to decide on something that may be personally troubling to him, such as defending his religious beliefs.

Mick's history may also cause him to be suspicious of authority figures, and he views Tom as a threat to his sense of personal control. Mick is under arrest and is being physically restrained. Even though the police officers are not directly applying any influence to Mick's choices concerning blood transfusion, their presence and his being handcuffed to the bed may be seen as enough coercive force to render limitations on his sense of autonomy.

Given these situational factors, could Tom reasonably consider Mick as being without sufficient capacity to make an informed decision? The difficulty here is the finding that Mick is, in fact, competent, because it refers to the legal definition of being able to perform certain functions, and based on his competency and the legal mandate to honor his right to self-determination, normally then Tom should not interfere with Mick's decisions (Van Norman, 1999). However, we are not sure that Mick has the decision-making capacity for this task—in fact, we have reason to believe he does not because he cannot, or is unwilling to, process the needed information. In Chapter 3, the case of the homeless person describes a failure of decision-making capacity for a given task. The determination of a patient's capacity to make healthcare decisions involves the patient's demonstration of receiving and understanding relevant information, as well as being able to verbalize consequences and alternatives (Van Norman, 1999). As we see in the case presented, the patient only communicates his wish not to be transfused, but he does not engage in further discussion of possible alternative interventions, and neither does he demonstrate his ability to fully understand the consequences of his decision. Even if Mick were to declare that he would rather die than be transfused, could his current circumstances be an overriding influence in this decision rather than a conscious decision based on religious principle?

This case brings forth two problems associated with informed consent for surgery and anesthesia. The first is the difficulty in determining if a patient truly understands the information given or has the capacity to fully understand relevant information, and the second is determining the responsibility of the practitioner in providing information that might counter the patient's decision (Van Norman, 1999). Canada and many states in the United States have adopted the "reasonable patient" standard as their legal model for requirement of informed consent, which focuses on "considering what a patient would need to know in order to understand the decision at hand" (Doyle, 2005). In the case given, the nurse anesthetist attempts to clarify the patient's request and explore alternatives but is unsuccessful because of the patient's apparent unwillingness to participate.

An additional problem seen with informed consent includes the disclosing of too much information, such as all the possible complications of tracheal intubation and general anesthesia, that confuses the patient or burdens the patient with unlikely scenarios that may cause undue anxiety. It's possible that a patient can take in only so much information during the preoperative period, and that even appropriate, mild anxiety makes it difficult for a patient to fully understand all that is told to him before surgery (Van Norman, 1999). Thus, it is very important to try to engage with the patient to determine what his or her particular needs are (see Chapter 3).

Last, it needs to be mentioned here that although a Jehovah's Witness's right to refuse blood products even at the risk of death is defended by legal precedence, there is no clear legal precedence established for the same condition to be applied to children. In fact, a U.S. Supreme Court ruling in 1944 declared that adults do not have the right to make their children martyrs for religious purposes until the child is of the age of full and legal discretion to make the choice for him- or herself (*Prince v. Commonwealth of Massachusetts*, 321 US 158). However, 39 states in the United States have laws that protect parents from prosecution when their children die as a result of not receiving medical care (Hickey & Lyckholm, 2004). The nurse anesthetist needs to be aware that in the event of a conflict between a parent or surrogate and healthcare professionals over the decision for a child to receive blood transfusion therapy, child protection services may need to be consulted. The rights of a parent or surrogate to make decisions for the child that appear medically harmful or negligent are severely limited by law (McNeil, 1997).

TRUTH TELLING IN THE OPERATING ROOM: THE OBLIGATION OF VERACITY

Telling the truth is a basic moral precept that is part of our social and moral development and is instilled in us during childhood. Few would question the wisdom of providing such moral lessons to a child, but as adults we understand that what constitutes the truth is not always so easily discerned and that some truths can be unpleasant and perhaps even harmful. The truth can be very emotionally upsetting for someone.

Nevertheless, as APNs, we have an obligation to be honest in our discourse with patients, and our information should be accurate and presented in a way that can be easily understood and cogent for the particularities of a patient's situation. This is a responsibility of good practice: that patients are assisted to make informed decisions concerning their medical care (Hebert, Hoffmaster, Glass, & Singer, 1997). However, in doing this, we must understand that situations will arise where our honesty will be distressing and possibly harmful to our patients and their families (Fry & Veatch, 2000). These situations require sensitivity and clinical judgment about the boundaries of information given and the manner in which it is given. The next section deals with the implications of truth telling during the perioperative setting.

Veracity in Therapeutic Relationships

Three concepts have been advanced to support the obligation of veracity in a therapeutic relationship. These are respect for individuals, fidelity and the keeping of promises, and productive therapeutic interaction and cooperation with patients (Beauchamp & Childress, 2001).

The healthcare practitioner respects the individual by providing the most accurate information for the patient to make an informed decision and then protects the individual's control over that information (Beauchamp & Childress, 2001). The keeping of promises is seen as a central element in the fiduciary relationship between a healthcare professional and a patient (see Chapter 2 for further discussion of fiduciary relationships). The fiduciary relationship is based on trust, and professionals have an implicit contract with patients to be honest in their discourse and faithful to their commitments (Beauchamp & Childress, 2001). Productive therapeutic relationships involve the execution of an effective therapeutic treatment plan based on the exchange with the patient of honest and accurate information and the instilling of confidence in the patient that such a care plan will be carried out (Beauchamp & Childress, 2001).

Veracity in Anesthesia Care

The therapeutic relationship between a nurse anesthetist and a patient is unique in that there is a critically short period of time in which to establish trust. This is often just a few minutes prior to surgery. It is still common practice that a surgical patient is evaluated by an anesthesia provider or a nurse practitioner for an anesthesia department to provide primary screening of a patient and address any problems or questions that a patient may have. However, this is certainly not the case for emergent or urgent cases, where there is no prescreening— even the prescreening process is not always successful at addressing all of the patient's concerns. It is also likely that the anesthesia provider involved with the prescreening process is not the one caring for the patient on the day of surgery. Because engendering trust is vital to establishing the sort of relationship in which there is an appropriate exchange of information, the patient must be assured that any and all information that she receives is honest, accurate, and directed toward meeting her needs. Any information that is perceived as deceptive or not an honest attempt to communicate the facts undermines trust. When trust is undermined, communication becomes even more difficult.

Yet patients often ask providers difficult questions. Some questions may be very direct and stark; for example, a moribund patient asks the CRNA if he could die from receiving general anesthesia and surgery, or a parent asks for assurances that nothing bad will happen to his or her child as a result of the surgery and/or anesthesia. The fact is, there are inherent risks with the performance of surgery and the delivery of anesthesia in almost all cases. However, when patients are very sick, having cardiac or respiratory conditions for example, surgery and anesthesia become even more risky to the extent that survival of surgery may be statistically problematic for some patients. Likewise, parents can't realistically be guaranteed a perfect outcome when their child undergoes anesthesia, especially if their child has serious health issues. The CRNA needs to find a way to remain honest but supportive. Information should be provided in a way that fits the situation and is both truthful and compassionate (Krizek, 2000). Families may need to know that their ongoing concerns can be addressed.

Some might argue that there may be some benefit to telling a moribund patient that he will be fine. For one thing, if he does die, he will not have had to face the loss of hope and experience unnecessary suffering, and if he dies during surgery, the anesthetist would not be confronted by the patient with his or her dishonesty. However, this patient may not be looking for a direct answer to this question; rather, he or she may be seeking to establish some relationship by perhaps testing the veracity of the anesthetist. Thus, loss of confidence in the anesthetist's honesty may undermine the patient's confidence in the anesthetist's integrity and competence for the anesthesia delivery process, causing the patient more suffering.

The parents of the child in the preceding example may actually be looking for some reassuring words to allay their anxiety and fear, and they may receive immediate benefit from hearing the words "everything is going to be just fine." But for the same reasons as mentioned earlier, if they are not convinced of the anesthetist's integrity, their confidence may be undermined. It is certainly understandable for the parents to desire reassurance, and for the nurse anesthetist to want to offer this promise to them, but the risks attendant upon violating veracity and supplying inaccurate information or by making a promise that can't be kept are too high. One possible long-term effect is that perceptions of deception or lack of truthfulness affect the ability of patients and their families to trust healthcare professionals with whom they interact in the future. Inability to trust, then, interferes with communication and ultimately necessary information exchanges. Patients will not be forthcoming, and providers will not be able to get the information they need to plan care that is appropriate for the patient.

Anesthesia, especially general anesthesia, provides a kind of veil of secrecy and silence over the patient. The patient is made unaware of the surroundings, and there is no familial or other representation for the patient normally allowed in the OR. The patient places implicit trust in the nurse anesthetist, as well as the other care team members, to see that his or her bodily integrity is maintained during surgery. Although the patient may be wide awake during surgery, such as during spinal or epidural anesthesia, the patient is immobile and his or her vision is obstructed by surgical drapes, and reliance on trust is no less acute.

Maintaining truthfulness and integrity is also important in nondirect patient care situations. The nurse anesthetist, along with allied caregivers, has professional responsibilities for truthfulness even when a particular patient is not the focus of care. CRNAs may feel pressured by colleagues, or others, to alter the details of a case, or hide certain information to protect certain parties from blame. For example, a CRNA may be asked to alter a chart to protect a fellow anesthetist who is at risk of losing his or her job as a result of having made a serious medication error or the CRNA may be asked not to report a surgeon's apparent intoxication during surgery for fear that his or her reputation would be irreparably harmed.

Even if there is no patient harm or adverse outcome in either case, not addressing such issues sensitively but honestly breaches our fiduciary obligations to this and future patients. Examples were given earlier about how "good-natured dishonesty" may be intended to relieve anxiety or lessen the fear of unknown consequences; however, it rarely has this desired effect, and even when it does, it calls into question the integrity of the professional as this pertains to other matters. Some have noted that worries about honesty related to revealing human error have arisen in the context of a medical and media culture of blame. An Institute of Medicine (IOM, 1999) report notes that systemic changes in the way healthcare institutions deal with the issue of error are warranted. A discussion of this is beyond the scope of this chapter, but it is an important topic for CRNAs to understand and involve themselves in. It would be a good class project for enterprising CRNA students.

Further questions, though, are, How honest should we be and, How can we be honest, yet not take away a person's hope? Some would still support the idea that sometimes telling the truth can be viewed as harmful and that direct honesty can be seen as the adversary of hope (Warm & Weissman, 2000). The next case study deals with the conflict between being honest and being compassionate when bad news must be given.

CASE STUDY 4: AN OBSTETRIC PATIENT WANTS THE TRUTH, BUT HER HUSBAND THINKS THE TRUTH WOULD BE HARMFUL TO HER

Kim is a 29-year-old healthy woman who is delivering her second child by elective cesarean section. Kim's husband, Bill, is with her in the OR and everything is thus far going well. Gail, her nurse anesthetist, who initiated epidural anesthesia for Kim's C-section, is monitoring Kim's anesthesia. Dr. Ross is Kim's obstetrician and announces the delivery of a baby girl, shows the baby to Kim and Bill, and then allows the nurses in the room to take the baby for initial neonatal care.

There seems to be some increased activity in the OR near Kim's baby, and Kim asks Bill to see what's going on. Without looking in the baby's direction, Bill assures his wife that everything is just fine and the baby is doing perfectly well. Bill gestures to Gail to keep silent by placing his finger up to his lips. A pediatrician is called immediately to the room, and the nurses take Bill aside and tell him that the baby is being transferred to the neonatal intensive care unit (NICU) immediately. Bill tells his wife that the baby is going for her first bath and some normal tests and that he is required to go with her, and there's nothing to worry about. Bill whispers to Gail that she absolutely must not tell Kim about the baby's condition right now because "she will have a nervous breakdown." Bill insists that this information is "not going to help my wife right now." Gail is aware that Kim's recent medical history involves psychiatric consultation for panic disorder and anxiety attacks.

One of the surgical residents working with Dr. Ross informs Gail quietly that there is a lot of bleeding right now and she should have blood in the room available to transfuse if Kim's bleeding continues at this rate. Kim asks Gail about her baby and what all the activity was really about. Gail responds, "I'm not sure. I need to focus on you right now, Kim." Kim becomes agitated and says, "I don't care about me. I want someone to tell me what is happening to my baby. Where's my husband?" Gail tries to calm Kim and manage her hemodynamic status during a larger-than-normal blood loss after a C-section. Kim's anxiety has caused her heart rate to increase and she appears distressed.

QUESTIONS

1. What should Gail tell Kim about the condition of her baby? What is her responsibility?
2. What would be the benefit of deceiving Kim? What would be the harm?
3. Does Gail have a responsibility to carry out the wishes of Bill? On what basis?
4. How does Kim's present condition of excessive bleeding relate to her need for information about her child's condition?
5. Under what circumstances, if any, might we honor Bill's request to withhold information from Kim?

DISCUSSION

Bill's request that Gail should deceive his wife seems rather unfair, even if he is correct that bad news would distress his wife. Gail's fiduciary obligation is to Kim, not Bill. But what if Gail were simply to say that the baby is "probably" fine and that babies are often taken to a specialty unit for evaluation immediately after a cesarean section? This is not really lying, and the truth is Gail is not really sure of the nature of the baby's problem because her primary responsibility is to Kim as her patient. Reassuring Kim might be enough to relieve some of Kim's distress and likely ensure a better outcome if it permits stabilization of Kim's vital signs.

Shopping for a right answer to a problem doesn't meet the requirement of veracity (complete honesty is a very tall order—what would complete honesty be?). However, clinical judgment demands that in this situation the benefits and risks of different courses of action (information exchanges are considered courses of action) are weighed to the extent that this is possible in an emergent situation. There is no universal agreement about the extent to which lying to or withholding information from a patient for the patient's perceived benefit is permissible (Beauchamp & Childress, 2001). It depends to a certain extent on knowledge of the patient and an understanding of her likely reactions, which isn't always possible when there is limited time for interaction.

The short-term benefit of calming Kim so that her present condition is not made worse is not unimportant. There is more at stake in this case than some temporary emotional strain. However, Kim's baby could possibly require extended neonatal care, and Kim is going to have to be emotionally prepared for that in the upcoming days. If her trust in medical professionals is damaged because of a well-intentioned breach of veracity, she could possibly find it very difficult to engage in meaningful, open therapeutic relationships with members of her baby's care team. On the other hand, if her situation is critical, it may be that we should do what is necessary to save her life and worry about accuracy or truth telling later.

When patients belong to a vulnerable population, for example, children, some elderly, and those with terminal illnesses, other factors may complicate the issue of veracity or truth telling. Children are developmentally immature and thus are not expected to have the emotional and mental ability to receive and interpret information in the same way as an adult. Perhaps patients in their final stages of life, as well as some terminally ill patients, might be looking for an approach to information exchange that focuses on their immediate quality of life and want an emphasis on hopeful short-term goals rather than unrealistic long-term goals that, within the realities of their present condition, offer no comfort (Warm & Weissman, 2000).

CONSCIENTIOUS OBJECTION IN ANESTHETIC PRACTICE

The Conflict Between Fetal- versus Maternal-Focused Ethical Obligations

The following are examples of another ethical quandary not uncommon in nurse anesthesia practice, that of determining the relative importance of a mother and fetus when a pregnant patient requires anesthesia for surgery or a procedure. During a preanesthesia interview, a nurse anesthetist is presented with a woman who is 28 weeks pregnant, has an acute appendicitis, and requires emergency surgery. The patient is very excited about being pregnant and refers to her fetus by name. She is, however, very anxious about the effects that anesthesia and surgery will have on her baby. How many patients are presented here? On a separate interview, a nurse anesthetist is presented with a 39-year-old female who is approximately 15 weeks pregnant and comes to the hospital to discuss her anesthesia for her elective termination of her pregnancy. How many patients are presented here?

Notice that these questions do not ask how many *lives* or how many *human entities* are presented, but specifically ask for the *number of patients*. This distinction is important in terms of the healthcare practitioner's ethical focus concerning maternal and fetal health issues.

We commonly think of maternal–fetal dilemmas or considerations as arising in reproductive health centers, obstetric health facilities, or in other centers where pregnancy termination procedures may be common. The nurse anesthetist who objects to elective pregnancy termination on moral or religious grounds may choose not to be employed there, with the intention of avoiding moral and ethical conflicts in practice. The AANA's code of ethics allows for a CRNA to withdraw from a case because of conflicting personal convictions, provided there is no harm to the patient or a breach of duty (AANA, 2005). In other settings, this problem has been referred to as refusal of care based on conscience (see Chapter 3).

Such practices and policies, initiated to avoid ethical conflict in anesthesia practice, have the potential to create access problems for patients who require certain services. An example of this currently in this country is when some pharmacists refuse to dispense the "morning after pill" on grounds that it constitutes providing an abortion, to which they object (Stein, 2006). Certain populations, because of economic or logistic reasons, do not have expansive access to many healthcare services and are subject to the decisions made by a relatively small number of healthcare providers, thus creating a conflict between a patient's right to equal healthcare treatment and the right of conscience for healthcare workers (Stein, 2006).

This is a justice problem. Professional autonomy to provide or withhold services based on personal moral principles conflicts with the ethical principle of justice. Justice, as discussed in Chapter 4, is about the equal distribution of health care and the balancing of inequalities in such a way that the least well off are not unduly disadvantaged. Patients in urban areas who have insurance coverage can usually access a large or several large medical centers that offer a variety of services and have good resources in terms of provider coverage, which makes it easier for a conscientious objector to find another provider who will agree to care for the patient. Whereas at smaller or rural health centers fewer practitioners are available and there may be no one to replace the provider who objects to providing a particular kind of care or service. This is an area of political concern for all providers in striving to provide good care but is of special concern to CRNAs, who provide most of the anesthesia care in many rural and semirural area institutions.

Besides the access problems, giving anesthesia in obstetrics cases can present the provider with a conflict of ethical obligations. In cases of conflict, the provider must answer the question of whose interests (maternal or fetal) prevail and under which circumstances. During a normal vaginal or cesarean delivery, the nurse anesthetist is mindful of the health and well-being of both the mother and the fetus when planning and managing an anesthetic care plan. When things go wrong, choices may need to be made, including where priorities rightly lie.

In other cases, where a woman's pregnancy has nearly come to term but complications have made a term delivery extremely dangerous to the woman's health and no realistic chance of fetal survival exists, pregnancy termination may be agreed upon by all involved as imperative for maternal survival. However, even in these seemingly less controversial cases, problems can arise. For example, what is the responsibility of the anesthesia provider if the woman asks that her fetus be given some sort of anesthetic to ensure that the fetus does not suffer during the termination? The patient has established a tremendous maternal bond with what she thinks of as her unborn "child" and is very protective of its interests. Anesthesia for a late-term fetus is theoretically possible, and there is some evidence that a fetus can sense painful stimuli after 11 weeks gestation. But no one can really say if a fetus feels pain, and fetal anesthesia in utero for abortive surgeries is not a common practice (White, 2001).

However, it seems that a humane approach to this problem is to further explore methods to reduce suffering in utero, even if there is only a probability that a fetus can experience pain. Is the anesthesia provider obligated to honor such a request based on the mother's autonomy to make her own decisions concerning her health care? Is this fetus now a patient, then, because the woman desires it to be cared for?

These matters of maternal- and fetal-focused ethical obligations are a key characteristic of obstetric ethics and are relevant for nurse anesthesia practice, although a truly in-depth consideration of this topic is beyond the scope of this chapter. "The concept of the fetus as a patient is shaped by the interaction of the principles of beneficence and respect for autonomy for the pregnant woman and the fetus" (Chervenak, McCullough, & Birnbach, 2003, p. 1483).

The anesthesia care plan for the parturient patient is created to benefit the patient according to accepted standards of anesthesia practice. The pregnant patient's autonomy is recognized based on her belief system and her values concerning her current health status. If we recognize that the woman has the right to autonomy based on her beliefs and values, then how do we recognize a fetus' autonomy if it is not believed to possess beliefs and values because of an insufficiently developed nervous system (Chervenak et al., 2003)? The lack of justification for fetal autonomy does not diminish the practitioner's obligation of beneficence toward the fetus, but this can only exist, in this example, if the fetus is considered our patient (Chervenak et al., 2003). Two criteria are proposed for determining whether a human being should be considered a patient: first, a human being must be presented for the purpose of medical treatment, and second, there must be a realistic set of goals that can be achieved via an effective medical treatment plan (Chervenak et al., 2003).

Some may argue on religious grounds that a fetus is a human being at the point of conception and should be considered so despite its inability to think and reason or make autonomous decisions. Others may claim that to be awarded independent personhood, the fetus must be considered viable, meaning that it is scientifically possible for the child to exist independent of its maternal host. Viability, however, is a function of the technological setting in which it exists, and this may vary from region to region (Chervenak et al., 2003).

It comes as no surprise that "there has been no agreement on a single authoritative account of the independent moral status of the fetus" for all the diverse opinions involved with this issue (Chervenak et al., 2003, p. 1483). Here we appear to be left with the only real justification of the fetus, especially the previable fetus, because a patient comes from the pregnant woman's autonomous decision to convey that status upon it.

Despite the problems of disparities with healthcare access, it is prudent for healthcare institutions to create policies that allow for caregivers to decline to participate in a practice because of caregivers' moral or religious beliefs because even the most carefully considered policy cannot eliminate moral disagreement in such a diverse cultural and religious milieu (Winkler, 2005). However, as discussed in Chapter 3, the decision to decline to participate should not be made lightly and the provider should both be convinced that a real threat to his or her personal integrity exists and seek an alternative provider for the patient. The case study for this section involves the principles of maternal beneficence and autonomy, fetal beneficence, and professional autonomy as these relate to a pregnant patient having minor surgery.

CASE STUDY 5: ELECTIVE SURGERY WITH A PREGNANT PATIENT

Sheila is a 29-year-old pregnant woman who presents to the ambulatory surgery center for repair of a large scar on her chest that occurred as a result of a poorly healed skin laceration. Tony is her nurse anesthetist and discusses with Sheila the implications of general anesthesia, which will be necessary for this surgery. Terry, Sheila's preop nurse, calls Tony aside and informs him that her pregnancy test is positive. Tony asks Sheila if she is aware of the results of this test and asks her if she doesn't mind repeating the test. Sheila admits to knowing that she is pregnant.

Sheila says, "Yes, I know. I really didn't think you guys would care. I'm having an abortion next week. I tried to get it done sooner, but next week is the earliest I could get and I have waited more than a month to get this surgery done."

Tony tells Sheila that he needs to mention this to the surgeon. Tony alerts the surgeon, who then chooses to cancel the procedure for today. The surgeon says, "Let's not mess around with this elective procedure. She can come back after her abortion." The surgeon informs Sheila that surgery can't take place today because it violates the center's policy to perform elective surgery on a pregnant patient. Eileen is another nurse anesthetist who hears about this case and informs Tony that she would be willing to stand in for him if he objects to it. Tony informs Eileen that he would choose to withdraw on moral grounds, but the case was canceled anyway.

QUESTIONS

1. Was this procedure rightfully canceled? Which conditions would you change to make this case justifiable/unjustifiable to cancel?
2. Whose interests were met with the decision to cancel?
3. Was this a case of a patient's autonomy losing out to professional autonomy?
4. Did Tony have an obligation to Sheila's fetus?
5. If the surgeon wanted to go ahead with the case, would Tony be justified in declining for moral reasons?
6. What do you think the real reason may have been for the surgeon to cancel this case?

DISCUSSION

Most anesthetic agents and sedatives that are used routinely in anesthetic practice are potentially harmful to the fetus, according to animal studies, although evidence of harm to the fetus has not been clearly established (Glosten, 2000). Aside from chemical agents, physiologic changes that can result from general or regional anesthesia such as tachycardia, bradycardia, hypotension, and hypovolemia may have deleterious effects on the fetus by impeding fetal oxygen delivery and fetal blood flow. For these reasons, pregnant women are advised to delay surgery until a time when they are no longer pregnant (Glosten, 2000).

One may view this approach of delaying elective surgery for pregnant women as a focus on fetal ethical obligations by avoiding the potential harmful effects of anesthesia to the fetus. Conversely, one may also argue that this approach supports the maternal responsibility to prevent harm to the fetus as part of the woman's body, and therefore this obligation serves maternal beneficence. It just also seems sensible to delay something that is not urgent until there is less risk to both the mother and her fetus.

In this case study, the woman is deciding to terminate her pregnancy at a later date, so there is no explicit or implicit maternally directed obligation to prevent harm to the fetus from anesthesia. Should her surgery take place, the obligation to provide optimal anesthesia care with concern for fetal health is purely practitioner-directed, meaning that the patient gives the directive to care for her fetus during her anesthesia.

If the woman were to reconsider her decision to have an abortion and carried this baby to term, the anesthetist and surgeon could conceivably face legal action if the baby suffered resulting defects, but they would also be morally accountable for the use of good clinical judgment. The legal risk for the anesthetist and the surgeon lies in the fact that each would have been complicit in placing the woman's fetus at risk for a nonemergent case. There are provisions whereby a woman is directed to sign a waiver limiting the liability of the anesthesia provider for alleged harm to a fetus if a woman refuses to take a pregnancy test and her pregnancy status in unknown (Bierstein, 2006). Here we see that her pregnancy status is known and is confirmed by the patient, so freedom from either moral or legal liability in this case can't reasonably be claimed or expected.

Tony's decision to withdraw from this case could have been based on potential medical legal implications, but he states that he has moral objections to giving this patient anesthesia, which probably indicates his concern about potential harm to the fetus from anesthesia. Tony's decision to withdraw could possibly have had some emotional impact on the patient, but no serious harm would have been inflicted. His withdrawal would have been much more difficult to justify, if not a breach of duty, if surgery was medically urgent and if finding someone to replace him was not possible.

The consideration of legal risk for the healthcare institution and the healthcare professionals over the patient's need for this particular elective surgery was likely the true impetus for canceling the surgery in this case study. Simply put, the patient's autonomy was not permitted to place the hospital and staff in any undue medical legal jeopardy. If one could imagine, hypothetically, that there was no risk at all that the patient would reconsider her abortion, and there was no justification for canceling her surgery because of legal risk, then the healthcare providers involved would have to decide, based on their own interpretations of their ethical obligations, whether to proceed with this case or not.

ANESTHESIA AND DISTRIBUTIVE JUSTICE

The Principle of Justice

Item 1.1 in the AANA's code of ethics states, "The CRNA renders quality anesthesia care regardless of the patient's race, religion, age, sex, nationality, disability, social or economic status" (AANA, 2005). The nurse anesthetist is obligated to provide optimal anesthesia care to everyone with medical indications for that care without regard to their ability to pay. But anesthesia care is expensive, and if anesthesia care is delivered without regard to incoming revenues or cost, then at some point, isn't it likely that these services will no longer be possible? Politics is about who gets what and at what expense. This is a reality of societal living (see Chapter 4). Human beings rely on one another to trade goods and services fairly to exist in a functioning society. When goods become scarce or difficult to obtain, there needs to be a system of deciding on what is fair distribution and which criteria should exist for society to determine who merits these goods.

Justice is a concept that is interpreted as fair, equitable, and appropriate treatment in light of what is owed to a person (Beauchamp & Childress, 2001). Justice is upheld, then, if someone receives something due to him or her for providing a service or producing a product or just by virtue of being human. (See Chapter 4 for a fuller discussion of justice and human rights.) Conversely, it is considered an injustice if something owed to a person is withheld or denied. This logical system of thought works adequately in many cases in our legal system but is more difficult to apply to our healthcare system, where defining the entitled recipient and the criteria by which that recipient receives what is due is much more complex.

Distributive Justice

The concept of distributive justice refers to fair, equitable, and appropriate distribution based on criteria that a society agrees to be ethical and justifiable (Beauchamp & Childress, 2001). For distributive justice to have any relevance, society is required to devise a morally correct system for allocating its resources (Waisel & Truog, 1997). This is obviously very difficult because we see individuals with vastly differing abilities to obtain certain resources based on economics and opportunity. Some individuals in our society cannot, or can barely, afford to pay a given co-payment for a certain health service, and some could purchase entire medical centers.

Armstrong and Whitlock (1998) propose six criteria for the justifiable distribution of resources: need, equity, contribution, ability to pay, effort, and merit. Although some have criticized these sorts of criteria as not addressing the needs of the oppressed, the criteria provide a useful framework for exploring the issue of resource allocation. *Need* refers to medical need and not individually determined need, such as with elective surgery, and *equity* refers to distributing the same level of service to all who are in need (Armstrong & Whitlock, 1998). *Contribution* means that an individual's entitlement is based on that person's potential contribution to society in the future, which makes sense for allocating larger resources for children, but the aged have made contributions for many years and could argue that they are entitled to the portion of the healthcare services they receive

(Maddox, 1998). Allocation based on the *ability to pay* for necessary healthcare resources contradicts the code of ethics for nurse anesthetists, as well as the generally accepted principle of charitable giving of needed health services to vulnerable populations (Armstrong & Whitlock, 1998). *Effort* refers to the commitment by the patient to follow through with medical treatment and comply with prescribed healthcare routines, and *merit* implies that evidence from research or current practice supports the use of particular resources because of the benefit they supply compared to their cost (Maddox, 1998).

Examining these criteria reveals just how complicated a process it is for a society to determine where and how resources are allocated, even with a logical system of determining need. Healthcare professionals bear an enormous burden to decide when medical care for patients becomes ineffective or futile and when the allocation of expensive resources would be better directed to patients with more promising prognoses (Boudreaux, 2001). It is essential for nurse anesthetists to take a global view of this dilemma because we are so often called upon to perform anesthesia care for the purpose of improving or sustaining a patient's quality of life during that person's final stages of life, even when such services may at times prove to have little benefit (Boudreaux, 2001).

Distributive Justice in Anesthesia Practice

To examine the matter of distributive justice in everyday anesthesia practice, let's explore this matter on the level of the individual practitioner. Ethical conflicts arise when the nurse anesthetist is compelled to deliver an anesthetic regimen based on questionable criteria, such as the personal connections of the patient or a patient's perceived economic, political, or celebrity status.

A prominent anesthesia provider was asked at a clinical conference what his recommended anesthetic regime would be to prevent postoperative nausea and vomiting (PONV). His reply was, "That depends on if the patient was the wife of the CEO of this hospital because then I would use . . . and for everyone else I would use . . ." Even though such a comment was said for mild comedic effect, it reveals a truth of the delivery of health care: as long as there is a human element in the decision-making process determining the delivery of treatment, there is potential for inequitable care.

For example, a nurse anesthetist withholds anti-nausea medication from a patient who requires surgery after being involved in a fatal automobile collision. In the collision, a young mother was killed. The patient who is at fault for the accident was driving while under the influence of alcohol and illicit drugs. The punitive action of the anesthetist is based on personal feelings and has no basis in any justifiable criteria of resource allocation or any regard for standards of safe and effective anesthesia practice for preventing PONV. This is an unethical action that is not based on sound clinical judgment.

This next case study involves just such a problem of a nurse anesthetist making decisions of resource allocation based on her personal views of equitable delivery of anesthesia care.

CASE STUDY 6: EQUALITY IN ANESTHESIA CARE

Glen is a nurse anesthetist who is employed by a large anesthesia company, which has multiple affiliations with hospitals and surgical centers throughout the city and surrounding suburban area. Today, he is working at a new ambulatory surgical facility that is housed in the city hospital, which caters to an economic and culturally diverse patient population. Most of the patients who use this surgical facility live in an urban setting.

Karl is the director of anesthesia services at this facility, and he has mandated that all patients who require a general anesthetic be given rapid-acting, IV anesthetic agents only, rather than more volatile agents, because of their ability to be metabolized quickly and their effect on preventing postoperative nausea. These pharmaceutical agents are far more expensive than traditional volatile agents are when comparing total patient hours under anesthesia. Karl has declared, however, that this mandate is necessary to ensure rapid turnover times of the rooms and to prompt patient discharge, ensuring an efficient surgical facility.

Glen refuses to comply with this mandate and continues to deliver traditional volatile anesthetics in conjunction with IV agents as adjuncts as his regimen for general anesthesia for all his patients. Glen argues that he is unable to provide such expensive anesthesia for his patients in the suburban facilities where he works. In those settings, fast-acting agents are simply not available because of cost-containment measures in place at these other facilities. Glen believes that it is unfair to allocate expensive anesthesia resources for patients who, as he says, can't pay for them or rely on "free-care" benefits to receive surgical services.

However, the patients who use the facilities in suburban locations have health insurance or pay out of pocket for their services. Glen also points out that his use of less-expensive agents is in no way a breach of duty to his patients because the use of traditional techniques and agents is in full compliance with current standards of safe and effective anesthesia practice. Karl argues that the purpose of the use of fast-acting anesthetic agents is necessary for the functioning of this facility and that Glen has no business making decisions based on cost of materials because such information is not salient to his practice. Glen states that all individual anesthesia providers have a responsibility to conserve medical resources and the liberal use of expensive resources is irresponsible.

QUESTIONS

1. Does Glen have any right to make such decisions?
2. Who is affected by his decision and what is the potential outcome?
3. Change the conditions to make Glen's position justifiable or unjustifiable.
4. Is Karl's mandate irresponsible in terms of use of resources?
5. Is Karl placing an unnecessary restriction on Glen's practice?
6. How can this dilemma be resolved?

DISCUSSION

Glen is in direct conflict with the AANA's code of ethics in that he is making a decision to formulate a care plan based on a patient's economic status. The AANA's code of ethics uses the term *economic status*, and we can probably imply that this means the ability to pay for anesthesia services. However, anesthesia services for certain elective cosmetic surgery cases are often legitimately denied to someone who cannot pay for such services. Denying such services is not considered discrimination because the surgery and thus the anesthesia are not medically necessary. But because Glen is not directly receiving payment from his patients for his services, he is not in a position to deny services to anyone because of an inability to pay, and, consequently, this is not a relevant argument for Glen's actions.

What's interesting here is the fact that Glen is not denying his patients adequate or safe anesthesia services. There is nothing incorrect or negligent about his choices of anesthetics to provide his patients. He has an opportunity to use more expensive agents because of a possibly different revenue or payment structure that allows this facility to operate without such tight restrictions on the use of anesthesia drugs, but he chooses not to use them. Karl justifies the use of these more expensive products for the benefit of a more efficient facility, which may, over time, prove more cost-effective than the cheaper, traditional anesthesia agents.

Glen probably makes a salient point by suggesting that all anesthesia providers have a responsibility to be conscious of cost containment and resource expenditure. It seems irresponsible to use resources as if it's on "someone else's dime." The balance possibly lies in the establishment of guidelines and policies set up for the purpose of guiding safe and effective anesthesia practice with regard to what is necessary and what may be excessive. For instance, there are medications that are routinely used by anesthesia providers and recovery room nurses to prevent, or treat, PONV. Because no healthcare provider wants his or her patient to be sick, we are compelled to give the most effective treatment when it's available. The truth is, there are many less-expensive agents that are shown to be effective in reducing the risk and incidence of PONV in some patients. Patients also have varying risk factors based on gender, age, smoking status, and history of PONV and may benefit from certain selections of medications.

Practice guidelines should take such information into account to develop effective and cost-efficient protocols for the use of anti-emetic therapy during the perioperative period. So, clinical judgment based at least in part on knowledge of the patient would be important in tailoring care. To avoid inconsistent and fragmented approaches to resource allocation, institutions, such as hospitals or other health-care delivery facilities, are obligated to develop standards and maintain them over time to ensure that a more consistent approach is used (Winkler, 2005). Coinciding with APNs' obligation to resolve injustices they encounter in their practice is the obligation to intervene in a broader sense, such as with political action, to explore and change practices that may be unjust or result in poor care. Refer to Chapter 3 for a more extensive discussion of the argument for APN responsibility to engage in political activity.

Glen's position, while seemingly based in logical reasoning, is not well thought out, and it is worrisome for patients and the person's colleagues because it is based in a prejudicial judgment that misses the deeper question of why some people have fewer resources than others do. Professional autonomy should not be used to ration care based on a patient's merit. Although in the case example, no harm is necessarily caused, neither is it necessarily true that Glen's patients suffer, but it is troubling that Glen is using his professional power in this potentially discriminatory manner. The ability of the individual patient with ample economic resources to dictate the very details of his or her anesthesia care is not commonly recognized in our healthcare system, but it is likely a topic for future consideration in nursing and medical ethics.

PROTECTING PATIENTS FROM INCOMPETENT AND IMPAIRED HEALTHCARE PROVIDERS

Fidelity and Advocacy in Anesthesia Practice

This section deals with the principle of fidelity as it pertains to the role of the nurse anesthetist as the protector or guardian of the patient's interests during anesthesia. *Fidelity* refers to being faithful to the obligation of keeping promises made in a therapeutic relationship (Beauchamp & Childress, 2001). Keeping promises is universally recognized as vital to the nurse–patient relationship, but it has a special meaning in nurse anesthesia practice because of the increase in vulnerability created by the process of using anesthesia.

Patient advocacy and protection of the patient's welfare (see Chapter 4 for a more extensive discussion) are hallmarks of nursing practice. The ANA's code of ethics calls for nurses to promote the health, safety, and rights of the patient in their care, and it directs nurses' roles as protectors of their patients (American Nurses Association, 2001). In most clinical settings, the nurse is often the first to establish a meaningful, therapeutic relationship with a patient and spends the most time in personal contact with the patient to develop that relationship. This relationship is based on the trust that the nurse will follow through with the patient's concerns and will keep that patient's interest as a foremost concern. This includes providing mediation between the patient and other healthcare team members or family members if necessary (Schroeter, 2002). Nurses take great pride in this role and have shown remarkable leadership in promoting patient rights and developing mechanisms for ensuring quality care. The dedication to protecting a patient's rights is born from a nurse's obligation to respect a patient's autonomy, prevent harm to the patient, and promote actions for the patient's benefit, the trust formed in a therapeutic relationship, and the commitment to be faithful in that relationship (Schroeter, 2000).

This role of being the guardian of a patient's well-being is vital in the clinical setting, whether inpatient or outpatient, because of the number of different healthcare providers that a patient is likely to come into contact with. In a large medical center, a patient is likely to have a number of different healthcare providers, all participating in different aspects of the patient's care. The nurse takes on the role of patient protector and primary advocate and attempts to ensure continuity of care for the patient. Responsibilities to guard against inconsistent treatment planning, harm from incompetent professionals, and the supervision of less experienced healthcare providers are all assumed by the ethical nurse. Recent surveys of registered nurses from New England and Maryland reveal that ethical conflicts around the protection of patient rights and patient advocacy rank highest among ethical conflicts encountered in their nursing practice (Fry & Damrosch, 1994; Grace, Fry, & Schultz, 2003). A recent survey of U.S. Army CRNAs had similar findings. The most frequently encountered ethical issues involved protecting patient rights and human dignity, and the personal conflict of working with incompetent or impaired colleagues (Jenkins, 2006).

The nurse anesthetist carries this role of patient guardian, protector, and advocate into the practice of anesthesia care. Advocacy has special meaning for the nurse anesthetist because it is during this period of anesthesia or deep sedation that the patient is most vulnerable (Schroeter, 2000). The need for patient advocacy during anesthesia stems from the fact that there can be no expression of autonomy or decision making by a patient who is anesthetized (Schroeter, 2002). The nurse anesthetist seeks to control the variables that can affect the patient under general anesthesia both at the time and after the anesthesia itself has dissipated. Patients are subject to noxious and possibly painful stimuli, immobility, and awkward positioning, and the physiologic depressive effects of most anesthetic agents. This commitment of being a patient guardian also applies to protecting patients from untoward actions of other health professionals in contact with the patient. This obligation is to patient advocacy, and protection from incompetent or impaired healthcare providers is central to the role and mission of the nurse anesthetist and is clearly stated in the AANA's code of ethics (AANA, 2005).

Incompetent and Impaired Healthcare Providers

An incompetent healthcare provider is one who engages in conduct that is unlikely to be beneficial to the patient and may even cause harm. The incompetent behavior may include such things as being inadequately skilled in an intervention, undertaking actions that are at odds with an agreed-upon treatment plan, or not engaging in an appropriate or thorough evaluation of the patient. The behavior may range from being ill advised and unlikely to provide benefit to overtly dangerous behavior that may jeopardize the health of the patient. Examples include the photographing or recording in any way of a patient's surgery without the patient's written consent to do so, or a blatant disregard of the patient's personal integrity and assault of the patient. Although all healthcare providers should be held responsible to uphold this commitment to the patient, it is the anesthesia provider who renders the patient defenseless and vulnerable by the inherent nature of CRNA practice. Thus, the obligation to defend the patient during this period of vulnerability is so much more acute.

The CRNA is also a member of a collaborative care team and, in many states, practices under the supervision of a physician anesthesiologist, which necessitates an ability to work harmoniously with others for a common purpose. CRNAs may feel pressured by a supervising physician or surgeon to comply with actions that are contrary to the patient's interests. Production pressure in the OR can unwittingly drive healthcare providers to place the economic and expediency concerns of the OR over concerns of the patient. For instance, a supervising anesthesiologist may convince a patient not to have a nerve block to alleviate knee pain after total joint surgery because it may slow down the turnover in the recovery room, or a surgeon may demand unsafe positioning of the patient for surgery, risking peripheral nerve damage, because diligence with proper patient positioning prolongs the time in the OR.

The abuse of narcotics and sedative drugs for personal use by anesthesia providers is a serious ongoing problem contemporarily. The incidence of healthcare providers who are substance abusers is overrepresented by anesthesia providers compared to other healthcare professionals, and this number is likely an underrepresentation because of the taboo of admitting to such a problem (Booth et al., 2002). The access to rapid-acting, highly potent narcotics enables an addicted practitioner to divert these agents for his or her personal addiction; for the most part this is accomplished in complete secrecy. One of the most frightening facts concerning addicted anesthesia providers is the insidiousness of this disease where the first signs of a problem may be overdose or death of the user (Quinlan, 1995). Because the addicted practitioner's narcotic use can go undetected, the practitioner may well be providing anesthesia care while impaired, placing the patient in enormous risk (Hudson, 1998). For fellow anesthesia providers to have knowledge of such actions and do nothing is unconscionable and violates the AANA code of ethics (2005), which states that a nurse anesthetist is obligated to protect patients from impaired healthcare providers. The code of ethics for nurse anesthetists calls for us to consider that the obligation to protect a patient's dignity and remain faithful to the delivery of safe anesthesia care pertains to all patients, not just the patients we are assigned to. However, confronting or reporting colleagues is no easy task.

Reporting of an impaired anesthesia provider may mean placing someone very close to you in great personal turmoil and will likely lead to disciplinary action by state boards of nursing (Quinlan, 1995). The revelation of such an addiction results in an immediate life change, and the person will need counseling and rehabilitation (Quinlan, 1995). Fortunately, there is a system of anonymous reporting for persons who are suspected to be practicing while impaired. The objectives of reporting are twofold: protection of the patient and assistance in resolving the anesthetist's problem. Successful treatment exists—the intention then is to assist the practitioner in returning to work, rather than permanently ending his or her career (Hudson, 1998). The term *impaired* here is not limited to the use of narcotics or alcohol (ETOH), but can refer to emotional stress, sleep deprivation, illness, depression, and injury (Schroeter, 2002).

These personal conflicts involved with attempting to protect and advocate for patients under the nurse anesthetist's care are cited in the survey of U.S. Army CRNAs referenced earlier in this section. The survey respondents noted that encountering such issues sometimes led to decreases in morale, less job satisfaction, and "burnout" (Jenkins, 2006). The responsibility of having to expose a colleague's secret addiction, and in the process upset fellow care team members or supervisors, is daunting. Keeping a focus on promoting the patient's good and protecting him or her from harm provides the motivation for appropriate action but can still take an emotional toll. This is a reality of assuming a professional responsibility for the care of another human and entails placing the needs of this individual above one's own and others'. The next two cases involve the personal conflict and the implications of protecting patients from impaired colleagues.

CASE STUDY 7: THE NURSE ANESTHETIST WITH A NARCOTIC ADDICTION

Joe and Steve are CRNAs working at the same hospital and have been close friends for more than 2 years. Steve was on a lunch break in the staff lounge when Joe entered, looking to put something into his duffle bag. Joe and Steve began to converse when Steve tried to help Joe by putting the bag back on the shelf behind him. Several small vials of fentanyl, a short-acting narcotic used in anesthesia, fell out of the bag onto the floor. Joe acted surprised to see them there and began making excuses of how he must have mistakenly placed them there, and then changed his story to say they must have fallen out of his scrub shirt pocket into his bag accidentally. Steve was not entirely shocked, however, because he had suspected Joe of diverting narcotics for some time. Joe has been acting strangely at work, taking frequent bathroom breaks, arriving to work extra early, and staying late on several occasions, despite many responsibilities at home.

Steve tells Joe that he needs to get some help and that he has a serious problem. Joe denies any illicit narcotic use initially, but as the conversation continues, he admits to Steve that he "took a few fentanyls for headaches he's been having and that's all." Steve persists gently that Joe should look into treatment for substance abuse. Joe pleads with Steve not to tell anyone about this and that he will never do this again. Steve asks Joe if he used any today, and Joe vehemently denies doing so. Joe claims that he has to return to do a case and repeats his plea to Steve to keep his confidence about this matter out of concern over losing his job and possibly his family.

QUESTIONS

1. What should Steve do next? What would you do next if you were Steve?
2. What ethical principles are involved here?
3. What is Joe obligated to do?

CASE STUDY 8: THE IMPAIRED SURGEON

The nurse in charge of the operating suite has been paging Dr. Pete for almost 3 hours with no return page. His patient, who is a 45-year-old woman who requires an appendectomy, has been waiting patiently this entire time but is beginning to get rather anxious and annoyed at the delay. Dr. Pete finally arrives, and he appears disheveled and sleep deprived. He appears confused when told his patient has been waiting for some time and that he has not returned any of his pages this evening. There does not appear to be any evidence of ETOH use, and Dr. Pete is known not to drink. He asks for the patient's chart and has difficulty reading it because he can't find his reading glasses. His conversation with his patient is very brief; in fact, he asks her what she is here to have done and tells her that he'll be ready shortly, and then leaves to change into surgical scrubs.

Denise is a nurse anesthetist, who is the CRNA manager of this facility, and has also been waiting for the surgeon to do this case. The patient calls Denise over to her and asks if the surgeon always looks so ill prepared for surgery. The patient then asks if Denise thinks that Dr. Pete is "fit to do surgery this evening." Denise is tempted to make light of this issue and give excuses for his appearance, but she knows that Dr. Pete has recently experienced some turmoil in his life that seems now to be intruding into his professional life. Dr. Pete is going through a very difficult divorce and has significant financial troubles that he has made known to Denise on a previous occasion.

The charge nurse confronts Denise and asks her to intervene with Dr. Pete to convince him to let someone else do this case. The charge nurse tells Denise that her nursing staff is concerned that Dr. Pete is not fit to perform surgery tonight because he seems too distracted and depressed. Dr. Pete is then seen coming from the changing room and without formally acknowledging Denise or the charge nurse simply says "Let's go" and makes his way toward the OR.

QUESTIONS

1. What should Denise do? What would you do?
2. What is the evidence that Dr. Pete is in any way impaired?
3. What ethical principles are involved here?
4. What are the implications for Denise if she insists that Dr. Pete not do this surgery?

DISCUSSION

Steve and Denise have been placed in very unenviable positions here, for which there are no easy choices. Steve's obligation is to see that Joe does not work today, or any future day, until he can resolve the matter about his bringing narcotics out of the OR, whereas Denise is obligated to protect her patient from Dr. Pete, who shows evidence of serious mental distraction resulting from an inability to successfully cope with life situations. Joe's impairment is more familiar and conceivable, because most everyone would agree that providing care to a patient under the influence of narcotics is unconscionable, but Dr. Pete's impairment appears to be from sleep deprivation and situational depression. Because many people in the healthcare profession sacrifice sleep to be available for their patients, some sleep deprivation is expected, and doesn't everyone get depressed sometimes?

If Denise and Steve act on behalf of their obligation to protect patients, whether in their care or not, their colleagues, Joe and Dr. Pete, are going to suffer some level of embarrassment, humiliation, and potential loss of finances. Joe may lose his current position, and there is no guarantee that his family will understand or sympathize with his situation. Dr. Pete will possibly face examination by hospital authorities because of his recent behavior and may be required to seek treatment and not perform surgery for a period of time. If Steve ignores this problem, a patient will be put at risk for errant practice if Joe is presently under the influence of narcotics. Ignoring this problem may also enable Joe to continue with his addiction and give him the false impression that his behavior is protected by the confidence of his colleague. If Denise does not act, she will have to give false assurance to her patient that Dr. Pete is "just fine" and she will also be negligent in keeping the promise of safely protecting her patient from harm, which is inherent in an effective nurse–patient relationship.

Nurse anesthetists need to take a global view of this commitment of protecting patients from unsafe practitioners and harmful situations while receiving anesthesia care. Patients should expect that nurse anesthetists of good moral conscience would intervene for their benefit even if there were no established nurse–patient relationship, as in the case of Steve with a patient that Joe may encounter. A patient has the right to believe that all nurse anesthetists will keep their promise of safeguarding patient interests during surgery.

SUMMARY

Ethical decision-making skills will continue to be a vital part of the skill set of the nurse anesthetist. The healthcare environment is becoming ever more complex as advances in biomedical and electronic technology allow many persons to live longer but with chronic diseases that require ongoing care. Difficult decision-making scenarios concerning all aspects of anesthesia care including the allocation of scarce, and increasingly expensive, medical resources will continue to challenge our practice. Our ability to meet these challenges will require an understanding of the nature and origins of our professional responsibilities, adequate preparation in ethical decision making, and ongoing knowledge development. Remaining up-to-date on current literature, sharing ethical conflicts and experiences with colleagues, participation in ethics-related policy creation and conflict resolution, and personal reflection and values clarification are all necessary ingredients for good practice.

REFERENCES

American Association of Nurse Anesthetists. (2004). *Considerations for development of an anesthesia department policy on do-not-resuscitate orders.* Park Ridge, IL: Author.

American Association of Nurse Anesthetists. (2005). *Code of ethics for the certified registered nurse anesthetist.* Park Ridge, IL: Author.

American Medical Association. (2001). *Principles of medical ethics.* Retrieved August 18, 2007, from http://www.ama-assn.org/ama/pub/category/2512.html.

American Nurses Association. (2001). *Code of ethics for nurses with interpretive statements.* Washington, DC: Author.

American Society of Anesthesiologists. (2001). *Ethical guidelines for the anesthesia care of patients with do-not-resuscitate orders.* Park Ridge, IL: Author.

Armstrong, C. R., & Whitlock, R. (1998). The cost of care: Two troublesome cases in health care ethics. *Physician Executive, 24*(6), 32–35.

Association of Perioperative Registered Nurses. (2004). *AORN position statement: Perioperative care of patients with do-not-resuscitate orders.* Denver, CO: Author.

Beauchamp, T. L., & Childress, J. F. (2001). *Principles of biomedical ethics* (5th ed.). New York: Oxford University Press.

Bierstein, K. (2006). *Preoperative pregnancy testing: Mandatory or elective?* Retrieved June 17, 2007, from http://www.asahq.org.

Booth, J. V., Grossman, D., Moore, J., Lineberger, C., Reynolds, J. D., Reves, J. G., et al. (2002). Substance abuse among physicians: A survey of academic anesthesiology programs. *Anesthesia and Analgesia, 95,* 1024–1030.

Boudreaux, A. (2001). *Ethics in anesthesia practice. 52nd annual refresher course lectures: Clinical updates and basic science reviews.* Retrieved June 10, 2007, from http://www.asahq.org.

Chervenak, F. A., McCullough, L. B., & Birnbach, D. J. (2003). Ethics: An essential dimension of clinical obstetric anesthesia. *Anesthesia and Analgesia, 96,* 1480–1485.

Cohen, C. B., & Cohen, P. J. (1991). Do not resuscitate orders in the operating room. *New England Journal of Medicine, 325,* 1879–1882.

Doyle, D. J. (2002). *American Journal of Therapeutics. Symposium, 9*(5), 417–424.

Doyle, D. J. (2005). *Autonomy, informed consent and the death of the therapeutic privilege: Lessons learned from the Jehovah's Witnesses.* Retrieved July 9, 2007, from http://www.en.wikibooks.org.

Fallat, M. E., & Deshpande, J. K. (2004). Do not resuscitate orders for pediatric patients who require anesthesia and surgery. *Pediatrics, 114,* 1686–1692.

Fry, S. T., & Damrosch, S. (1994). Ethics and human rights issues in nursing practice: A survey of Maryland nurses. *The Maryland Nurse, 13*(7), 11–12.

Fry, S. T., & Veatch, R. M. (2000). *Case studies in nursing ethics* (2nd ed.). Sudbury, MA: Jones and Bartlett.

Glosten, B. (2000). Anesthesia for obstetrics. In *Anesthesia* (5th ed., Vol. 2, pp. 2024–2068). New York: Churchill Livingstone.

Grace, P. J., Fry, S. T., & Schultz, G. S. (2003). Ethics and human rights issues experienced by psychiatric-mental health and substance abuse nurses. *Journal of the American Psychiatric Nurses Association, 9*(1), 17–23.

Hebert, P., Hoffmaster, B., Glass, K. C., & Singer, P. A. (1997). Bioethics for clinicians: Truth telling. *Canadian Medical Association Journal, 156*(2), 225–228.

Hickey, K., & Lyckholm, L. (2004). Child welfare vs. parental autonomy: Medical ethics, the law, and faith-based healing. *Theoretical Medicine and Bioethics, 25*(4), 265–276.

Hudson, S. (1998). Reentry using naltrexone: One anesthesia department's experience. *AANA Journal, 66,* 360–364.

Institute of Medicine. (1999). *To err is human: Building a safer health system.* Washington, DC: National Academy Press.

Jenkins, C. L. (2006). Identifying ethical issues of the department of the army civilian and army nurse corps certified registered nurse anesthetists. *Military Medicine, 171*(8), 762–769.

Jonsen, A. R., Siegler, M., & Winslade, W. J. (1998). *Clinical ethics* (4th ed.). New York: McGraw-Hill Health Professions Divisions.

Krizek, T. J. (2000). Surgical error: Ethical issues of adverse events. *Archives of Surgery, 135*(11), 1359–1366.

Maddox, P. J. (1998). *Administrative ethics and the allocation of scarce resources.* Retrieved June 17, 2007, from http://www.nursingworld.org.

Margolis, J. O., McGrath, M. J., & Kussin, P. S., et al. (1995). Do not resuscitate (DNR) orders during surgery: Ethical foundations for institutional policies in the United States. *Anesthesia and Analgesia, 80,* 806–809.

McNeil, S. B. (1997). Johnny's story: Transfusing a Jehovah's Witness. *Pediatric Nursing, 23*(3), 287–288.

Morgan, G. E., Mikhail, M. S., & Murray, M. J. (2002). *Clinical anesthesiology*. New York: McGraw-Hill.

Palmer, S. K., & Jackson, S. (2003). *Ethics: Hot issues in legally sensitive times*. Retrieved June 17, 2007, from http://www.asahq.org.

Patient Self-Determination Act. (1992, March 6). Public Law 101–508 Federal Register 57, page 341.

Prince v. Commonwealth of Massachusetts. 321 US 158.

Quinlan, D. (1995). The impaired anesthesia provider: The manager's role. *AANA Journal, 63*(6), 485–491.

Roberts, L. W., Geppert, C. M. A., Warner, T. D., Green Hammond, K. A., & Lamberton, L. P. (2005). Bioethics principles, informed consent, and ethical care for special populations: Curricular needs expressed by men and women physicians-in-training. *Psychosomatics, 46*, 440–450.

Schroeter, K. (2000). Advocacy in perioperative nursing practice. *AORN Journal, 71*(6), 1207–1218.

Schroeter, K. (2002). Ethics in perioperative practice—patient advocacy. *AORN Journal, 75*(5), 11–19.

Smith, K. A. (2000). Do-not-resuscitate orders in the operating room: Required reconsideration. *Military Medicine, 165*(7), 524–527.

Standards guidelines and statements. (2004). Retrieved June 17, 2007, from http://www.asahq.org.

Stein, R. (2006). *A medical crisis of conscience: Faith drives some to refuse patient's medication or care*. Retrieved July 17, 2007, from http://www.washingtonpost.com.

Van Norman, G. A. (1999). *Competence and informed consent: When is a patient not able to make decisions about medical therapy?* Retrieved July 9, 2007, from http://www.asahq.org.

Veatch, R. M., & Fry, S. T. (2005). *Case studies in nursing ethics*. Sudbury, MA: Jones and Bartlett Publishers.

Waisel, D. A., Jackson, S. B., & Fine, P. C. (2003). Should do-not-resuscitate orders be suspended for surgical cases? Ethics, economics and outcome. *Current Opinion in Anesthesiology, 16*(2), 209–213.

Waisel, D. B., & Truog, R. D. (1997). An introduction to ethics. *Anesthesiology, 87*, 411–417.

Warm, E., & Weissman, D. (2000). *Fast fact and concept #21: Hope and truth telling*. Retrieved July 16, 2007, from http://www.eperc.mcw.edu.

White, R. F. (2001). *Are we overlooking fetal pain and suffering during abortion?* Retrieved June 17, 2007, from http://www.asahq.org.

Winkler, E. C. (2005). The ethics of policy writing: How should hospitals deal with moral disagreement about controversial medical practices? *Journal of Medical Ethics, 31*, 559–566.

SUGGESTED READING

Calvin, S. (2000). *Ethical challenges of maternal-fetal practice in the United States*. Retrieved June 17, 2007, from http://www.med.umn.edu.

Keffer, M. J., & Keffer, M. J. (1992). Do not resuscitate in the operating room. *Anesthesia and Analgesia, 74*, 901–905.

Luck, S., & Hedrick, J. (2004). The alarming trend of substance abuse in anesthesia providers. *Journal of PeriAnesthesia Nursing, 19*(5), 308–311.

Ryan, M. A. (2004). Beyond a Western bioethics. *Theological Studies, 65*, 158–177.

CHAPTER 13

Nursing Ethics and Advanced Practice: Gerontology and End-of-Life Issues

Pamela J. Grace

To my way of thinking it is not the years in your life but the life
in your years that count in the long run
Adlai Stevenson (From "If I were twenty-one", Coronet, December 1955)

Death is beautiful when seen to be a law, and not an accident. It is as common as life.
Henry David Thoreau, 1842, letter to Ralph Waldo Emerson

INTRODUCTION

This chapter addresses two separate but often related areas of advanced practice nursing. The first area involves care of patients who are aging. That is, many advanced practice nurses (APNs) oversee the health care of patients who are in the latter part of their life spans. The aging of America has been well documented and has implications for nursing in that nursing practice in many settings consists of caring primarily for or for a good proportion of patients 65 years of age and older (Scholder, Kagan, & Schumann, 2004). Even when this is not the case, the population served may be caretakers of their aging relatives or be balancing childrearing with caretaking and thus seek the advice of APNs.

Persons as they age may need health promotion or health maintenance assistance, help in coping with a chronic illness, palliation for symptoms that alter the quality of their lives, or support in caregiving for significant others. Although the specialty practice of gerontology focuses on health problems related specifically to the impact of processes of aging, all APNs who work with older persons have responsibilities to understand both how the process of aging affects people and the ethical issues in trying to ensure a good for this population. Barriers to quality of life for aging persons may be economical, functional, and/or existential. The scope of responsibility for APNs in attending to this population's needs is correspondingly broad. It may require conceptualizing actions at the level of the individual or at broader institutional and social levels, as discussed in earlier chapters.

The second area this chapter addresses is that of ethical care for patients who are suffering from intractable symptoms of various sorts or who are facing the imminent end of their lives. Sometimes a patient must make a difficult decision about what care or treatment to accept, given that almost all treatments have aspects of uncertainty; sometimes a family member or guardian must make a decision on the person's behalf.

The need for palliative and/or end-of-life (EOL) care, of course, is not limited to the aging population. Thus, this chapter's discussion of ethical issues in end-of-life decision making is not limited to those practicing in gerontological settings. An important role of the APN (whether a clinical nurse specialist [CNS], nurse practitioner [NP], or other) involves preventive ethics. Preventive ethics, as discussed earlier in the book, is concerned with anticipating problems with the intention of preventing them from occurring or putting into place mechanisms for addressing them effectively. In all of the adult specialties, a crucially important preventive ethics strategy is to have ongoing discussions with patients about their desires for care should they become unable to make their own decisions temporarily or permanently. Knowing the patient as an individual and having an ongoing relationship with the person are facilitative of preventive ethics.

The preparation of advance directives for care or treatment including making an informed choice about who is a suitable proxy is one strategy of preventive ethics. Preparing an advance directive that can anticipate all eventualities of one's illness or incapacity is impossible. Nevertheless, advance directives, as the term suggests, do provide information for and direction to those who are charged with interpreting what the person would have wanted given the capacity to choose. In addition to written advance directives, it is helpful for patients to have chosen a designated proxy in advance with the expectation that this proxy will faithfully ensure that the person's wishes are respected and honored. However, choosing an appropriate person to interpret one's wishes may be difficult for patients, and the best person is not necessarily a spouse or close relative. In such cases where a person is socially isolated or without close family ties, assistance in identifying an appropriate legal representative or guardian is also important. These and other issues surrounding palliative or end-of life care are discussed in the second part of the chapter.

GERONTOLOGICAL ADVANCED PRACTICE

Definitions and Cautions

By definition, gerontology is the study and care of those who are aging. However, no satisfactory definition can distinguish an aged person from others, and persons vary in the rate at which they experience age-related physical changes. Thus, although knowledge of age-related physical changes and the possible impact of these on the health and/or resilience of an older person is an important part of a gerontological NP's skill set, it is equally important for NPs not to presuppose knowledge of persons' needs based purely on their age. Wide variations exist. For example, Ms. Jameson is a tall, well-built woman who is 75 years old. Her height is 5'9" and she weighs 165 pounds. Recently, she developed atrial fibrillation that resulted in a heart rate of approximately 130 beats per minute. Her primary care provider, believing that as persons age they lose renal function and experience a declining ability to clear medicines, prescribes a dose of digitalis that is half that recommended for adults with such problems. It had no effect upon her heart rate and she began to develop congestive heart failure. Although there are other things wrong with this case, for example, Ms. Jameson should have been referred relatively rapidly to an internist or cardiologist to see if medical or electrical cardioversion could be achieved, the real problem is that Ms. Jameson is not a frail 75-year-old. She still rides her bicycle, walks 2 to 3 miles every day, and has no other significant medical problems. All of this should have been taken into consideration in evaluating her needs and planning care with and for her. That is, the nursing perspective as argued in earlier chapters is to care for persons as whole individuals who are inseparable from their contexts and histories.

Multidisciplinary Approaches

Whereas gerontological APNs apply nursing knowledge and goals to the care of persons as they age, it is also widely recognized that both the promotion of healthy aging and the care of those experiencing an age-related loss of mental or physical function are facilitated by a multidisciplinary approach. Gerontological APNs are among those professionals who have received special education and preparation for the care of such patients and can serve as good resources for other nurses and allied professionals. Additionally, they often practice collaboratively with those in other disciplines when an aging person has a wide spectrum of possible needs. They understand what the appropriate resources are and how to access them. Their expertise also permits an understanding of the special challenges that can arise when trying to ensure good care in the face of barriers. As in other advanced practice settings, anything that gets in the way of assisting a patient in obtaining what clinical judgment (see Chapter 4, Table 4-1 on clinical judgment) determines is needed for well-being or comfort is an ethical issue.

Ethical Issues Related to Aging: Overview

Besides the more common or widely encountered ethical issues associated with healthcare delivery discussed in earlier chapters, such as those related to socioeconomic status, poverty, cultural misunderstandings, and the paternalistic attitudes of healthcare providers, older persons are at special risk for injustices that stem from ageist attitudes and age bias. This is true regardless of whether they are financially secure, sick or well, or have supportive relationships with those who can advocate for them or help them advocate for themselves.

Additionally, although not all older people experience many of the problems associated with the aging process such as physical and cognitive decline and many younger people do experience physical and cognitive problems that interfere with their functioning and/or quality of life, older people are susceptible to these problems in larger numbers. With advancing age, there is an increasing likelihood that people will experience some decline in physical functioning, multiple health problems, and a variety of losses, both physical and psychosocial (Grace, 2004).

Furthermore, losses are likely to be more existentially devastating to the elderly person. That is, the meaning of such losses is enduring and not likely to be lessened by other opportunities that become available. A person may lose his ability to transport himself independently because of sensory changes such as loss of eyesight or diminished reflexes or coordination. He may lose the ability to live alone and miss the companionship of friends and spouses who predecease him. Moreover, in the United States and other developed countries, women tend to outlive men and tend to be in the lower income groups. Many elderly from different cultures have not assimilated into the mainstream culture, making their problems even more difficult to address. All of these factors, in addition to cognitive changes, can lead to depression and anxiety about aging.

The experience of aging is unique to every individual. Some individuals who have profound cognitive changes may not be conscious of their surroundings or status. Thus, APNs' primary responsibility is to provide care for the person as a unique person with singular needs. In doing so, addressing the needs of that person's supports, caregivers, and/or significant others is also important.

Ageism and Age Bias

Ageism is a negative attitude toward older persons that results in treating them as less worthy of consideration for important goods than younger people are. It is a false generalization that lumps everyone into the same class. An ageist statement, for example, might assert that all elderly people are forgetful, fragile, or grumpy. Ageism, in a sense, allows us to separate them from us. Anytime a group is seen as unlike "us," they can be treated as if they are not fully human (see Chapter 4 for a more extensive discussion).

Sometimes ageism manifests in a way that may not be immediately recognized. For example, in the care setting, the use of affectionate terms such as "hon" or "sweetie" seems innocuous, but it is presumptuous and patronizing. It fails to treat the person as an individual or honor his or her dignity.

What it means to honor a person's dignity is itself debated. Gallagher (2004) has investigated the different historical and contemporary meanings of dignity. The meaning is subjective and contextual, for example, a person's experience or sense of personal dignity. As Shotton and Seedhouse (1998) note, "We lack dignity when we find ourselves in inappropriate circumstances, when we are in situations where we feel foolish, incompetent, inadequate or unusually vulnerable" (pp. 246–247). In the ethical or objective sense, dignity means being treated as a worthy individual, that is, as an individual whose needs are to be considered equally with the needs of other persons. This issue of dignity is discussed in more detail later in the chapter.

Other examples of ageist statements that demean aging persons both as a group and individually are "The elderly have trouble remembering things" or "the elderly are rigid in their thinking." The statements may be true of some elderly people but certainly not of all or even of most. Moreover, plenty of young people have trouble remembering things or are rigid in their thinking. Sometimes ageist attitudes result from a lack of thought about implications. For example, someone might say, "She is such a sweet little old lady" or "She is so cute" as if the person were a doll or a pet—the possession of another. Such attitudes fail to honor the dignity of the individual. In acute care settings, "evidence also suggests that when older patients are perceived as being cantankerous or complaining by nurses, the quality of care and the recovery of patients is affected" (Courtney, Tong, & Walsh, 2000, p. 66).

Age bias is the tendency to think that elderly people are not entitled to the same degree of health care or other societal benefits as younger people are either because they have already benefited or they cannot benefit as much from highly technologic care. Thus, age bias permits the rationing of health care, especially highly technologic advances or expensive care, in a way that favors younger persons over their older counterparts (Nelson, 2002; Wicclair, 1993).

Ironically, age bias might sometimes be expected to spare a person from overtreatment or treatment that is beyond what would be desired if the person was well informed about its goals and likelihood of benefit. Nevertheless, deciding what care and interventions are appropriate for an older person is best when decisions do not originate from a perspective of age bias. Rather, determinations about appropriate actions in a given situation should be predicated on other factors, such as how consistent these actions are with the person's situation, beliefs, values, and life goals. Additionally, APNs are in a good position to educate others who exhibit ageist attitudes or age bias about the need to treat each patient on his or her own merits, according to his or her own needs, and within the full context of his or her life.

Problems of Autonomy

Many of the ethical issues faced by APNs who care for older patients have to do with the person's temporary or permanent loss of autonomy and how this is best addressed. The ethical principle of autonomy has been discussed in great detail in earlier chapters, especially in Chapters 1 and 4. Autonomy may be lost in the sense that a person has diminished decision-making ability, that is, he or she is unable to make autonomous choices, or it may be lost in a second and more practical sense in that the person's range of choices is limited by dependence on someone else to meet her needs.

The ethical principle of autonomy as it is used in health care denotes a person's capacity to determine voluntarily which choices are acceptable. So, it is usually understood to be dependent upon cognitive capacity. However, it is also somewhat dependent upon a person's physical ability to enact choices or resist the actions of others. For example, physical incapacities can make persons reliant on others for their mobility and nutritional and other needs. As Castellucci (1998) notes, circumstances that interfere with an older adult's autonomy include "internal and external constraints" (p. 268). (Criteria for determining decision-making capacity along with a discussion of the implications of impaired decision making are found in Chapter 3.)

Loss of Independence

When a person who previously possessed autonomy in the sense of being self-reliant and independent loses some degree of independence, as happens more frequently in the aging population than in other cohorts, a whole other set of ethical issues is presented. How can the APN assist patients in maintaining integrity and a sense of well-being when they are reliant to varying degrees upon others for their transportation or other services? How can people be protected when their well-being is threatened by a caregiver? What do caregivers need to help them remain healthy while being stressed as a result of caregiving activities? APNs frequently encounter all of these problems.

A person's ability to act independently can be reduced by sensory or other physical changes. Sometimes the person recognizes his or her limitations and seeks assistance for needs. It is not unusual, though, for a person's judgment about his or her capabilities to be at odds with objective assessments. Thus, some people are unable or unwilling to recognize physical or sensory limitations.

Among the most difficult transitions for older adults to make is that of losing their ability to drive safely. A transition is described by Adams, Hays, and Hopson (1976) as a "discontinuity in a person's life space" (p. 5). Liddle, Carlson, and McKenna (2004) note that research has shown that "driving cessation is a major life transition for older people" and that it can result "in role loss, isolation and a loss of independence" (p. 1414). It is not surprising, then, that a relatively frequent request of healthcare providers made by an aging person's relatives is to help them persuade their loved one not to drive anymore. Loss of motor reflex acuity, visual losses, or cognitive changes can all endanger the individual in question and perhaps others who share the road. Thus, the provider must decide how to approach the issue in a way that is sensitive, understanding of the magnitude of the transition, and compassionate. He or she can envision and suggest alternatives means of transportation or even relocation based on an understanding of the individual's particular needs and available resources. For the elderly person, the loss of driving privileges represents an existential shift. Unlike a surgery or other transient loss of driving ability, this loss will be permanent.

Autonomy in Transport

In the United States, where automobiles are symbolic of individual freedom of movement, public transportation is limited in many areas, and most people are accustomed to using their own cars to go wherever and whenever they wish or need to. The loss of driving ability is experienced as a critical turning point, not just because of accessibility but also because it is bound up with personal identity. For example, Ms. Caro is 78 years old and lives in a small rural town. She has three children, but the closest one is 100 miles distant. She is relatively healthy and her only medical problem is hypertension, which has been well controlled with meds. She is active in the town, volunteers at the library and attends the local senior center activities, and she lives half a mile from her nearest neighbors. Until recently, she has been able to drive herself wherever she wishes. After her last eye test, however, her daughter telephoned Ms. Browning, an APN/general nurse practitioner (GNP) who has served as Ms. Caro's primary care provider for the past 10 years, to say that her mother has worsening macular degeneration and that she has been advised not to drive anymore. Ms. Caro does not want anyone to know and has forbidden her daughter to tell anyone. Her daughter appeals to Ms. Browning to help her talk to her mother because, if not, she is afraid that Ms. Caro will hurt herself or someone else. The following questions are posed to guide your analysis of this situation.

Questions to consider:

1. What are the ethical aspects of this situation?
2. What are the APN's moral and legal responsibilities and considerations?
3. What are the implications for Ms. Caro of no longer being allowed to drive?
4. What are the possible courses of action?
5. How might the impact of this transition be lessened?

Resources for envisioning alternative courses of action may also be found at the local elder services agency or the state agency on aging. A list of these can be found at http://www.aoa.gov/eldfam/How_To_Find/Agencies/Agencies.asp.

Impaired Mobility

When a person's mobility is impaired and it interferes with the ability to care for himself or herself, physical autonomy is limited and the person is forced to rely on others for assistance. APNs may be the crucial advocate for such persons, helping them to maintain as much autonomy as possible. This might require identifying resources for them, helping them talk to family members or friends, and helping them to explore options that will minimize their loss of physical independence leading to loss of decision-making independence. When one is dependent upon another person to meet one's needs, compromises may have to be made to achieve a balance or harmony among competing needs. The options for elderly people often are either to move in with a relative or friend who will provide assistance or to enter a long-term care facility. In either case, freedom to exercise personal autonomy further declines because many desired actions depend on the good will of the caregiver.

Caregiver Problems

Many people are happy to be in a position to provide care for their aging relative within the family setting. Any inconveniences are balanced by the benefits of a loving relationship, the ability to reciprocate for earlier assistances given by the person in question, and the knowledge that the loved one is well cared for. However, sometimes the motives for agreeing to provide care are not quite so open. The complexity of the care needed may not have been well anticipated or the consequences of caregiving can take their toll on the caregivers. Additionally, a person's care requirements may increase over time.

Problems arise when the caregiver's health starts to suffer, the caregiver's attitudes toward the relative deteriorate, or the aging person's needs are neglected. Upon evaluating an older person, APNs may begin to suspect that the person is being neglected or, worse, physically or mentally abused. The American Medical Association (AMA) defines abuse as follows:

> An act or omission which results in harm or threatened harm to the health or welfare of an elderly person. Abuse includes intentional infliction of physical or mental injury, sexual abuse, or withholding of necessary food, clothing, or medical care to meet the physical and mental needs of an elderly person by one having care, custody, or responsibility of an elderly person. (American Medical Association, 1990, p. 2460)

Neglect is thought to be the most common form of abuse. When people are physically neglected or become isolated, they often experience a slow decline. There are no comprehensive tools that measure abuse or neglect, but Fulmer and Paveza (1998) suggest that it is helpful to evaluate the vulnerability of the person along with the risk of abuse, whether physical or mental. Abuse or neglect may occur because the caregiver's resources are exhausted and not because of an intention to hurt or punish the dependent person. For this reason, APNs who suspect a problem may need to address it as a family issue, providing the appropriate care, interventions, and resources for the family unit.

A CASE OF NEGLECT?

John Longfellow is an 85-year-old man with residual left-sided weakness from a stroke that occurred 5 years previously. Although he is cognitively able to process information and can engage in conversation appropriately, his speech pattern is slow and he sometimes has to "search for words." He has been cared for at home by his wife, Janet, who is 76 years old. Brenda Fisk, a GNP, has been providing care for the couple since John's initial evaluation by the multidisciplinary gerontology clinic at the local hospital.

After discharge, John and Janet received home health services, and John attended rehabilitation to improve his ambulation and speech. Janet drives the couple to the health center for their check-ups and has always been very solicitous of John. At this current visit however, Brenda notices that John has lost weight, his clothes are slightly soiled, and his speech is more halting that usual. Janet, uncharacteristically, is talking for him. She tells Brenda within earshot of John that she is so tired of taking care of him—he is so ungrateful and miserable and she is weary; she never gets any time by herself. John does not meet Brenda's eyes when she asks him how he is doing and he seems very withdrawn. He has lost about 20 pounds in weight since their last visit. Brenda is worried that John is being neglected and wonders what her next steps should be.

Discussion

In most states, the Department of Adult Protective Services (APS) is charged with investigating reports of abuse or neglect. Whether reporting of suspected abuse is mandated or not (and what the associated criteria are) varies from state to state, and APNs must be familiar with their state law in this regard. However, in many cases good nursing evaluation, care, and the provision of adequate resources will result in a better outcome for the person and caregiver(s) than reporting will. Although the subject of abuse may fare better if an APS investigation determines that that person should be removed from a current situation for health and safety reasons, this is not the most frequent outcome.

In this case, Brenda must try to find out whether either John or Janet has any underlying physical or psychological problems that are exacerbating the situation. For example, is John depressed? If he is depressed, why or why now when previously he had been doing so well? Are his health changes negatively affecting Janet, or is Janet's attitude affecting his mental health? What is going on with Janet? The situation is complex, and the complexity must be acknowledged. Both John and Janet are in need of assistance.

Ethically, after a thorough investigation of the situation, Brenda must make a determination about the severity and imminence of any risks involved. In the absence of any immediate danger, she will include the couple in formulating a plan that is predicated on identified issues and needs and that will work for both John and Janet. Her job is to help preserve the dignity and autonomy of both parties. This may involve counseling, respite care, identifying family members who would be willing to offer assistance, or any number of other appropriate supports. When necessary, Brenda would help the couple talk to family members who could be helpful. She may help them decide whether alternative living arrangements, such as assisted living, could relieve Janet of her perceived burden. Further, to anticipate and prevent future problems, Brenda will discuss with the couple their preferences and desires for future living and healthcare arrangements should the health of either one of them deteriorate further (preventive ethics).

Long-Term Care

When persons become unable to care for themselves and have no one who is willing or able to assume responsibility for their care, they may need to enter a long-term care facility. APNs caring for this population often find themselves in the position of offering advice about how to choose an appropriate facility and thus should familiarize themselves with the types of facilities available. Also, many GNPs actually work for or have their practice in long-term care facilities.

Long-term care facilities have their own issues related to autonomy. Agich (1998) describes why "respecting the autonomy of elders in nursing homes is so difficult and why a reconceptualization of autonomy is so critical to enhancing their dignity and quality of life" (p. 200). Agich proposes a modified view of autonomy and sees autonomy as being compatible even with the varying degrees of physical dependence on others that is necessarily present in the nursing home setting. Agich (1998) argues that just because someone is in a nursing home and physically dependent does not mean that that person is "decisionally incapacitated" (p. 209). "Some elders clearly maintain decisional capacity even though their medical condition can limit their ability to execute or act on their choices . . . thus executional incapacity should not be mistaken for decisional incapacity" (p. 209). *Executional capacity* is the ability to carry out one's decisions.

Although no one, as noted earlier, is ever completely autonomous in actions or choices of action (even though we often think we are) because we are all susceptible to internal and external influences of which we are not always fully conscious, the problem of constraints on action in long-term care settings is even more obvious and worrisome. The institutional routines and order are, of course, important in terms of efficient uses of resources. Nevertheless, with creativity a balance that takes into consideration both the need for efficiency and the need to uphold the individual dignity of patients is possible. In understanding this as an ethical problem, APNs have the foundation for envisioning good care. In many cases, optimizing a patient's sense of control improves that person's well-being and facilitates autonomy.

It is important to make a distinction between capacity to make individual decisions (*informed voluntary choice*) and a more global determination of incompetence. When a person is incompetent to manage his or her affairs, a previously identified relative or friend may assume power of attorney. *Power of attorney* is a tool of the legal system whereby the legal authority over a person's affairs is granted to another. In the absence of a predetermined power of attorney, a guardian is appointed by the state. "Guardianship is a relationship created by state law in which a court gives one person or entity (the guardian) the duty and the power to make personal and/or property decisions for another (the ward or incapacitated person)" (Teaster et al., 2005, p. 1).

Guardianship Issues

Assigning guardianship to a designated person is for the purpose of protecting the ward's interests. Forty-eight states currently have public laws related to guardianship. In Massachusetts (the author's state of residence), the duties of guardians or conservators are as follows:

> Guardians and conservators have many duties in common and are subject to supervision of the Probate Court. Some of these duties are set forth below. The list is not complete, but rather a general indication of the scope of duties.

- Pay the ward's debts
- Represent the ward in all lawsuits
- Control and manage the ward's property
- Invest the ward's funds
- Collect funds due the ward
- Support the ward and his or her family from the ward's funds
- Sell, lease, or mortgage the ward's property, with the approval of the Probate Court

A guardian, unlike a conservator, has custody of the person of his or her ward. Also, a guardian must consent to such matters as medical treatment and where the ward will reside. The law gives no preference to any particular class of persons or relatives. Any person who is proper and fit is eligible. The paramount consideration of the Probate Court is the welfare of the ward and the appropriateness of the appointment to meet the ward's needs. (Massachusetts Bar Association, 2002)

In the comprehensive study by Teaster and colleagues (2005) of guardianship conditions across the states, many states reported that the number of wards in need of guardianship is large in proportion to the number of guardians. Thus, one can see that it may be difficult for a guardian to actually know the person as an individual or in reality serve that person's individual best interests. This is especially true when the guardian has many wards for whom he or she is responsible. Additionally, once a person has been deemed incompetent, it is very difficult to gain a reversal of the determination even when the person regains competency or has been wrongly judged incompetent to make his or her own decisions.

THE CASE OF ROSE DOYLE

In November of 2006, Rosie Doyle found herself in the hospital as a result of heart problems. Within a week, the hospital's attorney petitioned the county probate court to declare her mentally ill and thus incompetent. The required documentation from a hospital psychiatrist noted, "On exam, Ms. Doyle was calm, cooperative, and friendly. However, she had very little understanding of her medical problems; (was) unable to discuss any of the diagnoses mentioned above. She was unable to explain why she takes any of her medicines" (*Boston Globe*, January 13th, 2008). The judge, after deliberating for only a few minutes, declared Mrs. Doyle mentally ill.

Mrs. Doyle, however, on learning about this showed enough mental acuity to contact a lawyer. She was alarmed and angry about her unanticipated loss of freedom. Although the incompetency decision was eventually reversed, it was not in time to prevent her transferal to a nursing home, where she remained for 3 months. In a review of her hospital records prior to the case review, it was discovered that the only factor that pointed to a "behavior problem" was that she would not accede to the physician's recommendation for cardiac surgery. Additionally, by the time she was released from the nursing home, her property had been sold.

QUESTIONS TO CONSIDER

What went wrong in this case? In most states, before psychiatric patients can be committed for treatment, a rigorous evaluation must occur and the patient's status is reviewed periodically. Why do you think the standard in the case of an elderly person whose loss of freedom as a result may well be permanent is not at least as rigorous? What role might a CNS or NP have played in advocating for Mrs. Doyle? What sorts of policy or education is needed to assist nurses and others as they assess a patient's decision-making capacity? Imagine yourself in Mrs. Doyle's situation: what attitudes would you want the nurses and healthcare professionals around you to have and what actions would you want them to take?

Wrongful deprivation of one's rights to personal decision making is a serious constraint on freedom of action. It is only warranted if the risk of harm is high and there is reasonable evidence to show that the person does not understand implications of his or her actions and for this reason cannot adequately protect himself or herself from harm. However, there are other forms of restraint that are sometimes used on elderly people who become confused, agitated, and aggressive. The next section explores the ethical issues associated with the use of physical and chemical restraints.

Physical and Chemical Restraints

Hantikainen (2001) notes that "nursing staff who have difficulty in understanding and coping with the behavior of older people may be tempted to try and get to grips with the situation by means of control and manipulation" (p. 246). Although much has been written about the problems associated with restraint use for elderly people and strides have been made in raising awareness and even in changing standards of care in this regard, the practice of using chemical and physical restraints to manage perceived problematic behavior of elderly people has not been eradicated.

The underlying assumption in using restraints is that the person's safety is at issue and that restraining the person will protect him or her. In this sense, the use of restraints is seen to be guided by the ethical principle of nonmaleficence. Sometimes a person is also restrained if that person's actions are imminently likely to cause harm to another. In both long-term and acute care settings, restraints are mostly used to protect persons from harming themselves—although they are sometimes used to prevent persons' unruly behavior from harming others. Chemical restraints involve the use of drugs to calm behavior and/or to sedate the patient. Although restraints are ostensibly used to protect patients, often they are used for the expedience or relief of the caregivers, nurses, aids, or family members. Thus, their use is often harmful and unethical.

The prevalence of disruptive behaviors in nursing homes ranges from 43–93% (Voyer & Martin, 2003). Moreover, Voyer and Martin (2003) note that there is strong support for the idea that older persons who experience psychological problems, whether they are living in the community or reside in a nursing home, are not receiving optimal care. Previous studies have shown that instead of evaluating possible underlying causes of disruptive behavior such as depression, fear, confusion, and grief and initiating appropriate interventions, a focus on expedience, or a desire for rapid control of the situation, can lead to inappropriate treatment with antipsychotic drugs or other sedatives. Some studies have shown that nurses have influence over the prescribing practices of physicians in this regard (Simonson, 1984; Stevenson, Kellog, Ernst, & Whinney, 1989) and thus have contributed to the overuse and inappropriate use of chemical restraints. APNs with prescribing privileges could also be susceptible to the urging of nurses to medicate persons with disruptive behaviors. Furthermore, certain psychotropic drugs are addictive and when used on a regular basis cause dependency and problems with withdrawal (Voyer et al., 2004).

The implications for GNPs or CNSs are related to the professional ethical obligation to provide a good for patients (beneficence) and minimize harms (nonmaleficence). Proper evaluation of a patient's behavior and the use of clinical judgment to determine therapeutic actions are required. As nurse leaders, APNs may need to educate others who are urging inappropriate treatments and conceptualize policies that will facilitate patient well-being.

A CASE OF RESTRAINT

Bill Carr, 72 years old, is admitted to a long-term care facility as a result of the progression of his Alzheimer's disease. His family worries about his safety because he "is always trying to escape from the house." On one successful occasion, it took family members 3 hours to find him. His son reports him to be a very sociable person. On admission, Bill is very pleasant and amenable but obviously confused. He appears to settle in fairly well, although he does not like to stay in one place for any length of time. His son and daughter-in-law leave after settling him in his room, placing familiar objects on the bedside table, and hanging a picture of his deceased wife.

As night approaches, though, Bill starts to get increasingly agitated. The registered nurse Sara, who oversees the unit at night, is new to this facility, trained abroad, and although licensed in the United States, has been working at the nursing home for only 2 months. Although he is not aggressive, Bill is anxiously going in and out of the other residents' rooms, repeatedly calling his dead wife's name. When Bill refuses to take his meds, including a sedative that is prescribed to be taken as needed (PRN), Sara calls Marilyn, the GNP on call, and asks for an order to give an intramuscular (IM) antipsychotic drug.

QUESTIONS

1. Based on the discussions in this and previous chapters about nursing goals to provide a patient good, how should Marilyn respond?
2. What are the pertinent ethical principles involved in this case?
3. How do these direct or underpin Marilyn's decision making?
4. Assuming that Marilyn and Sara are able to formulate an ethical care plan and initiate effective interventions that further Bill's well-being, what is needed in the way of preventive ethics?

SUMMARY

The discussion in this section has centered on ethical care of persons as they age and the responsibilities of APNs related to care of this population. Nursing goals and ethical principles as well as knowledge of the special needs of aging persons guide the discussion about decision making. Among the responsibilities of APNs is the education and support of other nurses and allied health professionals as they provide care for this population. APNs can be influential in the education of other staff, in their collaborative relationships with physicians and nursing home administrators, and in formulating policies that facilitate the humane treatment of the residents and maximize their range of choices.

Upholding the principle of autonomy is crucially important and yet the most difficult to honor, especially in long-term care institutions where certain restrictions upon the personal freedom of residents are inevitable. Elders (and others) living in institutional settings are dependent to various degrees upon those who make the rules and uphold the routines. However, individuals' ability to make their own choices within the limits of the setting remains important for their well-being.

ETHICAL CARE AT THE END OF LIFE

APNs have important roles both in providing and improving end-of-life care for persons of all ages, including newborns (as discussed in Chapter 7). The importance to quality of life of nursing care for persons experiencing catastrophic, chronic, deteriorative, and/or terminal illnesses has been relatively well documented (Emnett, Byock, & Twohig, 2002; Oncology Nursing Society, 2003). The role of nursing is important because of the profession's emphasis on understanding patient experiences in response to life processes. Byock and Miles (2003) write that "quality of end-of-life care in the United States is seriously deficient" (p. 335) despite recent efforts to improve this aspect of health care. Many people do not communicate what their wishes for EOL care are via advance directives, and even when they do, their wishes may not be honored (see the discussion related to advance directives in Chapter 3).

Ethical issues that are associated with EOL situations include decision making under conditions of ambiguity, adequately informing patients and their families about treatments, balancing quality of life against extending suffering, managing intractable suffering, and futile treatments. Decisions around EOL care and who is involved in the decision making vary depending on the patient population, cultural beliefs, values, and other characteristics of the individual and setting. Other chapters in the book provide discussions related to EOL issues. For example, Chapter 7 describes the NICU and futility concerns, and Chapter 3 provides a discussion of advance directives and informed consent. This chapter does not repeat previous discussions but rather uses them as foundations for case exploration later. Some aspects of EOL care discussed in bioethics and applied philosophy literature provide a helpful background to discussions of futility, the ethical permissibility of withholding food and fluids at a patient's or patient surrogate's request, and the meaning and use of palliative sedation. These topics are discussed briefly in the following subsections.

The Meaning of Futility in EOL Decision Making

Lo (2005) notes that the "concept of futility" has seemed to many healthcare providers a good way to resolve certain dilemmas. That is, when biological and/or technologic advances can maintain physical function but it is unlikely or at best uncertain that the person can recover, a determination of futility can be made. This provides a definite answer to patients or to persons who are serving as a patient's decision-making proxy about whether treatment should continue. However, "the term 'futility' gives decision making power to physicians" (p. 61). *Futility* means that there is no meaningful purpose to the intervention, regardless of how many times the treatment is offered or how long it continues. The problem with this definition, of course, is that for many interventions we can have only a reasonable idea that the treatment is futile but no proof. So, care dilemmas cannot really be resolved in this way.

Further questions that must be answered are, What is the purpose of the treatment and is the treatment futile for that purpose? To answer these questions we must turn back to the patient (or surrogate). These questions focus the issue back on the person for whom the intervention is proposed, and then the question becomes: What does this patient want and how likely is this intervention to meet the patient's expressed or implied (by understandings of the person's previous life, values, beliefs, and so forth) needs? When the question is posed this way, it permits us to see that our responsibility is to help the person making the decision grasp the implications of the intervention as best we can.

Autonomy in EOL Decision Making

In decision making at the end of life, as in other circumstances, perhaps the most significant role of the APN is to assist patients and their relatives to conceptualize what they wish for themselves. That is, we can help them clarify their values and desires in relation to the options available. Little has been written about the nuances of the nurse–patient relationship in relation to choices about end-of-life care. Clover, Browne, McErlain, and Vandenberg's (2004) small qualitative Australian study found that "patient participation is highly dependent on professionals' skill in opening up negotiation" (p. 340). When nurses were able to facilitate patients' acquisition of necessary information, patients became less passive and more able to say what they really wanted.

Additionally, providing support for the relatives or close friends of a dying patient is an important role of the nurse. For many people, it might be their first time in encountering the death of someone close, and they must juggle personal feelings of grief with the need to make considered judgment related to care. Andershed's (2006) literature review of 94 studies is revealing. Themes that emerge include the significant person (relative or friend of the dying person) as "being exposed" and experiencing "increased vulnerability" (p. 1160); they themselves were often at risk from ill health and had to find ways to cope with the tensions between "burden and capacity" (p. 1161). Not surprisingly, it was important to relatives to see that their loved one was getting good care and was "content" (p. 1162). Among the study themes that emerged from this meta-analysis is the importance of well-structured care as occurred in palliative care and hospice settings. Another very important theme in many of the studies reviewed by Andershed (2006) was the relatives' need for effective communication and information about all aspects of care. Perhaps one of the most striking insights is that relatives have different needs from the patient and desire interactions with nurses that take this into consideration. That is, nurses need to approach relatives as people in their own right with their own needs.

Honoring Patient Wishes: Requests for Help with Dying

As more and more APNs assume the overall care of persons at the end of their lives, and with the gaining of prescriptive privileges, APNs are now more likely to be asked by their terminally ill patients for assistance in dying.

This may be one of the most difficult requests to which a nurse must respond because the situations of such patients making this request are usually dire and our relationship with the person makes us sympathetic to the request. Regardless of philosophical belief or emotional involvement with the patient, we must step back and be sure we understand the nature and complexity of the request.

As Brock (2008/1992) notes, "In the recent bioethics literature some have endorsed physician-assisted suicide but not Euthanasia" (p. 437). The term *euthanasia* means a good death. Most of us would agree that we would like a good death. In the end, death is not necessarily what we fear. It is the suffering before death and the not knowing what, if anything, will happen to us after we die that cause us the most anxiety.

It is beyond the scope of this chapter to trace the development of right-to-die legislation. Refer to any of a number of excellent ethics textbooks and the large body of literature related to euthanasia and assisted suicide for more information. Professional nursing organizations all oppose the idea of deliberately assisting a person in ending his or her own life. Some might argue that in certain cases the usual argument that effective palliation of symptoms makes the idea of assisted suicide or active euthanasia (legalized in the Netherlands) moot does not hold. I could describe several cases I encountered in my nursing career where a good argument for euthanasia could have been made; however, there are too many slippery slope worries that abuses would occur for me to readily agree that euthanasia should be legalized. For example, on one occasion, when I was supervising nursing students in their clinical rotation, a woman we were caring for was persuaded (against her wishes we later found out) by her family to accept palliative radiation treatment for her metastasized bone cancer. After the second treatment, she developed Stevens-Johnson syndrome, which resulted in extremely painful peeling of skin over large areas of her body. No amount of medication was able to palliate the pain she experienced, which worsened every time she moved. She died 6 days later. For the most part, though, good palliative care permits a person's pain and other symptoms to be well managed.

The American Nurses Association's (1994) position statement on assisted suicide is representative of the U.S. nursing profession's voice in regard to participation in assisted suicide or active euthanasia:

> The American Nurses Association (ANA) believes that the nurse should not participate in assisted suicide. . . . Nurses, individually and collectively, have an obligation to provide comprehensive and compassionate end-of-life care which includes the promotion of comfort and the relief of pain and, at times, forgoing life-sustaining treatments. (American Nurses Association, 1994)

Relief of Suffering

The ethical principle of double effect (Lo, 2005) is helpful in conceptualizing or rationalizing the permissibility of using high doses of drugs if necessary to alleviate a person's symptoms, even if it is known that the treatments used could shorten a person's life. "The doctrine of double effect distinguishes effects that are intended from those that are foreseen but unintended" (Lo, 2005, p. 107). Essentially, this principle asserts that the intent of an action is its most important aspect. The good effect is, of course, relieving the patient's suffering, and the unintended effect is the patient's death.

The doctrine of double effect originated within religious tradition. It is thought that when giving doses of analgesics or sedatives, maintaining a focus on the intent to alleviate suffering provides an important distinction that eradicates the need to talk in terms of intending the person's death. This focus on relieving suffering permits even those with deeply held beliefs against euthanasia to assist in ensuring a person's comfort. It is argued that making a distinction between passive euthanasia (i.e., withholding or withdrawing life-prolonging treatments) and active euthanasia (the intentional taking of someone's life) is important and can be maintained by the doctrine of double effect. In the ethics literature, there is debate about these distinctions and how important they really are. Nevertheless, for many people religious or philosophical beliefs make them uncomfortable with the idea of being involved in hastening someone's death, even if that person would prefer relief of suffering and finds the risk of death acceptable. The doctrine of double effect thus permits the patient's 'good' as conceived by that patient to be honored.

Palliative Sedation

Palliative sedation, also known as terminal sedation or total sedation, is the practice of titrating sedatives or analgesics to the point where a person no longer experiences symptoms (Davis & Ford, 2005). The goal of palliative sedation is the relief of suffering via the titration of medications to the cessation of symptoms—not the cessation of life.

The Hospice and Palliative Nursing Association position paper (Hospice and Palliative Nursing Association, 2003) titled "Palliative Sedation at the End of Life" provides guidelines for advanced practice and other nurses working in palliative care and hospice settings and has relevance for all nurses who work with those needing EOL care. It notes that "an array of physical and psychological symptoms and existential distress" (p. 235) may be experienced, and for the most part, they can be relieved by good care. Reports suggest that palliative sedation may be used in up to 30% of dying patients (Hospice and Palliative Nursing Association, 2003).

Relief of suffering is the goal of palliative sedation. Suffering includes a sense of helplessness or loss in the face of a seemingly relentless and unendurable threat to quality of life or integrity of self (Cassell, 1999). Additionally, Cherny, Coyle, and Foley (1994) propose that consciousness, or the ability to perceive and respond to the sense of loss and hopelessness, is a condition of suffering. For the most part, it is believed that suffering can be relieved with combinations of analgesia and other therapeutics—however, sometimes it cannot.

Some commentators have recommended that palliative sedation be used only when the person's death is expected within hours to a couple of days; other critics believe that palliative sedation can be used in other cases when intractable symptoms of various sorts occur, but that the drugs should be appropriate to the symptoms and titrated only to relief of symptoms, that is, not used in ever escalating doses (Cherny & Portnoy, 1994).

Guidelines for the use of palliative sedation have been developed by several scholars. General principles are that it is reserved for those who are imminently dying. The palliative sedation option should be discussed with patients and their families prior to the need for it (when possible). This permits patients and family members to ask questions and develop a plan. It also facilitates informed consent and thus upholds the principle of autonomy. Palliative care works best when an interdisciplinary team is available to assess the situation and collaborate both on care of the patient and support for the family. The collaborative team plans the therapeutics together (Rousseau, 2001). Team members may include a palliative care APN, the patient's physician or NP, a pain management specialist, and allied professionals as appropriate. Good documentation of the process and the rationale is needed.

A recent Public Broadcasting Service (PBS) television series offers an example of palliative sedation. In the third program of the PBS series featuring Bill Moyers titled "Dying in America: On Our Own Terms," a man is dying of liver cancer. He is very ill, with only a few days to live, and has been admitted back into a Virginia hospital for palliative care. Although he becomes quiet at times as a result of the sedation he is receiving, he becomes combative at night—during this time, the dose of the sedation is not enough to keep him calm and he needs more. Dr. Gomez and the man's wife discuss the issue. After a period of time, they agree that palliative sedation is the best approach. Dr. Gomez tells the man's wife that if they administer palliative sedation to the man, he will probably not wake up again. She says that they are both ready. "He wouldn't want this," she says. A few hours after starting the sedation, the man dies.

When APN graduate students in my class view the film and discuss it, there are varying perspectives. Not everyone is comfortable with palliative sedation. As noted earlier, nurses need to be self-reflective about the environments in which they work and whether their philosophy of care is congruent with the expectations of their role within that setting.

Patient Refusal of Nutrition and Hydration

Some patients with cancer or other terminal illnesses may refuse nutrition and hydration during their last few days of life. Indeed, voluntary refusal of sustenance "has been proposed as an alternative to physician assisted suicide for terminally ill patients who wish to hasten death" (Ganzini et al., 2003, p. 359).

It has been generally supposed that dying from dehydration is a terrible death, and thus it is worrisome when dying persons refuse food and fluids. The study by Ganzini and colleagues sought to discover whether this supposition could be validated. They surveyed 102 hospice nurses working in Oregon who reported having taken care of a patient in the prior 4 years who had stopped eating or drinking a few days prior to that person's death. "Nurses reported that patients chose to stop eating and drinking because they were ready to die, saw continued existence as pointless, and considered their quality of life as poor" (p. 359). Eighty-five percent of the patients died within 15 days of stopping food. The nurses assigned scores for their perception of the quality of the person's death. The median score was 8 on a scale of 1 to 10 where 10 represented a highest 'quality' death given the illness suffered.

APNs Responding to Requests to Die

APNs as well as other nurses who work in primary care, oncology, acute care, and hospice may receive requests from patients for assistance in dying. Hudson and colleagues (2006) collaborated on a project intended to result in some guidelines for addressing such requests in a therapeutic and humane way. They constituted an interdisciplinary team with members from "nursing, medicine, psychiatry, psychology, sociology, aged care and theology" (p. 703). Recommendations distilled from their work include the following:

1. Self-reflection about one's own reaction to such requests. Assume a non-judgmental pose.
2. A genuine willingness to listen to the person's feelings and perceptions. Be alert for cues and probe for more information.
3. Evaluate possible contributing factors—what pushed the person to this point. What else is going on? What are the psychosocial and physical problems? How severe are they? Is the person coherent, delirious, depressed?
4. Ascertain whether there are issues that can be addressed or turned around. Start planning strategies with the patient as amenable.
5. Review the situation with the patient. Ask if there are other issues. Reassure the patient that his or her confidentiality will be protected to the extent reasonable given the need of other team members to know (and in the absence of serious harm to others or self).
6. Document pertinent aspects using clinical judgment.

CONCLUSION

Many more issues are relevant to APN practice related to gerontology and care of patients at EOL than can be included here. Previous chapters provide the foundation for analyzing the issues and grasping the ethical nature of APN care in these settings. APNs have the knowledge, skills, and expertise to advocate for patients who may be vulnerable related to the aging process and to provide good care for those at the end of life.

DISCUSSION QUESTIONS

1. Barbara Jarvis a 64-year-old divorced woman who was diagnosed with Alzheimer's disease 3 years ago. She has been living with her daughter Jenny, who is 30 years old. Jenny recently got married, and Ben, the son-in-law, moved into the house after the marriage. They are expecting their first baby. Until now, Barbara, although increasingly forgetful, has not posed any problems. She has many friends in the area, and they have maintained contact and are a diversion for Barbara. Recently, though, Barbara has been having more difficulty with her memory and carrying out daily tasks. She is easily distracted, forgets to turn off the oven, leaves the front door open, and locks herself out of the house. Jenny is afraid to leave her home alone but has no choice because she has to work.

    a. How would you assist Jenny and Ben with their process of decision making about Barbara's future and whether they should continue to care for her at home?
    b. What are the important considerations?
    c. What are the possible roles of the APN in such situations?

2. "Advanced care planning ideally involves communication about values between patients, family members, and care providers" (Karel, Moye, Bank, & Azar, 2007).

    a. What values are important in advanced care planning?
    b. As a primary care APN, how would you initiate a conversation about advanced care planning?
    c. What strategies would you use to assist your patients and their families with decision making?

REFERENCES

Adams, J., Hayes, J., & Hopson, B. (1976). *Transition: Understanding and managing personal change*. London: Martin Robertson.

Agich, G. (1998). Respecting the autonomy of elders in nursing homes. In J. Monagle & D. Thomasma (Eds.), *Health care ethics: Critical issues for the 21st century* (pp. 200–211). Gaithersburg, MD: Aspen.

American Medical Association. (1990). White paper on elderly health: Report of the council on scientific affairs. *Archives of Internal Medicine, 150*, 2459–2472.

American Nurses Association. (1994). *Position statement on assisted suicide*. Washington, DC: Author.

Andershed, B. (2006). Relatives in end-of-life care—part 1: A systematic review of the literature the last five years, January 1999–February 2004. *Cancer and Palliative Care, 15*, 1158–1169.

Boston Globe. (2008). *Court strips elders of their independence*. Correspondents Kelly, J., Kowalski, M., & Novak, C. (January 13th). Accessed April 27th, 2008 from http://www.boston.com/news/local/articles/2008/01/13/courts_strip_elders_of_their_independence/.

Brock, D. (2008/1992). Voluntary active euthanasia. In T. Beauchamp, L. Walters, J. Kahn, & A. Mastroianni (Eds.), *Contemporary issues in bioethics* (7th ed., pp. 437–446). Belmont, CA: Thompson Wadsworth (Reprinted from the Hastings Center Report. *10*(10), 1992.)

Byock, I., & Miles, S. (2003). Hospice benefits and phase I cancer trials. *Annals of Internal Medicine, 138*(4), 335–337.

Castellucci, D. (1998). Issues for nurses regarding elder autonomy. *Nursing Clinics of North America, 33*(2), 265–274.

Cassell, E. (1999). Diagnosing suffering: A perspective. *Annals of Internal Medicine, 131*(7), 531–534.

Cherny, N., Coyle, N., & Foley, K. (1994). Suffering in the advanced cancer patient: A definition and taxonomy. *Journal of Palliative Care, 102*, 57–70.

Cherny, N., & Portnoy, R. (1994). Sedation in the management of refractory symptoms: Guidelines for evaluation and treatment. *Journal of Palliative Care, 10*(2), 31–38.

Clover, A., Browne, J., McErlain, P., & Vandenberg, B. (2004). Patient approaches to clinical conversations in the palliative care settings. Issues and innovations in nursing practice. *Journal of Advanced Nursing, 48*(4), 333–341.

Courtney, M., Tong, S., & Walsh, A. (2000). Acute-care nurses attitudes towards older patients: A literature review. *International Journal of Nursing Practice, 6*, 62–69.

Davis, M., & Ford, P. (2005). Palliative sedation: Definition, practice, outcomes. *Journal of Palliative Medicine, 8*(4), 699–701.

Emnett, J., Byock, I., & Twohig, J. (2002). *Advanced practice nursing: Pioneering practices in palliative care*. Missoula, MT: Promoting Excellence in End-of-Life Care.

Fulmer, T., & Paveza, G. (1998). Neglect in the elderly. *Nursing Clinics of North America, 33*(3), 457–466.

Ganzini, L., Goy, E., Miller, L., Harvath, T., Jackson, A., & Delorit, M. (2003). Nurses' experiences with hospice patients who refuse food and fluids to hasten death. *New England Journal of Medicine, 349*(4), 359–365.

Gallagher, A. (2004). Dignity and respect for dignity—two key health professional values: Implications for nursing practice. *Nursing Ethics, 11*, 587.

Grace, P. J. (2004). Advocacy of the elderly. One course in a 7 course continuing education series (Developed by Sharon Tennstedt, Series Editor-in-Chief Sara T. Fry) [Web-based continuing education course]. Watertown, MA: New England Research Institute. Funded by National Institute of Nursing Research of the National Institutes of Health (Grant #R44 NR05355). https://www.nursingethicsce.com/#1.

Hantikainen, V. (2001). Nursing staff perceptions of the behaviour of older nursing home residents and decision making on restraint use: A qualitative and interpretative study. *Journal of Clinical Nursing, 10*, 246–256.

Hospice and Palliative Nursing Association. (2003). Palliative sedation at the end of life. *Journal of Hospice and Palliative Nursing, 5*(4), 235–237.

Hudson, P., Scholfield, P., Kelly, B., Hudson, R., Street, A., O'Connor, M., et al. (2006). Responding to desire to die statements from patients with advanced disease: Recommendations for health. *Palliative Medicine, 20*, 703–710.

Karel, M., Moye, J., Bank, A., & Azar, A. (2007). Three methods of assessing values for advanced care planning. *Journal of Aging and Health, 19*(1), 123–151.

Liddle, J., Carlson, G., & McKenna, K. (2004). Using a matrix in life transition research. *Qualitative Health Research, 14*(10), 1396–1417.

Lo, B. (2005). *Resolving ethical dilemmas: A guide for clinicians* (3rd ed.). Philadelphia: Lippincott, Williams & Wilkins.

Massachusetts Bar Association. (2002). Family law: Guardians and conservators. Retrieved February 28, 2008, from http://www.masslawhelp.org/lawhelp/legal_info/?sw=3124&full_id=214.

Nelson, T. (2002). *Ageism: Stereotyping and prejudice against older persons.* Boston: MIT Press.

Oncology Nursing Society. (2003). *Statement on the scope and standards of advanced practice in oncology nursing* (3rd ed.). Pittsburgh, PA: Author.

Rousseau, P. (2001). Existential suffering and palliative sedation: A brief commentary with a proposal for clinical guidelines. *American Journal of Hospice and Palliative Care, 18*(3), 151–153.

Scholder, J., Kagan, S. H., & Schumann, M. J. (2004). Nursing competence in aging overview. *Nursing Clinics of North America, 39*(3), 429–442.

Shotton L., & Seedhouse, D. (1998). Practical dignity in caring. *Nursing Ethics, 3*, 246–255.

Simonson, W. (1984). *Medications and the elderly: A guide for promoting proper use.* Rockville, MD: Aspen.

Stevenson, G., Kellog, L., Ernst, V., & Whinney, P. (1989). *Medication use and elderly people. Senior drug action program.* British Columbia: Ministry of Health.

Teaster, P., Wood, E., Karp, N., Lawrence, S., Schmidt, W., & Mendiondo, M. S. (2005). *Wards of the state: A national study of public guardianship. Executive summary.* Retrieved February 28, 2008, from http://www.abanet.org/aging/publications/docs/wardsofstateexecsum.pdf.

Voyer, P., & Martin, L. (2003). Improving geriatric mental health nursing: Making a case for going beyond psychotropic medications. *International Journal of Mental Health Nursing, 12*, 11–21.

Voyer, P., McCubbin, M., Cohen, D., Lauzon, S., Collin, J., & Boivin, C. (2004). Unconventional indicators of drug dependence among elderly long-term users of benzodiazepines. *Issues in Mental Health Nursing, 25*(6), 603–628.

Wicclair, M. (1993). *Ethics and the elderly.* New York: Oxford University Press.

Glossary

Prepared with assistance from my undergraduate research assistant at the time,
Nora Sheehan, RN, BSN

Accountability   The responsibility of the professional for making sound clinical judgments, anticipating foreseeable harms, and being answerable for actions.

Advance directive   A person's instructions that name a proxy decision maker and/or delineate acceptable interventions and that are to be used if the person's decision-making capacity is lost. The legal status of these documents varies from state to state.

Advanced practice nursing   An advanced level of knowledge, skills, and experience applied to the nursing care of patients within primary care or specialty practice settings.

Aesthetics   Philosophical inquiry about art or beauty.

Altruism   Actions taken for or on behalf of another person that are not primarily self-serving. In the helping professions, altruism serves as a basis for ethical action along with an understanding of responsibilities incurred by assuming the professional role.

ANA *Code of Ethics with Interpretive Statements* (2001)   The written guidelines of the American Nurses Association that outline ethical action for all professional nurses practicing in the United States. The provisions are revised periodically as a result of societal changes and input from practicing nurses and nursing academics.

Applied ethics   The application of moral philosophy and moral theory to actual situations involving human action.

Assent   A child's affirmative agreement to participate in research or treatment after age- and developmentally appropriate information has been shared with and understood by the child. Failure to object to treatment or research is not the equivalent of assent.

Autonomy   An ethical principle that calls attention to a person's right to be treated with dignity and respect. It entails a right to self-determine both acceptable treatment and with whom information may be shared.

Beneficence   The ethical principle that enjoins healthcare professionals to remain focused on their professional goals in providing a good for individuals.

Caring   A concept that has been variously defined but that can best be described as a focused attention on and, when possible, engagement with a patient to determine that person's particular needs and the use of clinical judgment to meet those needs.

Case-based ethics or casuistry   An educational and analytic strategy whereby a landmark or epitome case (that has received some resolution or where improved understanding of nuances has occurred) is compared to and contrasted with a current problematic case or issue.

Confidentiality   The ethical requirement for professionals, institutions, and employees of institutions to disclose information only to those who need to know for the purposes of providing care; the patient's right to say with whom his or her healthcare information may be shared.

Cooperation   The responsibility to collaborate with others within and outside of the profession for the purposes of achieving a good for an individual or society related to health care.

Deprofessionalization   A phenomenon in which professionals lose their ability to govern their own practice, or professions lose the rights of self-regulation. It is a problem for society because the profession is less likely to be able to meet societal expectations of the practice or service.

Descriptive ethics   Observations of what human beings take to be good actions and/or the reasons people give to justify their actions as morally good; for example, research on practice behaviors.

Dilemma   A choice that must be made between two or more actions when it is not possible to be clear about which action is preferable. In healthcare settings, a dilemma usually involves negative choices or situations where no good action is available and one must choose among equally problematic alternatives.

Distributive justice   Fair, equitable, and appropriate allocation of goods, services, and resources based on criteria that a society agrees is ethical and justifiable.

Epistemology   Philosophical inquiry about knowledge. It explores questions such as *What is knowledge?*, *What counts as knowledge and why?*, and *What are salient characteristics of human beings related to knowledge?*

Ethical practice   The use of disciplinary knowledge, skills, experience, and personal characteristics to conceptualize and act upon what is needed either at the level of the individual or of society.

Ethical principles Rules, standards, or guidelines for action that are derived from theoretical propositions about what is good for humans.

Ethics Philosophical inquiry about the good; also called moral philosophy.

Feminist ethics An approach that takes the experience of women as a starting point by acknowledging that an individual lives in the context of societal, institutional, and interpersonal power structures. These structures give rise to injustices for women and other groups that are disadvantaged in some way.

Fidelity Refers to being faithful to the obligation of keeping promises made in a therapeutic relationship.

Fiduciary relationship An association based on trust. When there exists an inequality in knowledge, skills, or will, one party has to trust that the other—who has specialized knowledge or skills—will maintain a primary focus on meeting the first party's needs and interests.

Human rights Basic moral guarantees that a minimally good life is granted to all humans by virtue of their humanity (if granted to any), regardless of societal or political contexts. Some examples are provisions for education and health care, and protection from the effects of destitution.

Human subject A living individual about whom an investigator (whether professional or student) conducting research obtains (1) data through intervention or interaction with the individual, or (2) identifiable private information.

Implicit consent The implied permission given by the patient when entering a healthcare setting that the patient will accept certain routine evaluations and interventions, such as blood pressure measurement.

Informed consent The right of all patients—who are physically and cognitively able—to determine what is acceptable in the way of treatment and interventions. Implies that adequate information is given and is presented in a way that is comprehensible to that particular person.

Institutional review board A governmentally mandated committee charged with overseeing the protection of human subjects enrolled in research studies in an institution. The mandate for an institutional review board applies only to institutions that receive some government funding for research (almost all hospitals and research universities).

Legal rights Liberties or privileges that in democratic societies are conceived with the input of citizens and for which impingements warrant formal sanctions of some kind.

Maternal–fetal conflict A situation in which the well-being of the mother is taken to stand in opposition to the well-being of the fetus.

Medical model   A systems model that focuses on bodily functions and disturbances.

Moral reasoning   The application of theoretical understandings and reasoned assumptions to determine what is good action in complex situations where the best action is at least initially unclear.

Moral rights   Goods that are inherently granted to all persons in a society; these include such things as freedom to make one's own choices and freedom from state interference in personal affairs.

Moral theory   A systematic justified explanation of what good means in terms of how human beings do or should seek to live their lives.

Narrative ethics   An ethics framework that uses stories to explore hidden facts of morally worrisome cases.

Negative moral right   The right to be left alone and to be free from the interference of others or from the state.

Nonmaleficence   The ethical principle that enjoins us to avoid harm in the course of providing healthcare services. The duty of the nurse is to protect the patient from any avoidable harm caused in the course of providing care.

Nontherapeutic research   Research that aims to contribute more generally to the knowledge base for benefit to others rather than benefit to the subject.

Normative ethics   Reasoned and logically explored explanations of the moral purpose of human interactions or revealed truths about good action. Prescribes which actions ought to be taken, which actions are permissible, and which actions are forbidden.

Nursing theory   Describes and explains nursing care and provides a structure or framework that facilitates practice, guides research endeavors aimed at expanding nursing's knowledge base, and underpins practitioner development and education.

Nursing ethics   (1) The study of what constitutes good nursing practice, what obstacles to good nursing practice exist, and what the responsibilities of nurses are in relation to their professional conduct; (2) how nurses act to further professional goals in the practice of individual situations.

Paternalism   The intentional overriding of a person's preferences because these are determined by others not to be in the person's best interest.

Patient Self-Determination Act   Mandates that all hospitals accepting Medicare funding offer written information concerning a patient's right to make decisions concerning his or her health care and the right to consent to or refuse medical treatment.

Political action Activities informed by nursing knowledge and clinical judgment that are undertaken by the nurse, often in collaboration with others, for the purpose of influencing necessary changes in policy at the institutional, local, or societal levels.

Positive moral right A claim that can be made against someone or some institution for assistance or for the provision of goods and services.

Practical reason A type of reasoning that acts as a constraint on emotional and instinctual drives that can result in harmful actions, on the one hand, and lack of needed action or inadequate action, on the other hand.

Practical wisdom Permits a person to understand what is a good way to live and that living a good life means habitually moderating emotional impulses by using reason.

Preventive ethics Anticipating and addressing potential problems before they arise.

Privacy The right to be free from the interference of others and the freedom to grant or withhold access to information about oneself.

Private information Information about behavior that occurs in a context in which an individual can reasonably expect that no observation or recording is taking place, and information which has been provided for specific purposes by an individual and which the individual can reasonably expect will not be made public.

Profession A discipline that has an extensive and specialized knowledge base, takes responsibility for developing and using its knowledge, has a practice or action orientation that is used for the good of the population served, and autonomously sets standards for and monitors the actions of its members.

Professional advocacy Actions taken by a nurse or other professional to ensure good care at the level of the individual and at broader levels as necessary. Includes responsibilities both to address immediate situations of inadequate practice and to be active in addressing the environmental conditions that give rise to practice problems.

Professional autonomy A profession's warrant—granted by society—to be self-governing and self-regulating.

Professional judgment The nonlinear process of using knowledge, reasoning, tacit (experiential) knowledge, and interpersonal skills to determine—within the limits of available information—the probable best actions given the inevitable existence of some uncertainty about both the possession of adequate knowledge and the outcome of actions.

Proxy decision making   The act of deciding what healthcare actions are permissible for someone who temporarily or permanently has lost decision-making capacity, never had decision-making capacity (profound cognitive deficits), or is not yet considered sufficiently mature to make healthcare decisions (children).

Qualitative research   A form of social inquiry that is designed to understand the way people interpret and make sense of experienced phenomena.

Research   A systematic investigation—including research development, testing, and evaluation—designed to develop or contribute to generalizable knowledge.

Social contract   An agreement between an individual and society that assigns to both the individual and the society certain moral and political obligations.

Social justice   Formal systems that exist to decide who gets what in terms of social goods such as education, food, shelter, and health care.

Therapeutic research   Research that involves testing potential new treatments or therapies for a malady or condition experienced by the subject and that takes place as part of patient care.

Veracity   Truthfulness in giving patients information about their healthcare needs; facilitates autonomous choice and enhances patient decision making.

Verbal consent   The sanction given by the patient, after being educated and informed of the intended care, to be cared for by healthcare personnel, including evaluation, tests, therapeutics, and decisions about the best ways of managing chronic conditions.

Virtue ethics   In healthcare practice, the idea that a person can cultivate certain characteristics (virtues) that will predispose the person to good actions related to the profession's predetermined goals.

Virtues   Characteristics supposed to be essential for consistently good patient care and decision making. Some examples are empathy, veracity, transparency of purpose, cultural sensitivity, and motivation to act.

Written consent   The informed permission that the patient or the patient's designated proxy gives to the physician or advanced practice nurse to undertake a procedure. It consists of a signed legal document.

Index

413